a LANGE medical book

Correlative
Neuroanatomy

twenty-first edition

a LANGE medical book

Correlative Neuroanatomy

twenty-first edition

Jack deGroot, MD, PhD
Professor Emeritus, Anatomy and Radiology
University of California School of Medicine
San Francisco

With contributions by

Joseph G. Chusid, MD
Professor Emeritus, Neurology
New York Medical College
New York City

Director Emeritus, Department of Neurology
St. Vincent's Hospital and Medical Center
New York City

APPLETON & LANGE
Norwalk, Connecticut/San Mateo, California

0-8385-1332-8

Italian Edition: *Piccin Nuova Libraria, S.p.A., Via Altinate, 107, 35121 Padua, Italy*
Japanese Edition: *Kinpodo Publishing Co., Ltd., 34 Nishiteranomae-cho, Shishigatani, Sakyo-ku, Kyoto, 606, Japan*
Spanish Edition: *Editoral El Manual Moderno, S.A. de C.V., Av. Sonora 206 - Col. Hipodromo, 06100- Mexico, D.F.*
Portugese Edition: *Editora Guanabara Koogan S.A., Travessado Ouvidor, 11, 20 040 Rio de Janeiro - RJ, Brazil*
Polish Edition: *Panstwowy Zaklad Wydawnictw Lekarskich, P.O. Box 379, 00-950 Warsaw 1, Poland*
German Edition: *Springer-Verlag GmbH & Co. KG, Postfach 10 52 80, 6900 Heidelberg 1, West Germany*
Serbo-Croatian Edition: *Savremena Adminstracija, Crnotravska 7-9, 11000 Belgrade, Yugoslavia*
French Edition: *Masson, Editeur, 120 Boulevard Saint-Germain, F-75280 Paris, Cedex 06, France*
Indonesian Edition: *Yayasan Essentia Medica, P.O. Box 58, Yogyakarta D.I.Y., Indonesia*

93 94 95 / 10 9 8 7 6 5 4 3

Prentice Hall International (UK) Limited, *London*
Prentice Hall of Australia Pty. Limited, *Sydney*
Prentice Hall Canada, Inc., *Toronto*
Prentice Hall Hispanoamericana, S.A., *Mexico*
Prentice Hall of India Private Limited, *New Delhi*
Prentice Hall of Japan, Inc., *Tokyo*
Simon & Schuster Asia Pte. Ltd., *Singapore*
Editora Prentice Hall do Brasil Ltda., *Rio de Janeiro*
Prentice Hall, *Englewood Cliffs, New Jersey*

ISSN: 0892-1237
ISBN: 0-8385-1332-8

Production Editor: Sheilah Holmes
Cover Designer: Janice Barsevich

PRINTED IN THE UNITED STATES OF AMERICA

*To P.M., without whose help this book
would not have been completed.*

Table of Contents

SECTION VI. DISCUSSION OF CASES

Preface

Modern neuroanatomy, the study of the form and function of the nervous system, is part of an exciting array of rapidly developing disciplines that make up the neurosciences. *Correlative Neuroanatomy,* twenty-first edition, presents the latest knowledge in this evolving field in a practical clinical context and serves as a foundation for the study of the neurosciences.

This book is written as a basic text in neuroanatomy for students in medicine and other health sciences. It is intended for use in an initial course on the subject and as a review and reference in a variety of clinical courses, as well as in postgraduate studies.

ORGANIZATION

Correlative Neuroanatomy is divided into six sections. The first section covers the basic divisions, cellular elements, and signaling modes of the nervous system. The second section extensively describes the form and function of the spinal cord and spine. The third section discusses the functional anatomy of the brain and cranial nerves. The fourth section—expanded in this edition—summarizes the functional integration of the entire nervous system. The fifth section presents some diagnostic methods, including modern neuroradiology, and the sixth section discusses the clinical cases presented in earlier chapters.

FEATURES

The division of the material into compact units facilitates comprehension, retention, and ease of access. Information is presented in a logical order for study: a comprehensive overview of the subject is followed by discussions of cells and signaling, the anatomy of the spine and brain, and the functional systems of the central nervous system.

Clinical correlations throughout the book emphasize the clinical aspects of neuroanatomy. Numerous cases are included to provide a problem-solving format to assist students in preparing for clinical practice.

Many illustrations enhance and amplify the text. These include a large number of modern radiologic images that closely depict anatomic relationships.

Brief discussions of electrodiagnostic and neuroradiologic methods are included; the appendixes cover the neurologic examination, functional tests of principal muscles, and the spinal nerves and plexuses and provide questions and answers on the material covered in the text.

NEW TO THIS EDITION

This edition includes:

- Increased coverage of functional systems, with new chapters on somatosensory systems and the auditory, vestibular, and reticular systems.
- Additional information on chemical signaling.
- An expanded number of self-test questions and answers for each section of the book.
- A modernized art program with more than 100 new and modified line drawings and radiologic images.
- An appendix on spinal nerves and plexuses.
- Updated references throughout.

I owe many thanks to my colleagues who taught me and shared their material with me. Dr JG Chusid has been especially generous. Dr CM Mills graciously provided some of the MR images, and many of the line drawings were most ably prepared by Lena Lyons, MA.

San Francisco   Jack deGroot
March 1991

a LANGE medical book

Correlative Neuroanatomy

twenty-first edition

Section I.
Basic Principles

Fundamentals of the Nervous System

1

Modern scientific and technical advances have led to the development of sophisticated machines that might be compared to the human nervous system. The newest, most advanced mainframe computer is a simple, uncomplicated, clumsy machine compared with the human brain, which has a potentially much larger memory than any computer. The brain also has the ability to make complex decisions, think logically and creatively, draw conclusions, "feel" emotions, and select or preempt responses to stimuli and questions. "Minicomputers" at intervals along the spinal cord—and probably in other areas as well—are capable of initiating or receiving and modifying stimuli. Computers using artificial intelligence may someday be able to imitate to a small degree—but not equal—the complex functions of the human brain.

GENERAL PLAN OF THE NERVOUS SYSTEM

Main Divisions
A. Anatomy: Anatomically, the human nervous system is a complex of 2 subdivisions.
1. Central nervous system (CNS)-The CNS, comprising the brain and spinal cord, is enclosed in bone and wrapped in protective coverings (meninges) and fluid-filled spaces.
2. Peripheral nervous system (PNS)-The PNS is formed by the cranial and spinal nerves (Fig 1-1).
B. Physiology: Functionally, the nervous system is divided into 2 systems.
1. Somatic nervous system-This innervates the structures of the body wall (muscles, skin, mucous membranes).
2. Autonomic (visceral) nervous system (ANS)-The ANS contains portions of the central and peripheral systems. It controls the activities of the smooth muscles and glands of the internal or-

gans (viscera) and the blood vessels and returns sensory information to the brain.

Structural Units
The central portion of the nervous system consists of a large, complex **brain (encephalon)** and an elongated **spinal cord (medulla spinalis)** (Fig 1-2 and Table 1-1). The brain is further subdivided into the cerebrum, the brain stem, and the cerebellum. The **cerebrum (forebrain,** or **prosencephalon)** consists of the **telencephalon** and the **diencephalon;** the telencephalon includes the gray cerebral cortex, subcortical white matter, and the so-called basal ganglia, which are gray masses deep within the cerebral hemispheres. The major subdivisions of the diencephalon are the thalamus and hypothalamus. The **brain stem** consists of the **midbrain (mesencephalon), pons (metencephalon),** and **medulla oblongata (myelencephalon).** The **cerebellum** (the part of the metencephalon that lies behind the brain stem) includes the vermis and two lateral lobes. The brain, which is hollow, contains a system of ventricles; the spinal cord has a narrow central canal that is largely obliterated in adulthood. These spaces are filled with cerebrospinal fluid (CSF). (See Figs 1-3 and 1-4 and Chapter 10.)

Functional Units
The brain, which accounts for about 2% of the body weight, contains many billions (perhaps even a trillion) of neurons and glial cells (see Chapter 2). The **neurons,** or nerve cells, are specialized cells that receive and send signals to other cells through their extensions and connections (which contain nerve fibers). The information is processed and encoded in a sequence of electrical or chemical stimuli. Many neurons have relatively large cell bodies and long extensions that transmit the stimuli quickly over a considerable distance. While most large neurons can be readily identified in histologic sections and have been studied extensively, a far

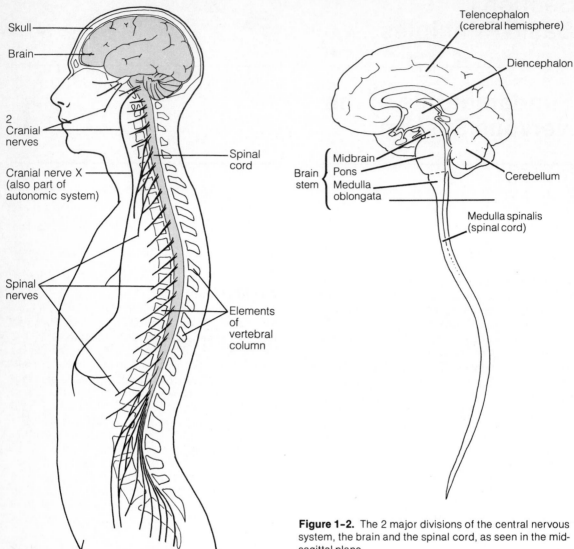

Figure 1-1. The structure of the central nervous system and the peripheral nervous system, showing the relationship between the CNS and its bony coverings.

Figure 1-2. The 2 major divisions of the central nervous system, the brain and the spinal cord, as seen in the mid-sagittal plane.

greater number of smaller cells (the interneuron pool) play a role in processing information in a way that is still poorly understood. Nerve cells with common forms, functions, and connections within the central nervous system are often grouped together into **nuclei.** These nuclei may originate, relay, modify, or multiply information signals within the nervous system. Nerve cells with common form, function, and connections outside the central nervous system are called **ganglia.**

Other elements that support and expedite the activity of the neurons are the **glial cells,** of which

there are several types; the glial cells outnumber the neurons 10:1.

Connections

Nerve cells convey signals to one another by means of synapses (see Chapters 2 and 3). The chemical transmitters found in most synapses are associated with the function of the synapse: excitation or inhibition.

The connections, or pathways, between groups of neurons in the central nervous system are in the form of fiber bundles, or tracts **(fasciculi);** they can also be diffusely distributed. Aggregates of tracts, as seen in the spinal cord, are referred to as columns **(funiculi).** Tracts may descend (eg, from the cerebrum to the brain stem or spinal cord) or as-

Table 1-1. Major divisions of the central nervous system.

Brain (encephalon)	Cerebrum (forebrain or prosencephalon)	Telencephalon	Cerebral cortex (gray) Subcortical white matter Commissures Basal ganglia (deeply placed gray masses)
		Diencephalon	Thalamus Hypothalamus Epithalamus Subthalamus
	Brain stem		Midbrain (mesencephalon) Pons (metencephalon) Medulla oblongata (myencephalon)
	Cerebellum		
Spinal cord (medulla spinalis)			

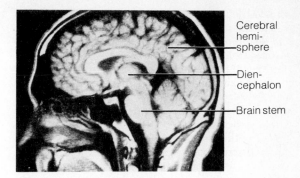

Figure 1-4. Magnetic resonance (MR) image of a midsagittal section through the head (short time sequence; see Chapter 22). Compare with Figs 1-3 and 11-9.

cend (eg, to the cerebrum). These pathways are vertical connections that in their course may cross **(decussate)** from one side of the central nervous system to the other. Horizontal (lateral) connections are called **commissures.**

The earliest tracts of nerve fibers appear at about the second month of fetal life; major descending motor tracts appear at about the fifth month. **Myelinization** (sheathing with myelin) of the spinal cord's nerve fibers begins about the middle of fetal life, some tracts are not completely myelinated for 20 years. The oldest tracts (those common to all animals) myelinate first; the corticospinal tracts myelinate largely during the first and second years after birth.

Although the structural organization of the brain is well established before neural function begins, there is evidence that most of the future connections are set before and shortly after birth. The maturing brain is susceptible to modification if an appropriate stimulus is applied or withheld during a critical period that can be a few days or even less (see Chapter 21).

PERIPHERAL NERVOUS SYSTEM

The peripheral nervous system consists of spinal nerves, cranial nerves, and their associated ganglia (groups of nerve cells outside the central nervous system). The nerves contain nerve fibers that conduct information to (afferent) or from (efferent) the central nervous system. In general, **efferent** fibers are involved in motor functions such as the contraction of muscles or secretion of glands; **afferent** fibers usually convey sensory stimuli from the skin, mucous membranes, and deeper structures.

EXPERIMENTAL METHODS

Early anatomists examined the nervous system in terms of gross appearance. Histologic examination with the light microscope added a great deal of new information that is now being amplified and

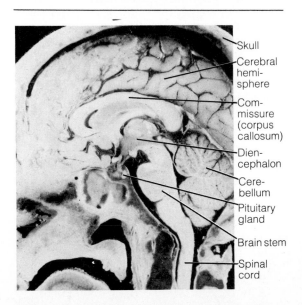

Figure 1-3. Photograph of a midsagittal section through the head and upper neck, showing the major divisions of the central nervous system. (Reproduced, with permission, from de Groot J: *Correlative Neuroanatomy of Computed Tomography and Magnetic Resonance Imagery.* Lea & Febiger, 1984.)

refined by ultrastructural procedures (freeze-fracture techniques, transmission electron microscopy, and scanning electron microscopy). Biochemical and physiologic analyses contribute to our understanding of the form and function of the brain, spinal cord, and nerves. Experimental methods are often needed to explain how the elements of the system interact; these include observation under varied experimental conditions, stimulation followed by the recording of reactions, and destruction of discrete parts followed by determining both deficits of function and changes in anatomy.

Stimulation (or irritation) and destruction of portions of the nervous system are processes that occur in disease. A loss of function is called a **lesion** or a **deficit**. Lesions may produce **signs** (observable abnormalities of function) or **symptoms** (subjective changes).

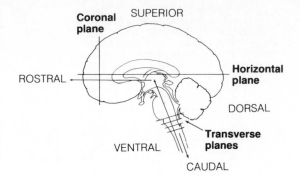

Figure 1–5. Planes (coronal, horizontal, transverse) and directions (rostral, caudal, etc) frequently used in the description of the brain and spinal cord. The plane of the drawing is the midsagittal.

STUDY OF THE NERVOUS SYSTEM

The nervous system can be studied in many ways and in the context of several disciplines collectively called **neurobiology,** or the **neurosciences.** Each field of study emphasizes different features, but all are rapidly expanding our understanding of the nervous system.

Neuroanatomy is the study of the form and function of the nervous system. Many thousands of special terms and identifications (language) are required to describe the processes and connections taking place almost continuously in the various parts of the nervous system (geography); some of these terms are listed in Table 1–2. This book discusses both normal anatomy and some changes caused by specific disorders and defects of the nervous system.

Neuroradiology, a modern specialty based on neuroanatomy, uses various refined methods of examination to depict normal or abnormal features of the brain, the spinal cord and nerves, and their coverings in order to locate and identify nervous system lesions—which are sometimes very small—as an aid to diagnosis. The planes of the section and the terms used in the study of neuroanatomy and neuroradiology are shown in Fig 1–5.

Neurology is the science and technique of deducing the location and nature of nervous system lesions from the signs and symptoms they give rise to; once determined (diagnosis), the abnormality can in many cases be treated (therapy).

Neuropathology is the study of the nature and extent of disease processes (lesions) through biopsies, autopsies, and chemical tests, using gross inspection and histologic and ultrastructural analyses of nervous tissue.

It is important to realize that in the human neurosciences, as nowhere else, the disciplines de-

Table 1–2. Terms used in neuroanatomy.

Ventral, anterior	On the front (belly) side
Dorsal, posterior	On the back side
Superior, cranial	On the top (skull) side
Inferior	On the lower side
Caudal	In the lowermost position (at the tail end)
Rostral	On the forward side (at the nose end)
Medial	Close to or toward the middle
Median	In the middle, the midplane (midsagittal)
Lateral	Toward the side (away from the middle)
Ipsilateral	On the same side
Contralateral	On the opposite side
Bilateral	On both sides

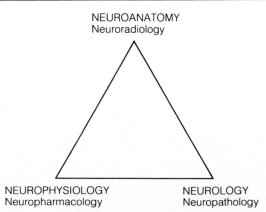

Figure 1–6. Triad of specialties related to neuroanatomy.

scribed are interrelated and interdependent (Fig 1–6). The study of the form of the nervous system is incomplete without considering the other aspects of the triad, that is, function and dysfunction.

REFERENCES

Barr ML, Kierman JA: *The Human Nervous System,* 4th ed. Harper & Row, 1983.

Brodal A: *Neurological Anatomy,* 3rd ed. Oxford Univ Press, 1981.

Carpenter MC, Sutin J: *Human Neuroanatomy,* 8th ed. Williams & Wilkins, 1983.

Heimer L: *The Human Brain and Spinal Cord.* Springer-Verlag, 1983.

Kandel ER, Schwartz JH: *Principles of Neural Science,* 2nd ed. Elsevier, 1985.

Martin JH: *Neuroanatomy.* Elsevier, 1989.

Netter FH: *Nervous System (Atlas and Connotations).* Vol 1: *The Ciba Collection of Medical Illustrations.* CIBA Pharmaceutical Company, 1983.

Romanes GJ: *Cunningham's Textbook of Anatomy,* 18th ed. Oxford Univ Press, 1986.

Romero-Sierra C: *Neuroanatomy: A Conceptual Approach.* Churchill Livingstone, 1986.

Elements of Nervous Tissue

CELLULAR ASPECTS OF NEURAL DEVELOPMENT

Early in the development of the nervous system, a hollow tube of ectodermal neural tissue forms at the embryo's dorsal midline. The cellular elements of the tube appear undifferentiated at first, but they later form various types of neurons (nerve cells) and supporting glial cells.

Layers of the Neural Tube

The embryonic neural tube has 3 layers (Fig 2–1): the **ventricular zone,** later called the **ependyma** around the lumen (central canal) of the tube; the **intermediate zone,** which is formed by the dividing cells of the ventricular zone (including the earliest radial glial cell type) and stretches between the ventricular surface and the outer (pial) layer; and the external **marginal zone,** which is formed later by processes of the nerve cells in the intermediate zone (Fig 2–1B). The intermediate zone, or mantle layer, increases in cellularity and becomes gray matter. The nerve cell processes in the marginal zone, together with other cell processes, become white matter when myelinated.

Differentiation & Migration

The largest neurons, which are mostly motor neurons, differentiate first. Sensory and small neurons and most of the glial cells appear later, up to the time of birth. Newly formed neurons may migrate extensively through regions of previously formed neurons. Because the axonal process of a neuron may begin growing toward its target during migration, nerve processes in the adult brain are often curved rather than straight. The newer cells of the future cerebral cortex migrate from the deepest to the more superficial layers; the small neurons of the future cerebellum migrate first to the surface and later to deeper layers; the latter process continues for several months after birth.

Once differentiated, neurons do not divide again. Any loss of neurons, whether from normal attrition or pathologic insult, is permanent.

NEURONS

Neurons vary in size and in complexity. The nuclei of one type of small cerebellar cortical cell (granular cell) are only slightly larger than the nucleoli of an adjacent large type (Purkinje cell; see Fig 6–19). Motor neurons are usually larger than sensory neurons. Nerve cells with long processes (eg, dorsal root ganglion cells) are larger than those with short processes (Figs 2–2 and 2–3).

Some neurons stretch from the cerebral cortex to the lower spinal cord, a distance of less than 2 feet in infants or 4 feet or more in adults; others have very short processes that reach only from cell to cell in the cerebral cortex, for example. The processes contain **neurofibrils** composed of thin **neurofilaments.** The receptive part of the neuron is the **dendrite,** or **dendritic zone** (see below); the conducting (propagating or transmitting) part is the **axon,** which may have one or more collateral branches. The downstream end of the neuron is called the **synaptic terminal, terminal zone,** or **arborization,** or **telodendrion.** The nucleus of the neuron and its surrounding cytoplasma are called the **perikaryon, soma,** or **cell body.** The chemical

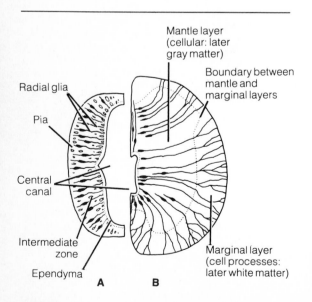

Figure 2–1. Two stages in the development of the neural tube (only half of each cross section is shown). *A.* Early stage with large central canal; *B.* Later stage with smaller central canal.

Radial glia

Pia

Central canal

Intermediate zone

Ependyma

Mantle layer (cellular: later gray matter)

Boundary between mantle and marginal layers

Marginal layer (cell processes: later white matter)

A   **B**

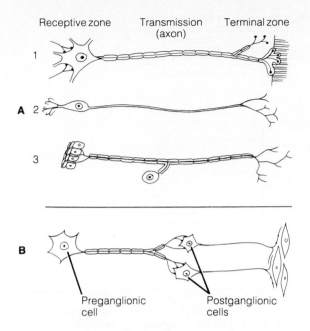

Figure 2-2. Schematic illustration of nerve cell types. *A.* central nervous system cells: *1:* motor neuron to striated muscle; *2:* special sensory neuron; *3:* general sensory neuron from skin. *B.* autonomic cells to smooth muscle. Note how the position of the nucleus along the axon varies.

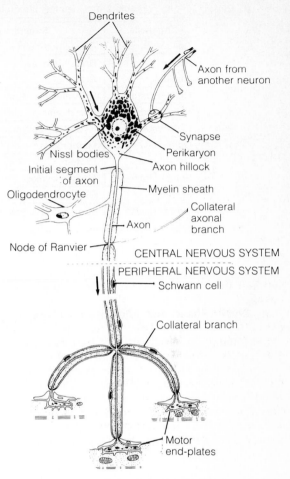

Figure 2-3. Schematic drawing of a Nissl-stained motor neuron. The myelin sheath is produced by oligodendrocytes in the central nervous system and by Schwann cells in the peripheral nervous system. Note the 3 motor end-plates, which transmit the nerve impulse to striated skeletal muscle fibers. Arrows show the direction of the nerve impulse. (Reproduced, with permission, from Junqueira LC, Cameiro J, Kelley RO: *Basic Histology,* 6th ed. Appleton & Lange, 1989).

structures and functions of neurons are shown in Table 2–1.

Cell Bodies

The cell body (see Fig 2–3) is the metabolic center of a neuron. Although its size varies greatly in different neuron types, the cell body makes up only a small part of the total volume of the neuron. The cell body contains a **nucleus,** a prominent **nucleolus,** and the **Nissl substance** (endoplasmic reticulum with ribosomes), a protein-synthesizing apparatus. Nissl substance is also involved in the synthesis of neurotransmitter substances used away from the cell body, in the synaptic terminal. Synapses from other cells or glial processes may cover the surface of a cell body (Fig 2–4).

Dendrites

Most neurons have many dendrites (see Figs 2–2, 2–3 and 2–5). The receptive surface area of the dendrites, the dendritic zone, is usually far larger than that of the cell body. Dendrites receive information via synapses from either the environment (sensory neurons) or other neurons (interneurons and motor neurons). To a large extent, the diversity among neurons depends on the complexity and position of the dendrites and on the position of the cell body.

Axons

A neuron has a single **axon** (formerly called a **neurite**), which is a cylindrical tube of cytoplasm covered by a membrane, the **axolemma.** The axon is a specialized structure that conducts electrical signals, normally from the initial segment to the synaptic terminals. The **initial segment** is an area of the axon near the cell body that has distinctive morphologic features; it differs from both cell body and axon. The initial segment does not contain Nissl substance (Fig 2–3). In large neurons, it arises conspicuously from the **axon hillock,** a cone-shaped portion of the cell body. Axons range in

Table 2-1. Chemical structures and functions of neurons.

Organelle	Structure	Function
Cell membrane	Glycolipoprotein complex	Excitation and transport
Nucleus	DNA, histones	Genetic information
Nucleolus	RNA	Protein synthesis
Nissl substance	RNA-membrane complex	Protein synthesis
Mitochondria	Enzyme-membrane complex	Energy metabolism
Lysosome	Hydrolytic enzymes	Degrading reactions
Golgi body	Membranes	Secretory
Neurofibril	Protein	Metabolic transport
Soluble fraction	Many enzymes	Glycolysis, etc
Myelin	Glycolipoprotein complex	Insulation
Synaptic vesicle	Transmitter substances	Synaptic transmission

length from a few micrometers to well over a meter and in diameter from 0.1 to more than 20 micrometers.

A. Myelin Sheathing: Many axons are covered by multiple concentric layers of **myelin,** a lipid-rich insulating material produced by Schwann cells in the peripheral nervous system (Figs 2-6 and 2-7) and by oligodendrocytes (a type of glial cell) in the central nervous system. The myelin sheath in peripheral nerves is divided into segments about 1 mm long by constrictions where myelin is absent; these are the nodes of Ranvier. The smallest axons are unmyelinated and are not very prominent in histologic preparations, even though they are far more numerous than the larger, myelinated axons.

B. Axon Transport: In addition to conducting action potentials, axons transport materials from the cell body to the synaptic terminals (**anterograde transport**) and from the synaptic terminals to the cell body (**retrograde transport**). Anterograde transport may be fast (up to 400 mm/d) or slow (about 1 mm/d). Retrograde transport is similar to rapid anterograde transport. Fast transport involves neurotubules (often called microtubules) extending through the cytoplasm of the neuron. Because of their threadlike appearance when seen in electron micrographs, microtubules have been given the name neurofilaments. In light microscopy, neurofibril is the term used to describe a group of neurofilaments.

Both anterograde and retrograde transport are being used experimentally to determine how groups of neurons are interconnected: Radioactive peptides injected in one area show up anterogradely in another after a few hours, and horseradish peroxidase is used in retrograde tracing experiments.

An axon can be injured by being cut or severed, crushed, or compressed. A typical reaction to severe nerve injury is discussed in Chapter 21.

Synapses

Communication between neurons usually occurs from the terminal of the transmitting neuron (presynaptic side) to the receptive region of the receiving neuron (postsynaptic side) (Figs 2-5, 2-8, and 2-9). This specialized interneuronal complex is a **synapse,** or **synaptic junction;** while it often is located between an axon and a dendrite, it may be between an axon and a nerve cell body or between 2 axons and 2 dendrites (Fig 2-9). Some large cell bodies may receive several thousand synapses (Fig 2-4).

Impulse transmission at most synaptic sites involves the release of a chemical transmitter substance (transmitter substances are discussed in Chapter 3); at other sites, current passes directly from cell to cell through specialized junctions called **electrical synapses,** or **gap junctions.** Chemical synapses have several distinctive characteristics: synaptic vesicles on the presynaptic side, a synaptic cleft, and a dense thickening on both the receiving cell and the presynaptic side (Fig 2-8).

Synapses are very diverse in their shapes and other properties: some are inhibitory and some excitatory; in some the transmitter is acetylcholine, in others it is a catecholamine or other substance (see Chapter 3). Some synaptic vesicles are large, some small; some have a dense core while others do not. Flat synaptic vesicles appear to contain an inhibitory mediator; dense-core vesicles contain catecholamines.

NEURONAL GROUPINGS & CONNECTIONS

Nerve cell bodies are grouped in characteristic ways in many parts of the nervous system. The patterns of grouping are studied by describing the **cytoarchitectonics** (the arrangement of cell in a tissue) of the nerve cell bodies. In the cerebral and

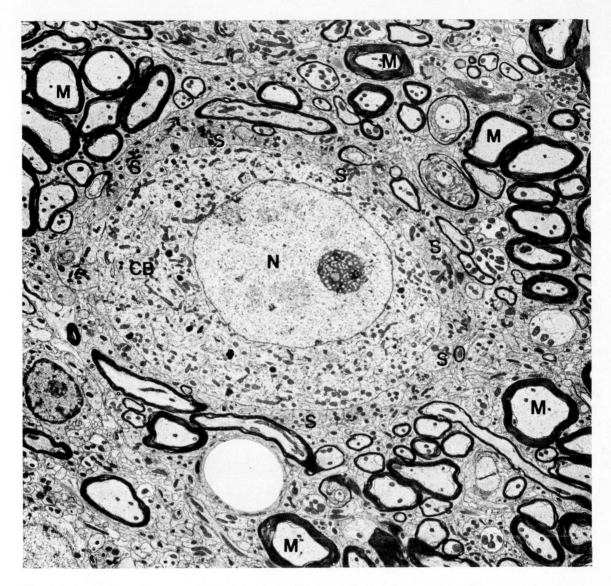

Figure 2-4. Electron micrograph of a nerve cell body (CB) surrounded by nerve processes. The neuronal surface is completely covered by either synaptic endings of other neurons (S) or processes of glial cells (G). Many other processes around this cell are myelinated axons (M). N, nucleus. × 5000. (Courtesy of Dr DM McDonald.)

cerebellar cortexes, cell bodies aggregate to form layers (laminas; see Fig 2–10). Nerve cell bodies in the spinal cord, brain stem, and cerebrum form compact groups, or **nuclei.** Within the nucleus, the nerve cells have a uniform shape and function. In the peripheral nervous system, these compact groups of nerve cell bodies are called **ganglia.**

Groups of nerve cells are connected by pathways formed by bundles of axons. In some pathways, the axon bundles are sufficiently defined to be identified as tracts, or fasciculi; in others, there are no discrete bundles of axons. Aggregates of tracts in the spinal cord are referred to as **columns,** or

funiculi (see Chapter 4). In some regions of the brain, axons are so intermingled that pathways are difficult to identify (**neural network,** or **neuropil;** see Fig 2–11).

NEUROGLIA

Astrocytes

There are 2 types of astrocytes, **protoplasmic** and **fibrillary,** but how they differ in function is unclear. Protoplasmic astrocytes are more delicate, they contain more protoplasm, and their

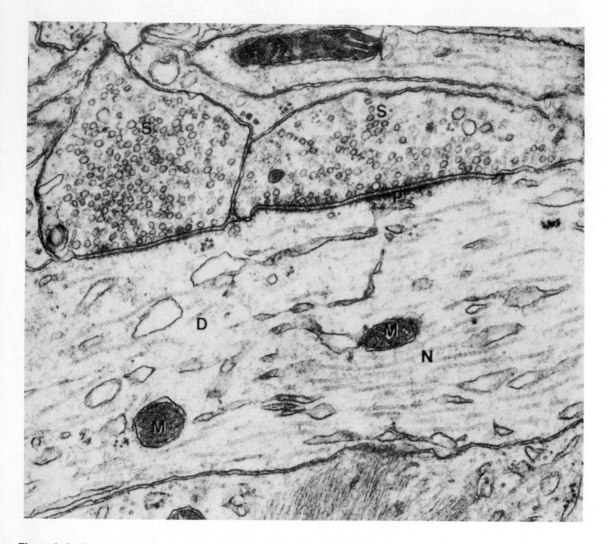

Figure 2–5. Electron micrograph of a dendrite (D) and 2 synaptic terminals (S). The dendrite contains 2 mitochondria (M) and several neurotubules (N). Note the presence of numerous vesicles within the terminals and the local thickening of the dendritic membrane at a postsynaptic site (P). × 20,000. (Courtesy of Dr DM McDonald.)

many processes are branched. They occur in gray matter or as satellite cells in dorsal root ganglia. Fibrillary astrocytes are more fibrous, and their processes (containing glial fibrils) are seldom branched. In light microscope preparations, an astrocyte is identified by its irregular oval nucleus without a distinct cytoplasm. Astrocytic processes radiate in all directions from a small cell body. They surround blood vessels in the nervous system, and they cover the exterior surface of the brain and spinal cord below the pia.

Astrocytes provide structural support to nervous tissue; they also play a role in synaptic transmission. Many synapses are closely invested by astrocytic processes, which may affect neurotransmitter function. Astrocytes also contribute to the formation of the blood-brain barrier (see Chapter 10). Although astrocytic processes around capillaries do not form a functional barrier, they can selectively take up materials in order to provide an environment optimal for neuronal function. Astrocytes act as regulators of electrolyte balance. They form

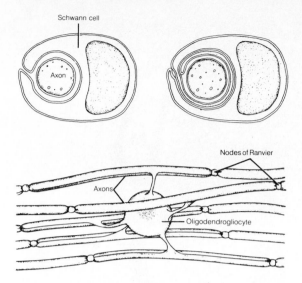

Figure 2–6. *Top:* Myelinization of axons in peripheral nerves. *Left:* Unmyelinated axon. *Right:* Myelinated axon. Note that the cell membrane of the Schwann cell has wrapped itself around the axon. *Bottom:* Myelinization of several axons in the central nervous system by an oligodendrogliocyte. (Reproduced, with permission, from Ganong WF: *Review of Medical Physiology,* 14th ed. Appleton & Lange, 1989.)

a covering on the entire central nervous system surface and proliferate to aid in repairing damaged neural tissue. These reactive astrocytes are larger, and are more easily stained. Chronic repair leads to a fibrillary gliosis, sometimes called glial scars.

Oligodendrocytes

These glial cells are identified in light microscope preparations by their round, rather dark nuclei without distinct cytoplasm. They have fewer processes than do astrocytes. Oligodendrites predominate in white matter; they form myelin in the central nervous system and may provide some nutritive support to the neurons they envelop. A single oligodendrocyte may wrap myelin sheaths around many axons (see Fig 2–6). All myelin sheaths are periodically interrupted by nodes of Ranvier. In the peripheral nerves, myelin is formed by the Schwann cells.

Microglia

Microglial cells (rod cells) have an elongated nucleus; they are the **macrophages,** or scavengers, of the central nervous system (Fig 2–12). When an area of the brain or spinal cord is damaged or infected, microglia migrate to the site of injury to remove cellular debris. Some microglia are always present in the brain, but when injury or infection occurs, others enter the brain from blood vessels.

Extracellular Space

There is some fluid-filled space between the various cellular components of the central nervous system. Studies with the electron microscope suggest that in adult central nervous systems, cellular processes and vascular elements are tightly packed, leaving little extracellular space (less than 2% per volume unit). The capillaries within the central nervous system are completely invested by glial or neural processes, so that no perivascular space is present.

Clinical Correlation

In **cerebral edema,** there is a definite and often rapid increase in the bulk of the brain. Cerebral edema, which tends to involve the white matter selectively, is either vasogenic (primarily extracellular) or cytotoxic (primarily intracellular). Electron micrographs may reveal massive expansion of the cytoplasm and of glial processes surrounding the capillaries. Therefore, an increase in the volume of the brain in cerebral edema may be caused by increases in the volume of not only the interstitial fluid but also of cells and their processes.

STAINING OF NEURAL TISSUE

The elements of nervous tissue are difficult to identify by light microscopy without fixation followed by staining. Many stains have been developed: some are specific for certain elements, while others are not (Table 2–2). Degenerating axons and myelin can be identified by specific staining procedures. Fluorescent microscopy is useful for identifying chemical tracers.

CHEMICAL COMPOSITION OF NEURAL TISSUE

Water

There is a high percentage of water in neural tissue. The adult brain is about 78% water; the spinal cord, about 75% (Table 2–3). Gray matter has a higher water content than white matter does. Most of the water is intracellular, only about 15% is extracellular. It appears to be freely and rapidly diffusible, serving as a solvent for metabolites and nutrients and contributing to the osmotic and hydraulic regulation of the nervous system.

Solids

Most neural tissue solids are proteins and lipids, with smaller fractions of inorganic salts and organic extracts.

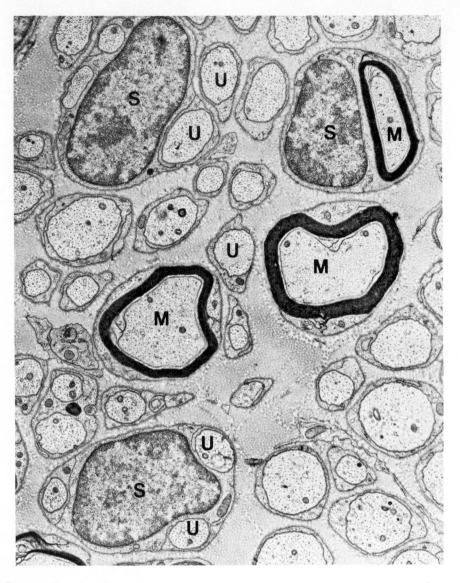

Figure 2–7. Electron micrograph of myelinated (M) and unmyelinated (U) axons of a peripheral nerve. Schwann cells (S) may surround one myelinated or several unmyelinated axons. × 16,000. (Courtesy of Dr. Dr DM McDonald.)

A. Proteins: These constitute up to 40% of the solids. Most protein in the brain is linked with lipids in the form of lipoproteins, compounds that resemble living protoplasm much more closely than do either free proteins or free lipids. Water-soluble liponucleoproteins (nucleoproteins combined with lipids) are present in the brain. The trypsin-resistant and pepsin-resistant protein fraction of liponucleoproteins is known as **neurokeratin.** Globulin and albumin are present in all nerve cells. A large fraction of brain protein is insoluble in water or saline solution but, unlike neurokeratin, is digestible by proteolytic enzymes.

The Nissl substance in cytoplasm is a center of protein production. Portions of the endoplasmic reticulum supply various enzymes and substrates, and the fine granular component of the cytoplasm supplies some of the components for protein synthesis. Oxidate and synthetic activities of the mitochondria and glycolytic activities of the fluid matrix may be coordinated by structural alterations within the cytoplasm (mitochodrial movement, cytoplasmic streaming, and changes from a soluble to a gel state, or vice versa, in the matrix). Microsomes, the particulates obtained from nerve cytoplasm by differential centrifugation, are rich in phospholipids and contain most of the ribonucleic acid of the cytoplasm.

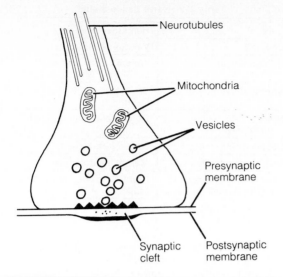
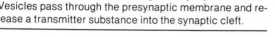

Figure 2-8. Schematic drawing of a synaptic terminal. Vesicles pass through the presynaptic membrane and release a transmitter substance into the synaptic cleft.

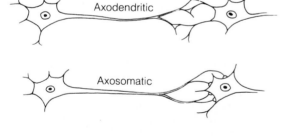

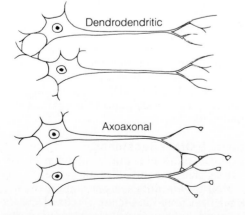

Figure 2-9. Schematic drawing of types of synapses.

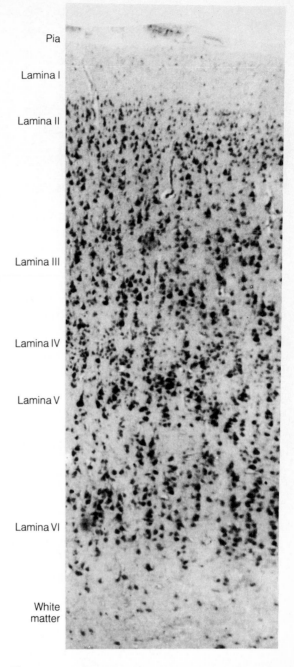

Figure 2-10. Light micrograph of cortical laminas. × 20. Nissl stain.

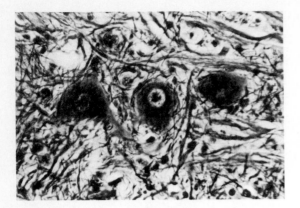

Figure 2-11. Light micrograph of a small group of neurons (nucleus) in a network of fibers (neuropil). × 800. Bielschowsky silver stain.

Table 2-2. Nerve tissue stains.

General	Hematoxylin-eosin
Cell body	Various Nissl stains
Normal myelin	Weigert with variants, Luxol Fast Blue
Normal nerve fibers	Bielschowsky, Bodian, Cajal
Normal cells with processes	Golgi metal impregnation
Degenerating axons	Nauta with variants
Degenerating myelin	Marchi (seldom used)
Chemical substances in cell or fibers	Darkfield or fluorescent microscopy

B. Lipids: Lipids make up a large part of the solid content of neural tissue (estimates range from 40 to 75%), but very little is simple lipid. The lipids of the central nervous system are highly complex and differ from those in the remainder of the body. Neutral fats and cholesterol esters are common to most body tissues but are not normally present in the central nervous system. Most lipids in the central nervous system are based on glycerol, sphingosine, or inositol, with added phosphate or hexose groups plus fatty acids and frequently amino acids. The abundant compound lipids include phospholipids (lecithins, cephalins, and sphingomyelin), cholesterol, cerebrosides or galactolipids (glycolipids), sulfur-containing lipids, and amino lipids. Lipids in the brain are synthesized there rather than being transported to the brain from other sources. The white matter contains more cholesterol, sphingomyelin, and cerebrosides than the gray matter. Neural tissue lipids may be unique in that certain of their important fatty acids (eg, 24-carbon fatty acids) have not been found elsewhere in the body. Lipids are metabolized faster during the early development of the brain than they are later. The turnover of fatty acids in the adult brain is slow, and they penetrate the brain very slowly, if at all.

C. Inorganic Salts: These salts are found in the combustion products of neural tissue. The principal inorganic salts found are potassium phosphate and potassium chloride. Sodium and other alkaline elements are found in lesser amounts. The intracellular potassium and magnesium concentrations are high, but there is little or no sodium or chloride; these are found extracellularly.

D. Nucleic Acids: The nuclei of nerve cells are rich in nucleic acids. Nucleic acids contain 2 general types of nucleotides: RNA and DNA. The tissue of the central nervous system contains about twice as much RNA as DNA. The DNA is confined to the nuclei of nerve and glial cells, with a considerable portion in the chromosomes. RNA is found in both the nucleus (mainly in the nucleolus) and the cytoplasm. RNA and DNA can be identified histologically by special stains or ultraviolet spectrophotometry.

Pigments & Other Substances

Histologic studies of neural tissue aid in identifying various pigments and other substances.

A. Neuromelanin: Neuromelanin is the deep black pigment found in the nerve cells of the substantia nigra and locus ceruleus, in some cerebrospinal and sympathetic ganglion cells, and in the

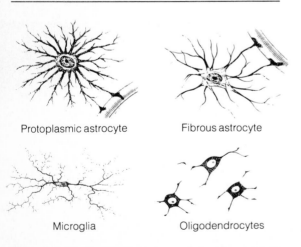

Protoplasmic astrocyte   Fibrous astrocyte

Microglia   Oligodendrocytes

Figure 2-12. Drawings of neuroglial cells specially stained by metallic impregnation. Observe that only the astrocytes exhibit vascular end-feet, which cover the walls of blood capillaries. (Reproduced, with permission, from Junqueira LC, Carneiro J, Kelley RO: *Basic Histology,* 6th ed. Appleton & Lange, 1989.)

Table 2-3. Fine chemical anatomy of neurons.*

Subdivision	Ultrastructure	% Water	Solids		
			% Lipid	% Protein	% Nucleic Acids†
1. Nucleolus	Chains or threads of 10–30 nm diameter granules	25	?	96	3.5(P)
2. Nucleolus-associated chromatin	(a) Nucleolar caps 0.5–2 μm diameter, numbering 2–4 (b) Satellite (sex chromatin) 1μm diameter in females (c) Chromocenter area—more prominent in females	... ...	... ...	... ...	...(D) ...(P) ...(P)
3. Nucleus	Double membranes, outer shows cytoplasmic projections and discontinuities up to 30 nm wide	77	25	74	0.5 P/D 2/1
4. Cytoplasm (perikaryon)	(a) Nissl bodies: (1) Endoplasmic reticulum of parallel tubules or vesicles 100–200 nm in diameter with walls 7–8 nm thick in continuous system of lacunae (2) Fine granules 10–30 nm in diameter in patterned rows and clusters along tubules (microsomal fraction—no succinoxidase, 50% pentose-type nucleic acid) (b) Fibrillar network: 6–10 nm in diameter and 200+ nm long, separating Nissl bodies (c) Mitochondria: 80% succinoxidase activity; 20% pentose-type nucleic acid (d) Lipid droplets and yellow pigment (e) Cell membrane: single, smooth	60	25	73	1.5 (P)
5. Dendrites	Similar appearance to perikaryon. Synaptic bulbs or end-feet on dendrites resemble simplified version of motor end-plate.	...	...	...	...
6. Axon hillock		85	?	±100	0
7. Axon: Axoplasm	(a) Extension of Nissl "endoplasmic reticulum" (b) Fibrillar network (c) Axoplasmic migration or flow	90	0(?)	±100	0
Sheath	Complex of concentric layers of protein interspersed with radially oriented bimolecular layers of lipid, each lamella separated by water spaces.	65	55	45	?

*Reproduced, with permission, from Harlow and Woolsey: *Biological and Biochemical Bases of Behavior.* Univ of Wisconsin, 1958.
†Nucleic acids: P = pentose type, D = deoxypentose type

chromatophore cells of the arachnoid and pia (see below). Neuromelanin is usually not present in the newborn; it appears toward the end of the first year, increases in amount until puberty, and remains more or less constant thereafter. Depigmentation of the substantia nigra is a frequent finding in parkinsonism (Fig 12-8).

B. Lipochrome (Lipofuscin): This yellow pigment appears in neurons of the spinal ganglia at about the sixth year of life, in the spinal cord a few years later, and in cerebrocortical neurons after the twentieth year. The amount of lipochrome increases with advanced age, and the pigment is quite marked in old age. It appears as droplets around the nerve cell nucleus, stains deeply with osmic acid and Sudan III, and is insoluble in the usual fat solvents.

C. Hemoglobin Derivatives: These are sometimes found in the central nervous system. Yellow-brown granules of hemosiderin, an iron-containing pigment, appear following extravasation of blood and in hemochromatosis. Hemofuscin, a light yellow granular substance containing no iron, is found in excessive quantities in hemochromatosis. Hematoidin, a decomposition product of heme, forms biliverdin, a green pigment that imparts a light green color to white matter surrounding a hemorrhagic site.

D. Calcium: Calcification occurs normally within the pineal body during adult life. Small granules or large masses of calcium phosphate and calcium carbonate may also occur pathologically in the central nervous system: Calcification occurs in the cerebral cortex in Sturge-Weber syndrome and within the vascular tree, meninges, and the choroid plexuses as a degenerative process. It also occurs in some brain tumors, such as meningiomas, oligodendrogliomas, and craniopharyngiomas.

E. Iron: Iron compounds are normally present in the globus pallidus and substantia nigra. Some of the iron in the brain has been found to be ferritin, a crystallizable protein containing 23% iron. The iron in the brain tissue is probably a product of iron metabolism in the brain, although it can also arise from extravasated red blood cells.

METABOLIC FEATURES OF THE BRAIN

Embryonic Brain

The metabolism of the embryonic brain is characterized by its great capacity to synthetize the proteins and lipids needed for growth. Although oxidative mechanisms are deficient, the brain is highly capable of utilizing carbohydrates by glycolysis. During fetal life, glucose-oxidation systems become more active, extending progressively from the lower to the higher centers and continuing after birth. As development proceeds, successive changes in the activity of individual enzymes take place, with new enzymes appearing, increasing in activity, and then declining.

Many studies have attempted to correlate functional brain status and enzymatic distribution. In early fetal life, the cerebral cortex of the guinea pig has been found to contain constant low concentrations of respiratory enzymes, cytochrome c, succinic dehydrogenase, and adenylpyrophosphatase (apyrase). The concentrations of these enzymes increase sharply at the time of morphologic differentiation and the onset of electrical activity in nerve cells. The adult level is reached or approximated at birth. In other vertebrate species, a similar close relationship has been noted between functional development and brain enzyme concentrations of cholinesterase and carbonic anhydrase.

Studies involving the induction of brain malformations in small laboratory animals have increased knowledge of the metabolic characteristics of mammalian embryonic tissues. Developing cells change their response to metabolic injury as they grow, and the organism changes metabolically as it develops. Although developmental patterns are primarily genetically determined and latent genetic abnormalities may be precipitated by injurious agents, different agents may produce different types of malformation at the same stage of development. In both late fetal and neonatal life, the brain is able to use glucose either aerobically or anaerobically for sustained periods. The capacity for anaerobic survival is lost in the second or third week, when embryonic cells have generally grown to their mature forms. The cerebrum becomes dependent upon an immediate supply of glucose and oxygen, although parts of the brain stem and midbrain may be less dependent than other tissues. Some drugs (cyanide, azide, and malonitrile) can cause damage, similar to that caused by anoxia, to the neurons of the cortex and striatum; they may also damage white matter. Certain parts of the hypothalamus, brain stem, and peripheral ganglia may be damaged by acetylpyridine; the damage can be prevented by its analogue, nicotinamide.

Various types of metabolic toxins or inhibitors can selectively damage primitive differentiating embryonal cells. These cells are susceptible to radiation during nucleic-acid and protein synthesis and the period of rapid growth to a more adult phase. Oxidizing compounds produced in water by radiation seem to affect enzymes with sulfhydryl groups, a type of enzyme that seems to be important at this early stage of cell differentiation. Effects similar to those of ionizing radiation may be produced by chemicals of nucleic acid metabolism (aminopterin and certain corticosteroids). Adult brain neurons are relatively radioresistant.

Adult Brain

The adult brain's ability to synthetize certain proteins and lipids is greatly reduced, but the dependence upon carbohydrate as its main fuel persists. The brain is characterized by a high overall oxygen consumption, with metabolic activity generally highest in the cortex and cerebellum. The high energy requirement of most portions of the brain is related to the transport of ions, the synthesis of acetylcholine, and the metabolism of glutamic acid. There are concomitant changes that affect phospholipids and nucleoproteins; however, the metabolic processes associated with the functional activity of the brain are poorly understood.

Carbohydrate, in the form of glucose, is the principal source of energy for tissue cells of the central nervous system; it serves as a major contributor in the building of amino acids and fatty acids and is a source of CO_2, which helps regulate pH. Carbohydrate metabolism of nerve tissue is similar to that of muscle. Lactic acid and pyruvic acid appear under anaerobic conditions; they disappear very slowly, and oxygen does not accelerate this process. Very little glycogen storage occurs in neural tissue, and brain extracts react more readily to glucose than glycogen. The respiratory quotient of neural tissue is 1.0, suggesting that ordinarily the tissues of the central nervous system use carbohydrate almost exclusively, burning sugar with oxygen and introducing energy into cells via high-energy phosphate esters. In some circumstances, however, the brain can apparently remain active without either extrinsic or intrinsic carbohydrates.

There is no evidence that high blood glucose levels affect nervous system function directly. The effects of low blood glucose levels, however, are better understood. Prolonged hypoglycemia depresses total brain metabolism, and patients may show confusion, excitement, combativeness, automatism, drowsiness, ataxia, incoordination, dysarthria, and diplopia. These symptoms are often preceded by marked sweating and sometimes hunger. Some patients pass rapidly into convulsions and coma.

A constant (rather than rich) supply of oxygen is considered essential for normal brain function. Quantitatively, the most important substance used for oxygen activation in the brain is probably cytochrome oxidase. The brain has a high anaerobic glycolytic rate, but its rate of aerobic glycolysis is small. Energy for the metabolic activities of the brain presumably comes largely from the oxidative breakdown of glucose. Two enzymes are of major importance in the degradation of glucose: hexokinase, which is probably responsible for initiating the metabolic reactions of glucose; and triosephosphate dehydrogenase, which controls the rate of energy production from glucose 6-phosphate.

REFERENCES

Bourne GH (editor): *The Structure and Function of Nervous Tissue.* Vol. 1. Academic Press, 1968.

Cajal S: *Histologie du Systeme Nerveux de l'Homme et des Vertebres.* Vol. 2. Librairie Maloine, 1911.

Junqueira LC, Carneiro J, Kelley RO: *Basic Histology,* 6th ed. Appleton & Lange, 1989.

Landon DN (editor): *The Peripheral Nerve.* Chapman & Hall, 1976.

Palay SL, Chan-Palay V: *Cerebellar Cortex, Cytology and Organization.* Springer-Verlag, 1974.

Peters A, Palay SL, Webster HF: *The Fine Structure of the Nervous System: The Neurons and Supporting Cells.* Saunders, 1976.

3 Signaling in the Nervous System

Neurons are the basic signaling units of the nervous system. They respond to stimuli by altering the electrical potential differences that exist between the inner and outer surfaces of their membranes. Modification of the electrical potential may be restricted to the place that received the stimulus or may be propagated throughout the neuron or to other neurons. This chapter describes the means by which neurons respond to and transmit stimuli.

RESTING MEMBRANE POTENTIAL

The membranes of cells, including nerve cells, are structured so that a difference in electric potential exists between the inside of the cell (negative) and the outside (positive); ie, there is **polarization.** This difference is called the **resting,** or **steady, membrane potential;** it is normally −70 mV.

The cell membrane is highly permeable to most inorganic ions but almost impermeable to proteins and many other organic anions. The difference (**gradient**) in ion composition inside and outside the cell is maintained by "pumps" in the membrane, which use metabolic energy to maintain a constant concentration of inorganic ions within the cell (Fig 3–1 and Table 3–1). This equilibrium is maintained by the combination of 2 opposite forces: a chemical force that moves ions outward, and an electrical force that keeps the same ions in. When the forces are equally strong, an **equilibrium potential** exists.

The **Nernst equation,** which describes the relationship between these forces, is used to calculate the magnitude of the equilibrium potential, ie, the membrane potential at which equilibrium exists. For example, normally there is relatively more potassium inside the cell and relatively more sodium outside. The Nernst equation for potassium ions (K^+) is as follows:

$$E_K = \frac{RT}{nF} \log_{10} \frac{[K^+]o}{[K^+]i}$$

where

E = equilibrium potential (no net flow across the membrane)

K = potassium

T = temperature

R = gas constant

F = Faraday constant (relates charge in coulombs to concentration in moles)

n = valence (for potassium, valence = 1)

$[K^+]i$ = concentration of potassium inside cell

$[K^+]o$ = concentration of potassium outside cell

When Na^+ (sodium ion) is substituted for K^+ in the equation, the equilibrium potential for sodium is much smaller.

The sum of the equilibrium potentials for potassium and sodium is the **resting membrane potential,** ie, the energy stored within the cell that can be used for signaling. Some cells can change the per-

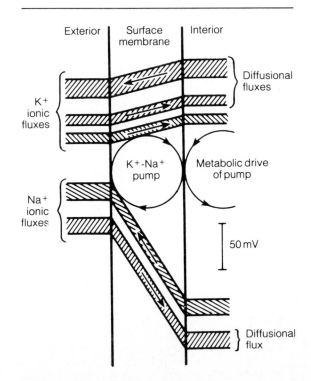

Figure 3–1. Na^+ and K^+ fluxes through the resting nerve cell membrane. (Reproduced, with permission, from Eccles JC: *The Physiology of Nerve Cells.* Johns Hopkins University Press, 1957.)

Table 3–1. Concentration of some ions inside and outside mammalian spinal motor neurons.*

Ion	Concentration (mmol/L H₂O)		Equilibrium Potential (mV)
	Inside Cell	Outside Cell	
NA⁺	15.0	150.0	+ 60
K⁺	150.0	5.5	− 90
Cl⁻	9.0	125.0	− 70
Resting membrane potential = −70 mV			

*Reproduced with permission, from Ganong WF: *Review of Medical Physiology,* 13th ed. Appleton & Lange, 1987. Data from Mommaerts WFHM, in: *Essentials of Human Physiology.* Ross G (editor). Year Book, 1978

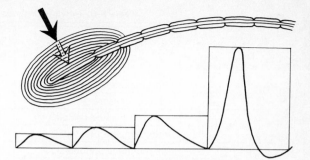

Figure 3–2. Demonstration of a generator potential in a pacinian corpuscle. The electrical responses to a pressure (black arrow) of 1x, 2x, 3x, and 4x are shown. The strongest stimulus produced an action potential in the sensory nerve, originating in the center of the corpuscle (open arrow).

meability of their cell membrane, however; when these cells are excited, they initiate a current that changes the resting membrane potential of the cell.

GENERATOR POTENTIAL

The **generator (receptor) potential** is a local, nonpropagated response that occurs in some sensory receptors (eg, muscle stretch receptors and pacinian corpuscles, which are touch-pressure receptors) where mechanical energy is converted into electric signals. The generator potential is produced in a small area of the sensory cell, the unmyelinated nerve terminal. In contrast to action potentials (see below), which are all-or-none responses, generator potentials are **graded**—the larger the stimulus (stretch or pressure), the larger the depolarization (decrease in negative voltage); and **additive**—2 small stimuli, close together in time, produce a generator potential larger than that produced by a single small stimulus. Further increase in stimulation results in larger generator potentials (see Fig 3–2). When the magnitude of the generator potential is increased to about 10 mV, a propagated action potential (impulse) is generated in the sensory nerve.

ACTION POTENTIAL

The entire sequence of electrical events that occurs when an impulse is propagated is called an **action potential.** When a sufficiently strong impulse approaches along a sensory or motor nerve fiber, the membrane begins to **depolarize,** ie, to decrease its negative voltage. When the initial depolarization reaches about 15 mV, the **firing level** is reached, and the rate of depolarization increases sharply to produce a spike: the **isopotential level (zero potential)** is overshot by about 35 mV (Fig 3–3). As the impulse passes, the charge reverses

and **repolarization** occurs, rapidly at first, then more slowly. The period of increased resistance to further impulses (**refractory period**—the rising and many of the falling phases of the spike) is characterized by **after-hyperpolarization.** The threshold for the action potential varies with experimental procedures, temperature, and type of axon; but once the impulse is strong enough to reach or pass

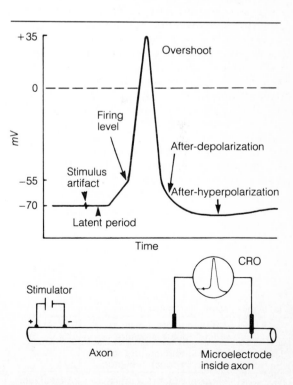

Figure 3–3. Action potential ("spike potential") recorded with one electrode inside cell. (Reproduced, with permission, from Ganong WF: *Review of Medical Physiology,* 14th ed. Appleton & Lange, 1989.)

Table 3-2. Nerve fiber types in mammalian nerve.*

Fiber Type		Function	Fiber Diameter (μm)	Conduction Velocity (m/s)	Spike Duration (ms)	Absolute Refractory Period (ms)
A	α	Proprioception; somatic motor	12–20	70–120		
	β	Touch, pressure	5–12	30–70	0.4–0.5	0.4–1
	γ	Motor to muscle spindles	3–6	15–30		
	δ	Pain, temperature, touch	2–5	12–30		
B		Preganglionic autonomic	<3	3–15	1.2	1.2
C dorsal root		Pain, reflex responses	0.4–1.2	0.5–2	2	2
sympathetic		Postganglionic sympathetics	0.3–1.3	0.7–2.3	2	2

*Reproduced, with permission, from Ganong WF: *Review of Medical Physiology,* 13th ed. Appleton & Lange, 1987.

the threshold, an action potential will follow in an all-or-none manner.

CONDUCTION OF SIGNALS

Types of Fibers

Nerve fibers have been divided into 3 types according to their diameters, conduction velocities, and physiologic characteristics (Table 3-2). **A fibers** are large and myelinated, conduct rapidly, and conduct various motor or sensory impulses. They are most susceptible to injury by mechanical pressure or lack of oxygen. **B fibers** are smaller than A fibers and are myelinated; they conduct slowly and serve autonomic functions. **C fibers** are the smallest and are unmyelinated; they conduct impulses most slowly, and they serve pain conduction and autonomic functions. Table 3-3 shows a numerical classification sometimes used for sensory neurons.

The large A fibers are least sensitive to local anesthetics and the small-diameter, poorly myelinated C fibers most sensitive. Conversely, large-diameter fibers are most easily excited by electrical stimuli and those with small-diameter fibers least easily.

Physiology

Because fibers with larger diameters have lower thresholds for electrical stimulation, only the large-diameter fibers (IA) are stimulated when a mixed peripheral nerve (one containing both sensory and motor fibers) is stimulated by a low-intensity electrical current. A stimulus of greater intensity affects the smaller efferent as well as the afferent fibers. The nerve itself is most sensitive to stimulation; the myoneural junction is intermediate in sensitivity, and the muscle is least sensitive.

The nerve-conduction velocity is normally 50–60 m/s in ulnar and median nerves and 45–55 m/s in the common peroneal nerve. The conduction velocity of a nerve may be markedly slowed by a decrease in temperature, compression, and other conditions: it may decrease by 2 m/s for each drop of 1 °C (1.8 °F) in temperature. The conduction velocity is highest in myelinated fibers (up to 50 times faster than in unmyelinated fibers; see Fig 3–4). In myelinated fibers, the insulating sheath is interrupted periodically by the unmyelinated nodes of Ranvier (Fig 2–3). Because the current flow through myelin is negligible, the depolarization in myelinated axons jumps from one node to the next (saltatory conduction; Fig 3–5).

SYNAPTIC TRANSMISSION

Individual nerve cells are in close contact at synapses, where functional connections between neurons occur (see also Chapter 2). Microelectrode techniques allow the detection of **excitatory** or **inhibitory postsynaptic potentials** in association with depolarization of the postsynaptic membrane. These potentials can be clearly differentiated from signals reaching the synapse (presynaptic poten-

Table 3-3. Numerical classification sometimes used for sensory neurons.*

Number		Origin	Fiber Type
I	a	Muscle spindle, annulospiral ending	A α
	b	Golgi tendon organ	A α
II		Muscle spindle, flower-spray ending; tough, pressure	A β
III		Pain and temperature receptors; some touch receptors	A δ
IV		Pain and other receptors	Dorsal root C

*Reproduced, with permission, from Ganong WF: *Review of Medical Physiology,* 13th ed. Appleton & Lange, 1987.

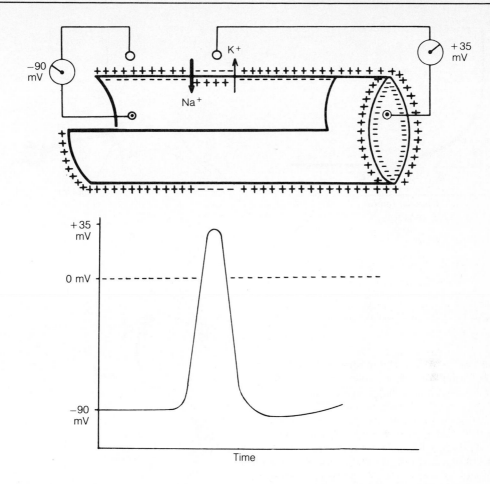

Figure 3-4. Conduction of the nerve impulse through an unmyelinated nerve fiber. In the resting axon, there is a difference of −90 mV between the interior of the axon and the outer surface of its membrane (resting potential). During the impulse passage, more Na$^+$ (thick arrow) passes into the axon interior than the amount of K$^+$ (thin arrow) that migrates in the opposite direction. In consequence, the membrane polarity changes (the membrane becomes relatively positive on its inner surface), and the resting potential is replaced by an action potential (+35 mV here). (Reproduced, with permission, from Junqueira LC, Carneiro J, Kelley RO: *Basic Histology,* 6th ed. Appleton & Lange, 1989.)

tials) and from the all-or-none impulses that originate in and are conducted from the postsynaptic element. The time interval (usually between 0.5 and 1 ms) required for an impulse to pass across a synapse is called the **synaptic delay.** The delay (latency) in reflexes is caused principally by the number of synaptic delays in a reflex arc. Transmission of signals at synapses may be facilitated or inhibited. Inhibition can be direct, presynaptic, or postsynaptic involving an interneuron (Fig 3–6).

End-Plate Potential

The motor nerve fiber axons terminate at a specialized portion of the muscle membrane called the **motor end-plate** (Fig 3–7), which represents localized specialization of the sarcolemma, the membrane surrounding a striated muscle fiber. The nerve impulse is transmitted to the muscle across

the **neuromuscular synapse (myoneural junction).** The end-plate potential is the prolonged negative electrical potential that occurs at the end-plate; it is not propagated but localized to the myoneural junction. Small amounts of acetylcholine are released randomly from the nerve cell membrane at rest; each release produces a minute depolarizing spike, a miniature end-plate potential, about 0.5 mV in amplitude. When a nerve impulse reaches the myoneural junction, however, substantially more transmitter is released. This causes a full end-plate potential that exceeds the firing level of the muscle fiber.

Clinical Correlations

A. Neuropathy: In neuropathies—diseases affecting the peripheral nerves—the conduction velocity of motor nerves may be reduced, frequently

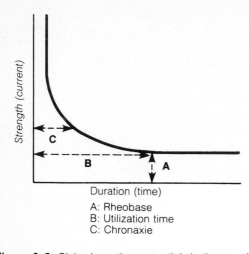

A: Rheobase
B: Utilization time
C: Chronaxie

Figure 3–5. Biphasic action potential; both recording electrodes are on the outside of the nerve membrane. (Reproduced, with permission, from Ganong WF: *Review of Medical Physiology,* 14th ed. Appleton & Lange, 1989.)

to less than 40 m/s. This reduction can be seen in increased conduction time between nerve stimulation and muscle stimulation and in the longer duration of the muscle action potential. Marked slowing in conduction velocity occurs in chronic neuropathies, during nerve regeneration following injury, and in a familial or hereditary form of progressive muscular atrophy. There is little or no reduction in nerve conduction velocity in diseases affecting the anterior horn cells, eg, amyotrophic lateral sclerosis.

B. Myasthenic Reaction: In myasthenia gravis, myasthenic syndrome, and some other types of neural disorders, the involved muscles rapidly become fatigued upon repeated electrical stimulation and finally do not respond at all. Excitability usually returns after a rest period.

C. Myotonic Reaction: In disorders characterized by myotonia (eg, myotonia congenita or atrophica), the affected muscles may show a prolonged response to a single stimulus.

D. Tetanic Reaction: In tetany, a disorder characterized by intermittent tonic muscle contractions, the muscles may be hyperexcitable.

NEUROTRANSMITTERS

One of the most exciting areas of study in the neurosciences is the effects of neurotransmitters; the discovery of an increasing number of transmitter agents is drawing a new type of chemical brain map that enriches the traditional pathways map.

A large number of chemical compounds act as neurotransmitters at chemical synapses (see also

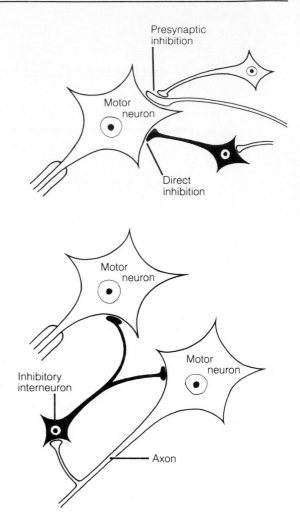

Figure 3–6. *Top:* Schematic illustration of two types of inhibition in the spinal cord. In direct inhibition, a chemical mediator released from an inhibitory neuron causes hyperpolarization (inhibitory postsynaptic potential) of a motor neuron. In presynaptic inhibition, a second chemical mediator released onto the ending (axon) of an excitatory neuron causes a reduction in the size of the postsynaptic excitatory potential. *Bottom:* Diagram of a specific inhibitory system involving an inhibitory interneuron (Renshaw cell).

Chapter 2). Such substances are present in the synaptic terminal, and their action may be blocked by pharmacologic agents. Some presynaptic nerves can release more than one transmitter; differences in the frequency of nerve stimulation probably control which transmitter is released. Common transmitters that consist of relatively small molecules are listed with their main areas of concentration in the nervous system in Table 3–4.

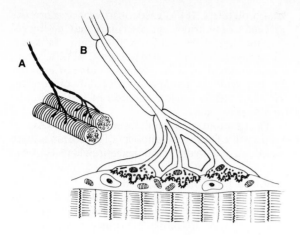

Figure 3-7. Schematic illustrations of a myoneural junction. *A:* Motor fiber supplying several muscle fibers. *B:* Cross section as seen in an electron micrograph.

It has been shown that some neurons in the central nervous system not only make and store the common transmitters but also accumulate a variety of peptides (Table 3–5). Some of these peptides act much like conventional transmitters; others appear to be hormones. A few are both classic transmitters and hormone-type neuropeptides.

Acetylcholine

Acetylcholine is synthesized by the enzyme choline acetyltransferase and broken down by the enzyme acetylcholinesterase. The transmitter ACh has, in general, a short, sudden excitatory or stim-

Table 3-4. Areas of concentration of common neurotransmitters.

Neurotransmitter	Areas of concentration
Acetylcholine (ACh)	Neuromuscular junction, autonomic ganglia, parasympathetic neurons, motor nuclei of cranial nerves, caudate nucleus and putamen, basal nucleus of Meynert, portions of the limbic system
Norepinephrin (NE)	Sympathetic nervous system, locus ceruleus, lateral tegmentum
Dopamine (DA)	Hypothalamus, midbrain nigrostriatal system
Serotonin (5-HT)	Paraysmpathetic neurons in gut, pineal gland, nucleus raphe magnus of pons
Gamma-aminobutyric acid (GABA)	Cerebellum, hippocampus, cerebral cortex, strionigral system
Glycine	Spinal cord
Glutamic acid	Spinal cord, CNS

Table 3-5. Mammalian neuropeptides.

Hypothalamic-releasing hormones
  Thyrotropin-releasing hormone (TRH)
  Gonadotropin-releasing hormone
  Somatostatin
  Corticotropin-releasing factor (CRF)
  Growth-hormone-releasing hormone
  Luteinizing-hormone-releasing hormone (LHRH)
Pituitary peptides
  Corticotropin (ACTH)
  Growth hormone (GH), somatotropin
  Lipotropin
  Alpha melanocyte-stimulating hormone (alpha MSH)
  Prolactin
  Luteinizing hormone
  Thyrotropin
Neurohypophyseal hormones
  Vasopressin
  Oxytocin
  Neurophysin(s)
Circulating hormones
  Angiotensin
  Calcitonin
  Glucagon
  Insulin
Gut brain peptides
  Vasoactive intestinal peptide (VIP)
  Cholecystokinin (CCK)
  Gastrin
  Motilin
  Pancreatic polypeptide
  Secretin
  Substance P
  Bombesin
  Neurotensin
Opioid peptides
  Dynorphin
  Beta-endorphin
  Met-enkephalin
  Leu-enkephalin
  Kyotorphin
Others
  Bradykinin
  Carnosine
  Neuropeptide Y
  Proctolin
  Substance K
  Epidermal growth factor (EGF)

ulatory effect on its receptors. It is found in many areas of the nervous system as well as in ganglia and myoneural junctions. It has an inhibitory effect on heart muscle.

Catecholamines

Norepinephrine, epinephrine, and dopamine are formed by hydroxylation and decarboxylation of the essential amino acid phenylalanine. Phenylethanolamine-N-methyltransferase, the enzyme responsible for converting norepinephrine to epinephrine, is found in high concentration only in the adrenal medulla. Dopamine is the immediate precursor of norepinephrine, and its distribution in the brain parallels that of norepinephrine except in the caudate nucleus and putameu, where there is a very high concentration of dopamine and a low concentration of norepinephrine. Dopamine, like norepinephrine, is inactivated by monoamine oxidase and catechol O-methyltransferase (COMT). The biochemical events that occur in cholinergic and noradrenergic junctions have been well analyzed (Fig 3–8). Norepinephrine secretion, in general, has an inhibitory, slow, long-lasting effect on its receptors. In parkinsonism, the dopamine content of some brain areas (the caudate nucleus and the putamen) is greatly reduced; this may be related to secondary degeneration of nerve endings on degenerating cells in another area (the substantia nigra). The connections between these two areas are called the nigrostriatal system (see Chapter 12). Other aminergic pathways have been analyzed in experimental animals. There is evidence that similar systems occur in humans. These include a pathway from the midbrain to the cerebral cortex (medial or limbic portion) and pathways from the hypothalamus to the gray matter of the spinal cord and to the pituitary gland.

Serotonin

Serotonin (5-hydroxytryptamine), like histamine, epinephrine, and norepinephrine, may be one of the most important regulatory amines of the body. Serotonin is present in high concentration in the hypothalamus, the brain stem (raphe nuclei and locus ceruleus), the caudate nucleus, and in descending tracts in the spinal cord. It can also be found in the mammalian gastrointestinal tract and

blood platelets. It has vasoconstrictor and pressor effects. Some drugs, eg, reserpine, may act by releasing bound serotonin in the brain. In small doses, lysergic acid diethylamide (LSD), a structural analogue of serotonin, is capable of evoking mental symptoms similar to those of schizophrenia. The vasoconstrictive action of LSD is inhibited by serotonin.

The tissue enzyme **monoamine oxidase (MAO)** is responsible for the metabolism of serotonin and its excretion as **5-hydroxyindoleacetic acid (5-HIAA).**

Gamma-aminobutyric Acid

Gamma-aminobutyric acid (GABA) is present in relatively large amounts in the gray matter of the brain. It is an inhibitory substance and probably the mediator responsible for presynaptic inhibition. GABA and glutamic acid decarboxylase (GAD), the enzyme that forms it from L-glutamic acid, occur in the central nervous system and the retina.

Endorphins

This is a general term used for some endogenous morphinelike substances whose activity has been defined by their ability to bind to opiate receptors in the brain. Endorphins (brain polypeptides with actions like opiates) may act as synaptic transmitters or modulators. When injected into animals, endorphins can be analgesic and tranquilizing.

Enkephalins

Two closely related polypeptides (pentapeptides) found in the brain that also bind to opiate receptors are **methionine enkephalin (met-enkephalin)** and **leucine enkephalin (leu-enkephalin).** The amino acid sequence of met-enkephalin has been found in alpha-endorphin and beta-endorphin, and that of beta-endorphin has been found in beta-lipotropin, a polypeptide secreted by the anterior pituitary gland.

Histamine

Histamine in large amounts has been found in the pituitary gland and the adjacent median eminence of the hypothalamus and in mast cells in blood. In injured tissues, histamine released from damaged cells increases capillary permeability and is therefore probably responsible for some of the swelling in areas of inflammation.

Substance P

This polypeptide, formed of 11 amino acids, is found in the hypothalamus, substantia nigra, and dorsal roots of the spinal nerves. There is evidence that substance P is a transmitter in primary sensory afferent neurons ending in the dorsal horn of the spinal cord.

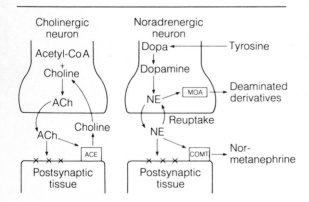

Figure 3–8. Comparison of the biochemical events at cholinergic endings with those at noradrenergic endings. ACh, acetylcholine; ACE, acetylcholinesterase; NE, norepinephrine; X, receptor. Because monoamine oxidase (MAO) is intracellular, some norepinephrine is constantly being deaminated in noradrenergic endings. Catechol-O-methyltransferase (COMT) acts on norepinephrine after it is secreted. (Reproduced, with permission, from Ganong WF: Review of Medical Physiology, 14th ed. Appleton & Lange, 1989.)

Other Peptides

Peptides such as cholecystokinin and vasoactive intestinal polypeptide, which were first known as intestinal hormones, have been found in the brain. In some cases, it appears that a peptide may occur together with a classic transmitter in the same neuron. About 30 small peptides have been found in neurons in the mammalian central nervous system.

CASE 1

Six months before presentation, a 35-year-old unmarried woman began to complain that she occasionally saw double when watching television. The double vision often disappeared after she had some bed rest. Subsequently, she felt that her eyelids tended to droop during reading, but after a good night's rest, she felt normal again. Her physician referred her to a specialty clinic.

At the clinic, the woman said she tired easily and her jaw muscles became fatigued at the end of the meal. No sensory deficits were found. A preliminary diagnosis was made, and some tests were performed to confirm the diagnosis.

What is the differential diagnosis? Which neuroradiologic procedures, if any, would be useful? What is the most likely diagnosis?

Cases are discussed further in Chapter 24. Questions and answers pertaining to Section I (Chapters 1–3) can be found in Appendix D.

REFERENCES

Amaral DG, Sinnamon HM: The locus coeruleus: Neurobiology of a central noradrenergic nucleus. *Prog Neurobiol* 1977;**9**:147.

Hokfelt T, Bjorklund A: Classical transmitters and the transmitter receptors in the CNS. In: *Handbook of Chemical Neuroanatomy,* Vol 3, Part 2. Elsevier, 1989.

Kaczmarck L, Levitan I: *Neuromodulation.* Oxford University Press, 1987.

Kandel ER, Schwartz J: *Principles of Neural Science.* Elsevier, 1981.

Krieger DT: Brain peptides: What, where and why? *Science* 1983;**222**:975.

Krnjevic K: Chemical nature of synaptic transmission in vertebrates. *Physiol Rev* 1974;**54**:418.

Shepherd GM: *The synaptic organization of the brain,* 2nd ed. Oxford University Press, 1979.

Starke K, Gothert M, Kilbinger H: Modulation of neurotransmitter release by presynaptic receptors. *Physiol Rev* 1989;**69**:864.

Section II.
Spinal Cord & Spine

The Spinal Cord

4

DEVELOPMENT OF THE SPINAL CORD

Differentiation

At about the third week of prenatal development, the ectoderm of the embryonic disc forms the **neural plate,** which folds at the edges into the **neural tube (neuraxis).** A group of cells migrates to form the **neural crest,** which gives rise to dorsal and autonomic ganglia, the adrenal medulla, and other structures (Fig 4–1). The middle portion of the neural tube closes first; the openings at each end close later.

The cells in the wall of the neural tube divide and differentiate, forming an ependymal layer that encircles the central canal and is surrounded by intermediate (mantle) and marginal zones of primitive neurons and glial cells (Figs 4–1 and 4–2). The mantle zone differentiates into 2 regions, an **alar plate** that contains mostly sensory neurons and a **basal plate** that is mostly motor neurons. These 2 regions are demarcated by the **sulcus limitans,** a groove on the wall of the central canal. The alar plate differentiates into a dorsal gray column; the basal plate becomes a ventral gray column. The processes of the mantle zone and other cells are contained in the marginal zone, which becomes the white matter of the spinal cord (Fig 4–2).

An investing layer of ectodermal cells around the primitive cord forms the 2 inner meninges: the arachnoid and pia (pia mater) (Fig 4–2). The thicker outer investment, the dura (dura mater), is formed from mesenchyma.

Clinical Correlations

Failure of the neural tube to close at the cranial end results in **anencephaly,** a type of maldevelopment of the brain and skull that is incompatible with life. Failure of closure at the caudal end results in **spina bifida,** which is associated with maldevelopment of the vertebrae (see Fig 5–9). Sometimes the meninges balloon out to form a sac, or **meningocele,** associated with a defect in the

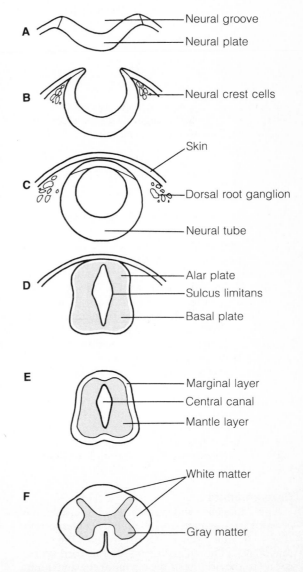

Figure 4-1. Schematic cross sections showing the development of the spinal cord.

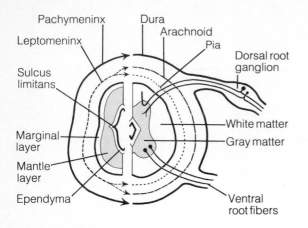

Figure 4-2. Cross section showing 2 phases in the development of the spinal cord (each half shows one phase). *A:* Early phase. *B:* Later phase with central cavity.

overlying vertebra. If such a sac contains nervous tissue, it is a **myelomeningocele** and is associated with severe disturbances of function.

EXTERNAL ANATOMY OF THE SPINAL CORD

The spinal cord (**medulla spinalis,** or **myelon**) is an elongated, cylindrical mass of nerve tissue that occupies the upper two-thirds of the adult spinal canal within the vertebral column (Fig 4–3). The cord is normally 42–45 cm long in adults and is continuous with the brain stem at its upper end. The **conus medullaris** is the conical distal (inferior) end of the spinal cord; the **filum terminale** extends from the tip of the conus and attaches to the distal dural sac. The filum terminale consists of pia and glial fibers; it often contains a vein.

The **central canal** extends the length of the spinal cord during development. It is lined with ependymal cells and filled with cerebrospinal fluid. It opens upward into the inferior portion of the fourth ventricle in the lower brain stem. In adults, the canal usually disappears except at cervical levels; nests of ependymal cells are found elsewhere in the cord.

Enlargements

The spinal cord widens laterally in 2 regions: the **cervical enlargement** and the **lumbar enlargement** (Fig 4–3). The latter tapers off to form the conus medullaris. The enlargements of the cord correspond to the origins of the nerves of the upper and lower extremities. The nerves of the brachial plexus originate at the cervical enlargement; the nerves of

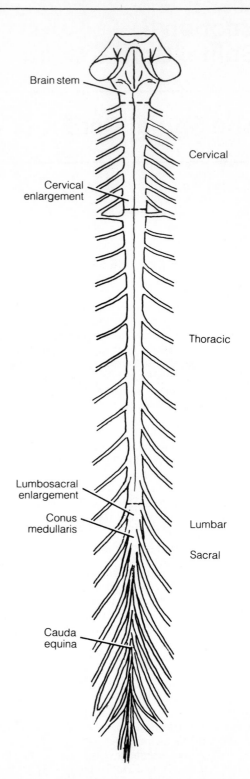

Figure 4-3. Schematic dorsal view of isolated spinal cord and spinal nerves (roots of nerves not shown).

the lumbosacral plexus arise from the lumbar enlargement.

Segments

The spinal cord is divided into approximately 30 segments (see Fig 4–3 and Appendix C)—8 cervical (C) segments, 12 thoracic (T) segments, 5 lumbar (L) segments, 5 sacral (S) segments, and a few small coccygeal (Co) segments—that correspond to attachments of groups of nerve roots (Figs 4–3 and 4–5). Individual segments vary in length; they are about twice as long in the midthoracic region as in the cervical or upper lumbar area. There are no sharp boundaries between segments within the cord itself.

Longitudinal Divisions

A cross section of the spinal cord (Fig 4–4) shows a deep anterior **median fissure** and a shallow **posterior median sulcus,** which divide the cord into symmetric right and left halves that are joined in the central midportion. The anterior median fissure contains a fold of pia and blood vessels; its floor is the **anterior white commissure** (a misnomer, since the fibers decussate here). The dorsal nerve roots are attached to the spinal cord along a shallow vertical groove, the **posterolateral sulcus,** which lies a short distance anterior to the posterior median sulcus. The ventral nerve roots exit in the **anterolateral sulcus.**

SPINAL ROOTS & NERVES

Each segment of the spinal cord pertains to 4 roots: a ventral and a dorsal root of the left half, and a similar pair of the right half (Fig 4–4). The first cervical segment usually lacks dorsal roots.

Each of the 31 pairs of spinal nerves that arise from the spinal cord has a ventral root and a dorsal root (Fig 4–5); each root is made up of 1–8 rootlets. Each root consists of bundles of nerve fibers. In the dorsal root of a typical spinal nerve, close to the junction with the ventral root, lies a **dorsal root (spinal) ganglion,** a swelling that contains nerve cell bodies. The portion of a spinal nerve outside the vertebral column is sometimes referred to as a peripheral nerve. The spinal nerves are divided into groups that correspond to the spinal cord segments (Fig 4–5).

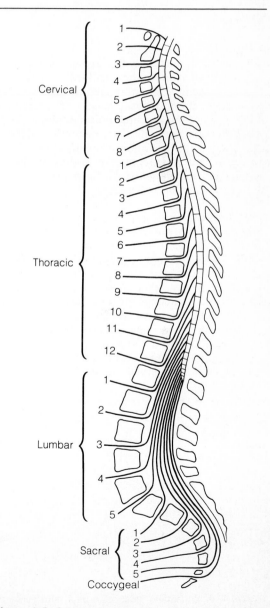

Figure 4–5. Schematic illustration of the relationships between the vertebral column, the spinal cord, and the spinal nerves.

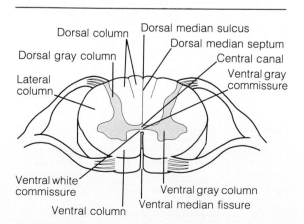

Figure 4–4. Anatomy of the spinal cord shown in cross section.

Direction of Roots

Until the third month of fetal life, the spinal cord is as long as the vertebral canal. After that point, the vertebral column elongates faster than the spinal cord, so that at birth the cord extends to about the level of the third lumbar vertebra. In adults, the tip of the cord normally lies at the level of the first or second lumbar vertebra. Because of the different growth rates of the cord and spine, the cord segments are displaced upward from their corresponding vertebrae, with the greatest discrepancy in the lowest cord segments (Fig 4–5). In the lumbosacral region, the nerve roots descend almost vertically below the cord to form the **cauda equina.**

Ventral Root

The ventral roots carry the large-diameter alpha motor neuron axons to the extrafusal striated muscle fibers; the smaller gamma motor neuron axons that supply the intrafusal muscle of the muscle spindles (Fig 4–6); preganglionic autonomic fibers at the thoracic, upper lumbar, and midsacral levels (see Chapter 19); and a few afferent, small-diameter axons that arise from cells in the dorsal root ganglia and convey sensory information from the thoracic and abdominal viscera.

Dorsal Root

Each dorsal nerve root (except usually C1) contains afferent fibers from the nerve cells in its ganglion. The dorsal roots contain a variety of fibers from cutaneous and deep structures (see Table 3–2): The largest fibers (Ia) come from muscle spindles and participate in spinal cord reflexes; the medium-sized fibers (A-beta) convey impulses from mechanoceptors in skin and joints. Most of the axons in the dorsal nerve roots are small (C, nonmyelinated; A-delta, myelinated) and carry information of noxious (eg, pain) and thermal stimuli.

Branches of Typical Spinal Nerves

A. Posterior Primary Division: This usually consists of a medial branch, which is in most instances largely sensory, and a lateral branch, which is mainly motor.

B. Anterior Primary Division: Usually larger than the posterior primary division, the anterior primary divisions form the cervical, brachial, and lumbosacral plexuses. In the thoracic region they remain segmental, as intercostal nerves.

C. Rami Communicantes: The rami join the spinal nerves to the sympathetic trunk. Only the thoracic and upper lumbar nerves contain a white ramus communicans, but the gray ramus is present in all spinal nerves (Fig 4–7).

D. Meningeal or Recurrent Meningeal Branches: These are quite small; they carry sensory and vasomotor innervation to the small meninges.

Types of Nerve Fibers

Nerve fibers can be classified on a physioanatomic basis (Table 4–1):

A. Somatic Efferent Fibers: These motor fibers innervate the skeletal muscles. They originate in large cells in the anterior gray column of the spinal cord and form the ventral root of the spinal nerve.

B. Somatic Afferent Fibers: These fibers convey sensory information from the skin, joints, and muscles to the central nervous system. They originate in unipolar cells in the spinal ganglia that are interposed in the course of dorsal roots (dorsal root ganglia). The peripheral branches of these ganglionic cells are distributed to somatic structures; the central branches convey sensory impulses through the dorsal roots to the dorsal gray column and the ascending tracts of the spinal cord.

C. Visceral Efferent Fibers: The **autonomic fibers** are the motor fibers to the viscera. **Sympathetic** fibers from the thoracic segments and L1 and L2 are distributed throughout the body to the viscera, glands, and smooth muscle. **Parasympathetic** fibers, which are present in the middle 3 sacral nerves, go to the pelvic and lower abdominal viscera.

D. Visceral Afferent Fibers: These fibers convey sensory information from the viscera. Their cell bodies are in the dorsal root ganglia. Re-

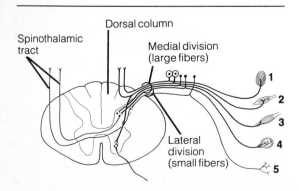

Figure 4–6. Schematic illustration of a cord segment with its dorsal root, ganglion cells, and sensory organs. *1:* Golgi organ; *2:* muscle spindle; *3:* tendon organ; *4:* encapsulated ending; *5:* free nerve endings.

Table 4–1. Anatomic relationships of spinal cord and bony spine in adults.

Cord Segments	Vertebral Bodies	Spinous Processes
CB	Lower C6 and upper C7	C6
T6	Lower T3 and upper T4	T3
T12	T9	T8
L5	T11	T10
S	T12 and L1	T12 and L1

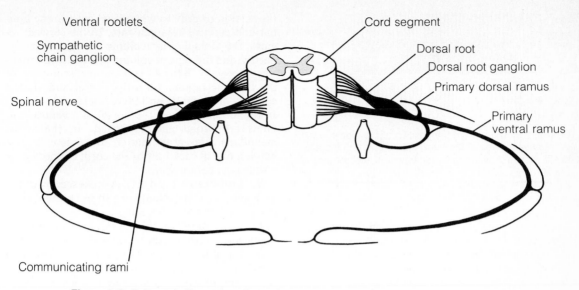

Ventral rootlets

Sympathetic
chain ganglion

Spinal nerve

Cord segment

Dorsal root

Dorsal root ganglion

Primary dorsal ramus

Primary
ventral ramus

Communicating rami

Figure 4–7. Schematic illustration of a cord segment with its roots, ganglia, and branches.

cent experimental evidence suggests that the visceral afferent fibers enter the cord through the ventral roots.

Dermatomes

The sensory component of each spinal nerve is distributed to a dermatome, a well-defined segmental portion of the skin. The pattern of cutaneous innervation generally follows the segmental distribution of underlying muscle innervation (Fig 4–8). Testing the motor functions (see Appendix B) and the sensation of the skin is very useful in determining the extent of a lesion in the nerve, spinal cord segment, or tract. The territories of dermatomes tend to overlap (Fig 4–9), however, making it difficult to determine the absence of a single segmental innervation.

INTERNAL DIVISIONS OF THE SPINAL CORD

Gray Matter

A. Columns: A cross section of the spinal cord shows an H-shaped internal mass of gray matter surrounded by white matter (Fig 4–4). The gray matter is made up of 2 symmetrical portions joined across the midline by a transverse connection (commissure) of gray matter that contains the minute central canal or its remnants. The **ventral gray column** (in cross-section, the **anterior,** or **ventral, horn**) is in front of the central canal. It contains the cells of origin of the fibers of the ventral roots. The **intermediolateral gray column** (or **horn**) is the portion of gray matter between the dorsal

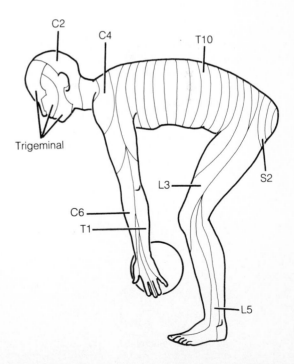

Figure 4–8. Segmental distribution of the body viewed in the approximate quadruped position.

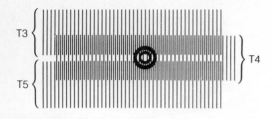

Figure 4-9. Diagram of the position of the nipple in the sensory skin fields of the third, fourth, and fifth thoracic spinal roots, showing the overlapping of the cutaneous areas.

and ventral gray columns; it is a prominent lateral triangular projection in the thoracic and upper lumbar regions, but not in the midsacral region. It contains preganglionic cells for the autonomic nervous system. The **dorsal gray column** (in cross section, the **posterior,** or **dorsal, horn**) reaches almost to the posterolateral (dorsolateral) sulcus; a compact bundle of small fibers, the **dorsolateral fasciculus (Lissauer's tract),** part of the pain pathway, lies on the periphery of the spinal cord.

The form and quantity of the gray matter vary at different levels of the spinal cord (Fig 4–10). The proportion of gray to white is greatest in the lumbar and cervical enlargements. In the cervical region, the dorsal gray column is comparatively narrow and the ventral column is broad and expansive, especially in the 4 lower cervical segments. In the thoracic region, both the dorsal and ventral columns are narrow, and there is a lateral column. In the lumbar region, the dorsal and ventral columns are broad and expanded. In the conus medullaris, the gray matter looks like 2 oval masses, one in each half of the cord, connected by a wide gray commissure.

B. Laminas: (Fig 4–11). A cross section of the gray matter of the spinal cord shows a number of laminas (layers of nerve cells).

1. Lamina I-This thin marginal layer contains many neurons that respond to noxious stimuli.

2. Lamina II-Also known as **substantia gelatinosa,** this lamina is made up of small neurons, some of which respond to noxious stimuli.

3. Laminas III and IV-These are referred to together as the **nucleus proprius.** Their main input is from fibers that convey position sense.

4. Lamina V-This layer contains cells that respond to both noxious and visceral afferent stimuli.

5. Lamina VI-The deepest layer of the dorsal horn, it contains neurons that respond to mechanical signals from joints and skin.

6. Lamina VII-This is a large zone that contains the cells of the **dorsal nucleus (Clark's column)** medially, as well as a large portion of the ventral gray column.

7. Laminas VIII and IX-These layers repre-

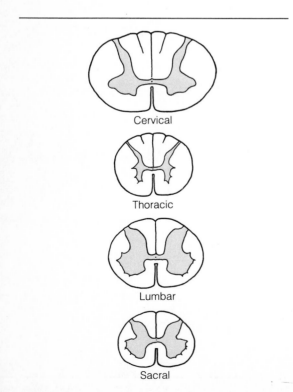

Figure 4-10. Transverse sections of the spinal cord at various levels.

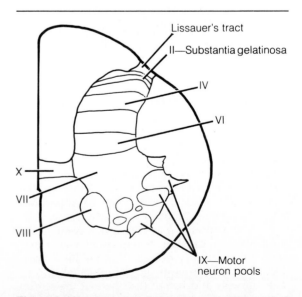

Figure 4-11. Laminas of the gray matter of the spinal cord (only one half shown).

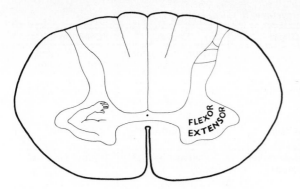

Figure 4-12. Diagram showing the functional localization of motor neuron groups (flexor extensor) in the ventral gray horn of a lower cervical segment of the spinal cord.

sent motor neuron groups in the medial and lateral portions of the ventral gray column. Innervation of extensor muscles is from the peripheral groups of neurons; flexors are represented more centrally in the ventral horn (Fig 4–12).

8. Lamina X–This represents the small neurons around the central canal or its remnants.

White Matter

A. Columns: Each lateral half of the spinal cord has white columns (funiculi)—dorsal, lateral, and ventral—around the spinal gray columns (Fig 4–4). The dorsal column lies between the posterior median sulcus and the posterolateral sulcus. In the cervical and upper thoracic regions, the dorsal column is divided into a medial portion, the **fasciculus gracilis,** and a lateral portion, the **fasciculus cuneatus.** The lateral column lies between the posterolateral sulcus and the anterolateral sulcus. The ventral column lies between the anterolateral sulcus and the anterior median fissure.

B. Tracts: The white matter of the cord is composed of myelinated and unmyelinated nerve fibers. The fast-conducting myelinated fibers form bundles (fasciculi) that ascend or descend for varying distances. Glial cells (mostly oligodendrocytes) lie between the fibers. Fiber bundles with a common function are called tracts. The lateral and ventral white columns contain tracts that are not well delimited, and may overlap in their cross-sectional areas; the dorsal column tracts are sharply defined by glial septa. Slow-conducting unmyelinated fibers form ill-defined bundles at the margin of the white matter. Their function is poorly understood.

PATHWAYS IN WHITE MATTER

Descending Fiber Systems

A. Corticospinal Tract: Arising from the cerebral cortex in a hemisphere, this large bundle of myelinated fibers descends through the brain stem, then crosses over (decussates) into the opposite half of the spinal cord to course downward in the lateral white column (Fig 4–13, Table 4–2). A small number of fibers cross at lower levels in the cord. Most of the fibers in this tract are less than 6 μm in diameter, but there are some very large fibers that arise from the giant Betz cells in the motor cortex. The fibers terminate throughout the ventral gray column and at the base of the dorsal column. The motor neurons supplying the muscles of the distal extremities have direct monosynaptic input from the corticospinal tract; other motor neurons are innervated by interneurons (polysynaptic connections).

About a third of the fibers of the corticospinal tract project to the dorsal gray column to function as modifiers of afferent information, allowing the brain to suppress certain incoming stimuli and pay attention to others (see Chapter 13).

B. Vestibulospinal Tract: The fibers of this tract arise from the lateral vestibular nucleus in the brain stem and course downward uncrossed in the

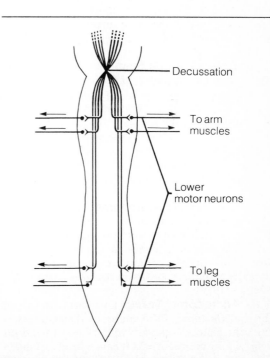

Figure 4-13. Schematic illustration of the course of corticospinal tract fibers in the spinal cord (only 4 cord segments are shown on each side). This and following similar illustrations show the cord in an upright position.

Table 4–2. Descending fiber systems in the spinal cord.

System	Function	Origin	Ending	Location in Cord
Corticospinal pyramidal	Origin of motor function Modulation of sensory functions	Cortex	Anterior horn cells, interneurons	Lateral column Ventral column
Vestibulospinal	Postural reflexes	Lateral vestib. nucleus	Anterior horn motor neurons (for extensors)	Ventral column
Rubrospinal	Motor function	Red nucleus	Ventral horn interneurons	Lateral column
Reticulospinal	Modulation of sensory transmissions (especially pain) Spinal reflexes (fibers)	Brain stem reticular formation	Dorsal and ventral horn	Tractus proprius
Descending autonomic	Modulation of autonomic functions	Hypothalamus, brain stem nuclei	Preganglionic autonomic neurons	Tractus proprius
Tectospinal	Reflex head turning	Midbrain	Ventral horn interneurons	Ventral column
Medial longitudinal fasciculus	Coordination of head and eye movements	Vestibular nuclei	Cervical gray	Tractus proprius

ventral white column of the spinal cord. Fibers of this tract project directly to the motor neurons for extensor muscles. This system facilitates quick movements in reaction to sudden changes in body position (eg, falling). The fibers also influence the discharge of gamma motor neurons.

C. Rubrospinal Tract: This fiber system arises in the contralateral red nucleus in the brain stem and courses in the lateral white column. The tract projects to interneurons in the spinal gray columns and plays a role in motor function (see Chapter 6).

D. Reticulospinal System: This tract arises in the reticular formation of the brain stem and descends in both the ventral and lateral white columns. The fibers terminating on dorsal gray column neurons may modify the transmission of sensation from the body, especially pain (some of these fibers are serotoninergic; see Chapter 13). Those that end on ventral gray neurons influence gamma motor neurons and, thus, various spinal reflexes.

E. Descending Autonomic System: Arising from the hypothalamus and brain stem, this poorly defined fiber system projects to preganglionic sympathetic neurons in the thoracolumbar spinal cord (lateral column) and to preganglionic parasympathetic neurons in sacral segments (see Chapter 19).

F. Tectospinal Tract: This tract arises from the roof (**tectum**) of the midbrain, then courses in the contralateral ventral white column to end on ventral gray interneurons. It causes head turning in response to sudden visual or auditory stimuli.

G. Medial Longitudinal Fasciculus: This tract arises from vestibular nuclei in the brain stem; some of its fibers descend into the cervical

spinal cord to terminate on ventral gray interneurons. It coordinates head and eye movements.

These last two descending fiber systems are present on each side only in the cervical segments of the spinal cord.

Ascending Fiber Systems

All afferent axons in the dorsal roots have their cell bodies in the dorsal root ganglia (Table 4–3).

A. Dorsal Column Tracts: These tracts, the **medial lemniscal system**, convey well-localized sensations of fine touch, vibration, 2-point discrimination, and proprioception (position sense) from the skin and joints; they ascend, without crossing, in the dorsal white column of the spinal cord to the lower brain stem (Fig 4–14). The **fasciculus gracilis** courses next to the posteromedian septum; it contains input from the lower half of the body, with fibers that arise from the lowest, most medial segments. The **fasciculus cuneatus** lies between the fasciculus gracilis and the dorsal gray column; it contains input from the upper half of the body, with fibers from the lower (thoracic) segments more medial than the higher (cervical) ones. Thus, one dorsal column contains fibers from all segments of the ipsilateral half of the body arranged in an orderly fashion from medial to lateral; such an arrangement is called **somatotopic organization** (Fig 4–15).

B. Spinothalamic Tract: Small-diameter fibers conveying the sensations of sharp (noxious) pain, temperature, and crudely localized touch course upward for one or two segments at the periphery of the dorsal gray horn. These short, ascending stretches of incoming fibers, the dorsolateral fasciculus, or Lissauer's tract (Fig 4–16), then synapse with dorsal column neurons, especially in

Table 4-3. Ascending fiber systems in the spinal cord.

Name	Function	Origin	Ending	Location in Cord
Dorsal column system	Fine touch, proprioception, 2-point discrimination	Skin, joints, tendons	Dorsal column nuclei, brain stem	Dorsal column
Spinothalamic tract	Sharp pain, temperature, crude touch	Skin	Dorsal horn, then to contralateral thalamus	Ventrolateral column
Dorsal spinocerebellar tract	Movement and position mechanisms	Deep tendons, joints	Cerebellar paleocortex	Lateral column
Ventral spinocerebellar	Movement and position mechanisms	Deep tendons, joints	Cerebellar paleocortex	Lateral column
Spinoreticular tract	Deep and chronic pain	Deep somatic structures	Reticular formation of brain stem	Diffuse in tractus proprius

laminas I, II, and V (Fig 4–11). After one or more synapses, subsequent fibers cross to the opposite side of the cord, to ascend steeply as the spinothalamic tract, or ventrolateral system, located in the lateral and ventral columns. This system also shows somatotopic organization (Fig 4–15).

C. Clinical Correlations: It should be emphasized that the second-order neurons of both the spinothalamic and dorsal column tracts cross, those of the former at every segmental level in the spinal cord and those of the latter in the lower brain stem. This fact aids in determining whether a lesion is in the brain or the spinal cord: With brain stem lesions, deficits in pain perception, touch sensation, and proprioception are all contralateral; with spinal cord lesions, the deficit in pain perception is contralateral while the others are ipsilateral.

D. Spinoreticular Pathway: The ill-defined spinoreticular tract courses within the ventrolateral portion of the spinal cord, arising from cord neurons and ending (without crossing) in the reticular formation of the brain stem. This tract plays an important role in the sensation of pain, especially deep, chronic pain (see Chapter 13).

E. Spinocerebellar Tracts: Two ascending pathways (of lesser importance in human neurology) provide input from the spinal cord to the cerebellum (Fig 4–17 and Table 4–3).

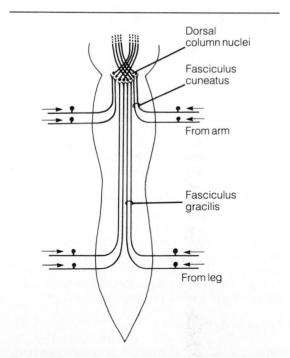

Figure 4-14. Schematic illustration of the course of fibers of the dorsal column system in the spinal cord (only 4 segments are shown on each side).

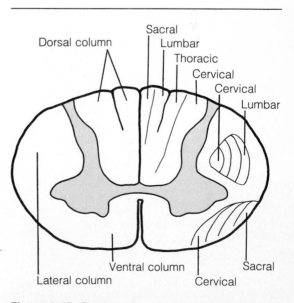

Figure 4-15. Somatotopic organization (segmental arrangement) in the spinal cord.

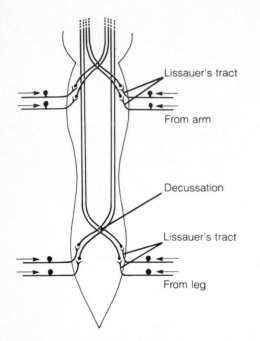

Figure 4-16. Schematic illustration of the course of fibers of the spinothalamic (ventrolateral) system in the spinal cord (only 4 segments are shown on each side).

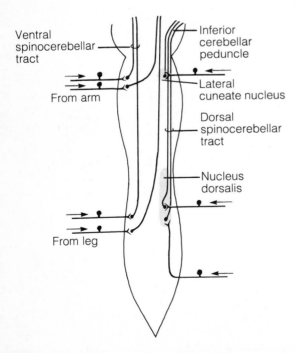

Figure 4-17. Schematic illustration of the course of some fibers of the spinocerebellar systems in the spinal cord.

1. Dorsal spinocerebellar tract–Afferent fibers from muscle and skin carry information about joint position and other sensory information via first-order neurons in the dorsal root ganglia and the second-order neurons of the nucleus dorsalis (Clarke's column). Fibers of sacral and lower lumbar origin ascend within the cord to reach the lower portion of the nucleus dorsalis. Fibers of cervical origin ascend to the brain stem, to synapse in the lateral (external) cuneate nucleus. The second-order neurons from the nucleus dorsalis form the dorsal spinocerebellar tract; second-order neurons from the lateral cuneate nucleus form the cuneocerebellar tract. Both tracts stay on the ipsilateral side of the spinal cord, ascending via the inferior cerebellar peduncle to terminate in the paleocerebellar cortex.

2. Ventral spinocerebellar tract–This system is involved with movement control. Second-order neurons ascend through the superior cerebellar peduncle to the paleocerebellar cortex. Because the neurons ascend bilaterally, this tract is of little value in localizing lesions in the spinal cord.

REFLEXES

Reflexes are subconscious stimulus-response mechanisms. The instinctive behavior of lower animals is governed largely by reflexes; in humans, behavior is more a matter of conditioning, and reflexes act as basic defense mechanisms. The reflexes are, however, extremely important in the diagnosis and localization of neurologic lesions (see Appendix B).

Simple Reflex Arc

Several structures are involved (Fig 4-18): a **receptor,** eg, a special sense organ, cutaneous end organ, or neuromuscular spindle, whose stimulation initiates an impulse; the **afferent neuron,** which transmits the impulse through a peripheral nerve to the central nervous system, where the nerve synapses with an intercalated neuron; one or more **intercalated neurons (interneurons)** which relay the impulse to the efferent nerve; the **efferent neuron,** which passes outward in the nerve and delivers the impulse to an effector; and an **effector,** eg, the muscle or gland that produces the response.

Note that interruption of this simple reflex arc at any point will abolish the response.

Types of Reflexes

The reflexes of importance to the clinical neurologist may be divided into 4 groups: superficial (skin and mucous membrane) reflexes, deep tendon (myotatic) reflexes, visceral (organic) reflexes, and pathologic (abnormal) reflexes (Table 4-4).

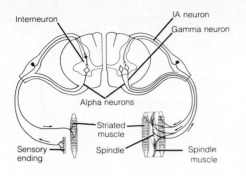

Figure 4–18. Schematic illustration of the neurons involved in the simple reflex arc (left half) and the stretch reflex (right half).

Reflexes can also be classified according to the level of their central representation, eg, as spinal, bulbar (postural and righting reflexes), midbrain, or cerebellar reflexes.

Spinal Reflexes

The segmental spinal reflex involves the afferent neuron and a motor unit at the same level (Fig 4–18). Simple reflex reactions involve patterns of movement rather than specific muscle contractions. The delay between stimulation and effect is caused by the time needed for propagation of the impulse along the nerve fibers concerned and the synaptic delay (5 ms at each synapse).

A. Flexor Reflex: The flexor reflex represents a withdrawal mechanism that removes an extremity from a harmful stimulus. Much experimental work has been done in vertebrate animals, severing

Table 4–4. Summary of reflexes.

Reflexes	Afferent Nerve	Center	Efferent Nerve
Superficial reflexes Corneal	Cranial V	Pons	Cranial VII
Nasal (sneeze)	Cranial V	Brain stem and upper cord	Cranials V, VII, IX, X, and spinal nerves of expirate
Pharyngeal and uvular	Cranial IX	Medulla	Cranial X
Upper abdominal	T7, 8, 9, 10	T7, 8, 9, 10	T7, 8, 9, 10
Lower abdominal	T10, 11, 12	T10, 11, 12	T10, 11, 12
Cremasteric	Femoral	L1	Genitofemoral
Plantar	Tibial	S1, 2	Tibial
Anal	Pudendal	S4, 5	Pudendal
Deep reflexes Jaw	Cranial V	Pons	Cranial V
Biceps	Musculocutaneous	C5, 6	Musculocutaneous
Triceps	Radial	C6, 7	Radial
Periosteoradial	Radial	C6, 7, 8	Radial
Wrist (flexion)	Median	C6, 7, 8	Median
Wrist (extension)	Radial	C7, 8	Radial
Patellar	Femoral	L2, 3, 4	Femoral
Achilles	Tibial	S1, 2	Tibial
Visceral reflexes Light	Cranial II	Midbrain	Cranial III
Accommodation	Cranial II	Occipital cortex	Cranial III
Ciliospinal	A sensory nerve	T1, 2	Cervical sympathetics
Oculocardiac	Cranial V	Medulla	Cranial X
Carotid sinus	Cranial IX	Medulla	Cranial X
Bulbocavernosus	Pudendal	S2, 3, 4	Pelvic autonomic
Bladder and rectal	Pudendal	S2, 3, 4	Pudendal and autonomics
Abnormal Reflexes Extensor plantar (Babinski)	Plantar	L3–L5, S1	Extensor hallucis longus
Oppenheim	Superficial peroneal	L5, S1	Extensor hallucis longus

the spinal cord from the brain stem. The animals subsequently exhibit prominent flexion responses that involve several segments. A single afferent nerve can stimulate many motor units; the smaller nerve branches to the skin are usually more effective than the deep sensory nerves in exciting flexor motor units. The postures seen in some forms of prolonged pathologic irritation are probably caused by flexor reflexes. A patient with peritonitis assumes a doubled-up attitude, for example, and stiffness and retraction of the neck occur in irritation of the meninges by infection, blood, or tumor cells.

B. Extensor Reflex: Extensor (deep tendon, stretch) reflexes are concerned with resisting the action of gravity upon body posture. The stretch (myotatic) reflex, with its receptors within the muscle, is the basis for the extensor reflex (Fig 4–18, right half). When extensor muscles contract, antagonistic flexor muscles relax. A sensory organ and stretch receptor, the **muscle spindle,** is present in the muscle; its sensory nerve fiber is the fast-conducting Ia fiber, which becomes excited when the muscle is stretched suddenly. The muscle spindle is connected to short intrafusal muscles at each end and innervated by gamma motor fibers from neurons in the anterior horn of the spinal cord. Through innervation, the gamma fibers maintain a constant tension on the muscle spindle, keeping the tone of the muscle constant by way of the Ia-gamma loop: Stretching the spindle causes a discharge of an afferent Ia fiber in the dorsal root, which (monosynaptically or via interneurons) activates both the efferent alpha and gamma motor neurons. Alpha fiber discharge causes the extrafusal muscle to contract, while gamma efferent discharge keeps the spindle taut.

If the alpha motor neuron fibers in a ventral root or peripheral nerve are cut, the muscle's resistance to stretching is reduced: the muscle becomes flaccid and has little tone. Hyperactive stretch reflexes can lead to hypertonic, spastic muscles.

The large extensor muscles that support the body are kept constantly active by coactivation of alpha and gamma motor neurons. The fact that transection of the spinal cord reduces muscle tone indicates that supraspinal descending axons modulate the alpha and gamma neurons.

Clinical correlations. Experimental interruption of both corticospinal and rubrospinal tracts results in a state of extreme extensor rigidity. This type of extensor rigidity has been called gamma rigidity because the rigidity disappears if the dorsal roots (in which the Ia fibers course) are subsequently cut. If the anterior portion of the cerebellum is then removed, the rigidity returns; this is alpha rigidity and occurs when the gamma loop is bypassed and the alpha motor neurons are excited directly.

C. Polysynaptic Reflexes: In contrast to the extensor stretch reflex (eg, patellar, Achilles ten-

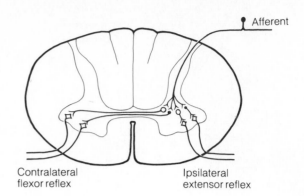

Figure 4–19. Schematic illustration of a polysynaptic reflex.

don), polysynaptic, crossed extensor reflexes (Fig 4–19) are not limited to one muscle; they usually involve many muscles on the same or opposite side of the body. These reflexes have several physiologic characteristics.

1. Reciprocal action of antagonists–Flexors are excited and extensors inhibited on one side of the body; the opposite occurs on the opposite side of the body.

2. Divergence–Stimuli from a few receptors are distributed to many motor neurons in the cord.

3. Summation–Consecutive or simultaneous subthreshold stimuli may combine to initiate the reflex.

4. Hierarchy–When 2 antagonistic reflexes are elicited simultaneously, one will override the other.

LESIONS IN THE MOTOR PATHWAYS

Lesions in the motor pathways, the muscle or its myoneural junction, or the peripheral nerve all result in disturbances of motor function (Fig 4–20; see also Chapter 12). Two main types of lesions—of the upper and lower motor neurons—are distinguished in spinal cord disorders.

Lower-Motor-Neuron Lesions

A lower motor neuron (LMN), the motor cell concerned with striated skeletal muscle activity, consists of a cell body (located in the anterior gray column of the spinal cord or brain stem) and its axon, which passes to the motor end-plates of the muscle by way of the peripheral nerves. Motor neurons are considered the final common pathway because many neural impulses funnel through them to the muscle; ie, they are acted upon by the corticospinal, rubrospinal, olivospinal, vestibulospinal, reticulospinal, and tectospinal tracts as

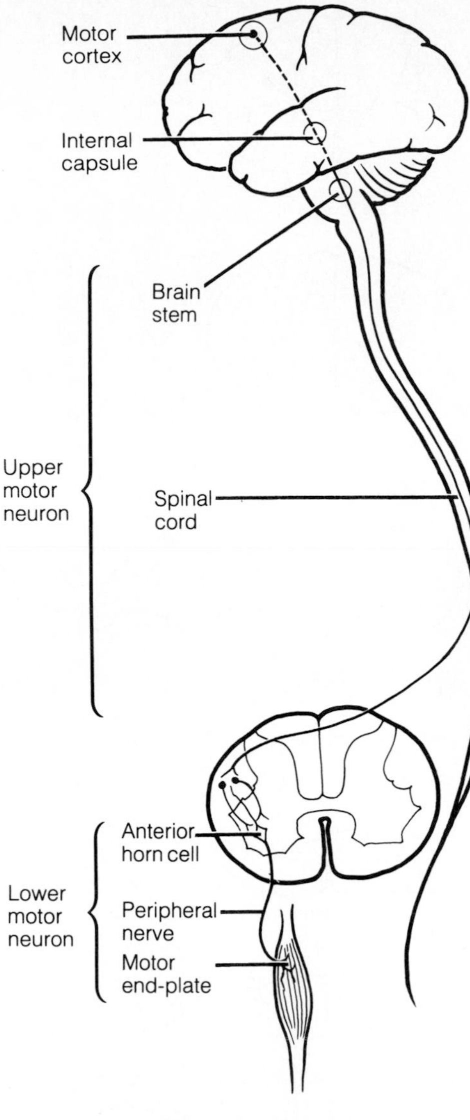

Motor
cortex

Internal
capsule

Brain
stem

Upper
motor
neuron

Spinal
cord

Anterior
horn cell

Lower
motor
neuron

Peripheral
nerve

Motor
end-plate

Figure 4–20. Motor pathways divided into upper- and lower-motor-neuron regions.

ical reaction of degeneration (10–14 days after injury; see *Electromyography,* Chapter 23); diminished or absent deep tendon reflexes of the involved muscle; and the absence of pathologic reflexes (see below).

Upper-Motor-Neuron Lesions

Damage to the lateral white column of the spinal cord can produce signs of upper-motor-neuron (UMN) lesions. These signs include spastic paralysis or paresis (weakness) of the involved muscles, little or no muscle atrophy (merely the atrophy of disuse), hyperactive deep tendon reflexes, diminished or absent superficial reflexes, and pathologic reflexes and signs. Withdrawal responses, especially the extensor plantar reflex (Babinski's sign), are common after stimulation of the sole of the foot (Fig 4–21). The corticospinal, rubrospinal, and reticulospinal tracts lie close together or overlap within the lateral white column; interruption of the corticospinal tract is accompanied by interruption of the other 2 tracts, resulting in spasticity caused by hyperreflexia. Isolated lesions of the corticospinal tract therefore usually result in normal reflexes and flaccid paralysis.

Disorders of Muscle Tissue or Neuromuscular Endings

Abnormal muscle tissue may be unable to react normally to stimuli conveyed to it by the lower motor neurons. This may manifest as weakness, paralysis, or tetanic contraction caused by disturbances in the muscle itself or at the myoneural junction. **Myasthenia gravis, myotonia congenita,** and **progressive muscular dystrophy** are typical disorders characterized by muscular dysfunction in the presence of apparently normal nerve tissue.

Localization of Spinal Cord Lesions

Before the site of spinal cord lesions can be found, the anatomic substrate for each sign and symptom must be determined. The side on which there is a lesion should be decided, then the level

well as by inter- and intrasegmental reflex neurons.

Lesions of the lower motor neurons may be located in the cells of the ventral gray column of the spinal cord or brain stem or in their axons, which constitute the ventral roots of the spinal or cranial nerves. Lesions can result from trauma, toxins, infections, vascular disorders, degenerative processes, neoplasms, or congenital malformations. Signs of lower-motor-neuron lesions include flaccid paralysis of the involved muscles; muscle atrophy with degeneration of muscle fibers after some time has elapsed; electrical manifestations of a typ-

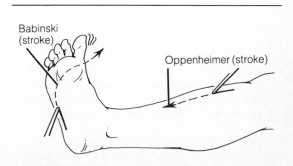

Figure 4–21. Testing for extensor plantar reflexes.

and extent of each lesion. The area where all findings converge is the site of the lesion.

Types of Spinal Cord Lesions

1. A **small central lesion** (Fig 4–22A) almost always affects the spinothalamic tract on both sides at the site of decussation.

2. A **large central lesion** (Fig 4–22D) involves, in addition to the pain pathways, portions of adjacent tracts, adjacent gray matter, or both.

3. An **irregular peripheral lesion** (Fig 4–22B) (eg, stab wound, compression of the cord) involves long pathways and gray matter; functions below the level of the lesion are abolished.

4. **Complete hemisection** of the cord (Fig 4–22E) causes Brown-Sequard syndrome (see below and Fig 4–23).

Lesions outside the cord (extramedullary lesions) may affect the functions of the cord itself:

5. A **tumor of the dorsal root** (Fig 4–22C), eg, a **neurofibroma,** or **schwannoma,** involves the first-order sensory neurons of a segment.

6. A **tumor** of the meninges or the bone (Fig 4–22F) may compress the spinal cord against a vertebra, causing interruption of the functions of the ascending and descending fiber systems.

EXAMPLES OF SPINAL CORD DISORDERS

Brown-Sequard Syndrome

This syndrome is caused by hemisection of the spinal cord as a result of syringomyelia, spinal cord tumor, hematomyelia, bullet or stab wounds, etc. Signs and symptoms (see Fig 4–23) are ipsilateral lower-motor-neuron paralysis in the segment of the lesion; ipsilateral upper-motor-neuron paralysis below the level of the lesion; an ipsilateral zone of cutaneous anesthesia in the segment of the lesion; an ipsilateral loss of proprioceptive, vibratory, and 2-point discrimination sense below the level of the lesion; and a contralateral loss of pain and temperature sense below the lesion. Hyperesthesia may be present in the segment of the lesion or below the level of the lesion, ipsilaterally or on both sides.

Tabes Dorsalis

Tabes dorsalis, a form of tertiary syphilis, is characterized by marked ataxia caused by loss of the proprioceptive pathways (dorsal roots and dorsal column). Subjective sensory disturbances known as tabetic crises consist of severe cramping pains in the stomach, larynx, or other viscera.

Syringomyelia

Syringomyelia is characterized by loss of pain and temperature senses at several segmental levels (Figs 4–24 and 4–25) although the patient usually

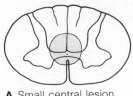

A. Small central lesion

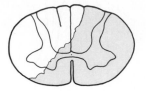

B. Incomplete hemisection

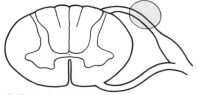

C. Dorsal root tumor

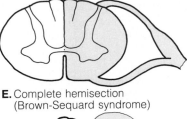

D. Large central lesion

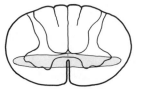

E. Complete hemisection (Brown-Sequard syndrome)

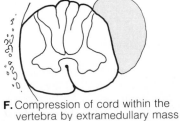

F. Compression of cord within the vertebra by extramedullary mass

Figure 4–22. Schematic illustrations of various types of spinal cord lesions.

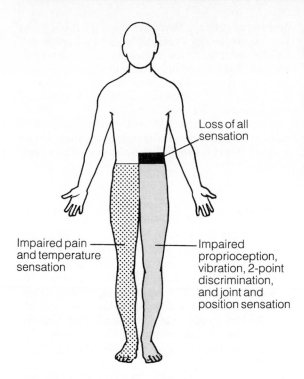

Loss of all
sensation

Impaired pain
and temperature
sensation

Impaired
proprioception,
vibration, 2-point
discrimination,
and joint and
position sensation

Figure 4–23. Brown-Sequard syndrome with lesion at left tenth thoracic level (motor deficits not shown).

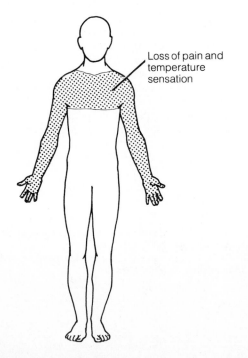

Loss of pain and
temperature
sensation

Figure 4–24. Syringomyelia involving the cervico-thoracic portion of the spinal cord.

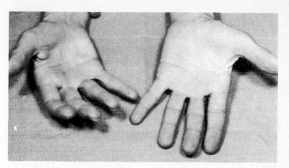

Figure 4–25. Wasting of the small muscles of the hands in a woman with syringomyelia.

retains touch and pressure senses in the affected parts **(dissociated anesthesia).** The syndrome may be caused by abnormal enlargement of the central canal **(hydromyelia)** or by a cleft **(syrinx)** formation in the spinal cord itself. The syrinx may involve the ventral gray matter, resulting in lower-motor-neuron lesions.

Subacute Combined Degeneration (Posterolateral Sclerosis):

Extreme deficiency in intake (or utilization) of vitamin B_{12} (cyanocobalamin) may result in degeneration in the dorsal and lateral white columns (Fig 4–26). There is a loss of position sense, 2-point discrimination, and vibratory sensation. Ataxic gait, muscle weakness, hyperactive deep muscle reflexes, spasticity of the extremities, and a positive Babinski sign are seen. Almost a fourth of the patients with acquired immunity deficiency syndrome (AIDS) suffer from this syndrome.

Spinal Shock

This syndrome results from transection of or severe injury to the spinal cord, from sudden loss of stimulation from higher levels, or from an overdose of spinal anesthetic. All body segments below the level of the injury become paralyzed and have no sensation; all reflexes, including autonomic reflexes, are suppressed. Spinal shock is usually transient; it may disappear in 3–6 weeks and is followed by a period of increased reflex response.

CASE 2

A 15-year-old girl was referred for evaluation of a weakness of the legs that had progressed for 2 weeks. Two years earlier, she had begun to have pain between the shoulder blades. The pain, which radiated into the left arm and into the middle finger of the left hand, could be accentuated by

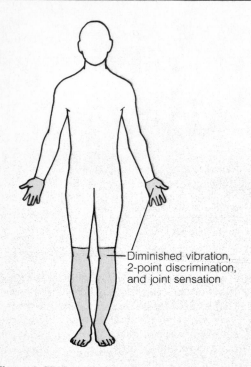

Diminished vibration, 2-point discrimination, and joint sensation

Figure 4–26. Posterolateral sclerosis (motor deficits not shown).

coughing, sneezing, or laughing. She had seen a chiropractor, who had manipulated the spine; however, mild pain persisted high in the back. The left leg and, more recently, the right leg had become weak and numb. In the last few days, the patient had found it difficult to start micturation.

Neurologic examination showed a minimal degree of weakness in the left upper extremity and wrist. Voluntary movement was markedly decreased in the left leg, less so in the right leg. The joints of the left leg showed increased resistance to passive motion, and clonus was present. The biceps

and radial reflexes were decreased on the left but normal on the right side; knee jerk and ankle jerk reflexes were increased bilaterally. Both plantar responses were extensor. Abdominal reflexes were absent bilaterally. Pain sensation was decreased to the level of C8 bilaterally; light touch sensation was decreased to the level of C7.

Where is the lesion? What is the differential diagnosis? Which neuroradiologic procedures would be most informative? What is the most likely diagnosis?

CASE 3

A 66-year-old photographer was referred for evaluation of progressive weakness of both legs, which had started some 9 months earlier. Two months previously, his arms had become weak, but to a lesser degree. The patient had recently begun to have difficulty swallowing solid food, and his friends had noted that his speech had become "thick," as though his tongue did not move. He had also lost almost 14 kg (30 lbs) during the 9-month period.

Neurologic examination showed loss of function in the muscles of facial expression, poor elevation of the uvula, a hoarse voice, and loss of mobility of the tongue. Widespread muscular atrophy was noted about the shoulders, in the intrinsic hand muscles, and in the proximal leg muscles—more on the left than on the right. All 4 extremities showed fasciculations at rest. Strength in all extremities was poor. Cerebellar tests were normal. All reflexes were reduced, and some were absent; both plantar responses were extensor. All sensory modalities were intact everywhere.

Muscle biopsy revealed various stages of denervation atrophy.

What is the most likely diagnosis?
Cases are discussed further in Chapter 24.

REFERENCES

Brown AG: *Organization in the Spinal Cord.* Springer-Verlag, 1981.

DeMyer W: Anatomy and clinical neurology of the spinal cord. In: *Clinical Neurology.* Vol 3. Baker AB, Baker LH (editors). Harper and Row, 1981.

Rexed BA: Cytoarchitectonic atlas of the spinal cord. *J Comp Neurol* 1954;**100:**297.

Williams PL, Warwick R: *Functional Neuroanatomy of Man.* Saunders, 1975.

Willis WD, Coggeshall RE: *Sensory Mechanisms of the Spinal Cord.* Plenum, 1978.

The Spinal Cord in Situ; Imaging

5

INVESTING MEMBRANES

Three membranes surround the spinal cord: The outermost is the dura (dura mater), the next is the arachnoid, and the innermost is the pia (pia mater) (Figs 5–1 and 5–2). The dura is also called the **pachymeninx,** and the arachnoid and pia are called the **leptomeninges.**

Dura

The dura mater is a tough, fibrous, tubular sheath that extends from the foramen magnum to the level of the second sacral vertebra, where it ends as a blind sac (Fig 5–1). The dura of the spinal cord **(theca spinalis)** is continuous with the cranial dura. The epidural, or extradural, space separates the dura from the bony vertebral column; it contains loose areolar tissue and a venous plexus. The subdural space is a narrow space between the dura and the underlying arachnoid.

Arachnoid

The arachnoid is a thin, transparent sheath separated from the underlying pia by the subarachnoid space, which contains cerebrospinal fluid.

Pia

The pia closely surrounds the spinal cord and sends septa into its substance. The pia also contributes to the formation of the **filum terminale internum,** a whitish fibrous filament that extends from the conus medullaris to the tip of the dural sac. The filum is surrounded by the cauda equina, and both are bathed in cerebrospinal fluid. Its extradural continuation, the **filum terminale externum,** attaches at the tip of the dural sac and extends to the coccyx. The filum terminale stabilizes the cord and dura lengthwise.

Dentate Ligament

The dentate ligament is a long flange of whitish, mostly pial tissue that runs along both lateral margins of the spinal cord, between the dorsal and ventral rootlets (Fig 5–2). Its medial edge is continuous with the pia at the side of the spinal cord, and its lateral edge pierces the arachnoid at intervals (21 on each side) to attach to the inside of the dura. The dentate ligament helps to stabilize the cord from side to side. It is also an important landmark in neurosurgery.

Spinal Nerves

There are 8 pairs of cervical nerves: The first 7 emerge above each respective cervical vertebra; the eighth (C8) lies below vertebra C7 and above the first thoracic vertebra (Fig 5–1). Each of the other spinal nerves (T1–12, L1–5, S1–5 and—normally—2 coccygeal nerves, Co1 and Co2) emerges from the intervertebral foramen below the vertebra of its type and number. The cauda equina is made up of dorsal and ventral roots from both sides of the lower cord. The composition of a typical spinal nerve (eg, a thoracic nerve) is discussed in Chapter 4.

Investment & Support of Spinal Nerves

As the ventral and dorsal roots (on each side) at each segmental level converge to become a spinal nerve, they are enclosed in sleeves of arachnoidal and dural tissue (Fig 5–2). The dorsal root sleeve contains the dorsal root ganglion near the point at which both sleeves merge to become the connective tissue sheath **(perineurium)** of a spinal nerve. The dorsal root, with its ganglion, and the ventral root of the nerve, surrounded by fat and blood vessels, course through the intervertebral foramen—except in the sacral segments, where the dorsal root ganglia lie within the sacrum itself (see below).

Clinical Correlations

Abnormal masses (tumor, infections, hematomas) may occur in any location in or around the spinal cord. Tumors are most often located in the intradural extramedullary compartment. Epidural masses, including bone tumors or metastases, displace the dura locally (Fig 5–3). Intradural extramedullary masses, most often in the subarachnoid space, may push the spinal cord away from the lesion and may even compress the cord against the dura, epidural space, and vertebra (Fig 4–22 E, F). Intramedullary, and therefore intradural, masses expand the spinal cord itself (Fig 4–22A–D). An epidural mass is usually the least difficult to remove neurosurgically; however, resection of an intramedullary mass is a very difficult and delicate procedure.

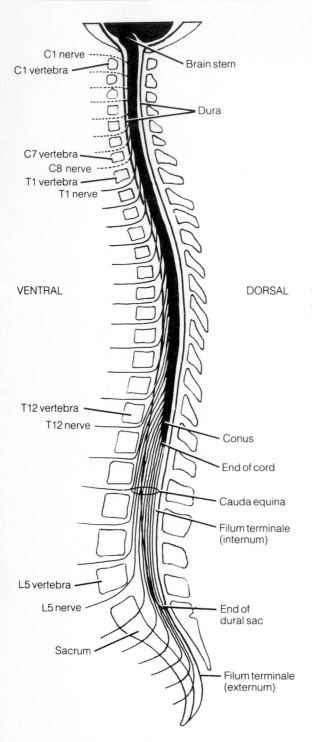

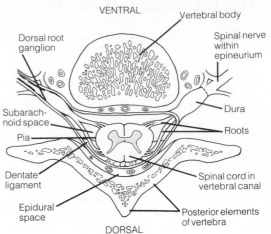

Figure 5-2. Drawing of a horizontal section through a vertebra and the spinal cord, meninges, and roots. Veins (not labeled) are shown in cross section. The vertebra and its contents are positioned as they customarily would be with CT and MR imaging procedures.

SPINAL CORD CIRCULATION

Arteries

A. Anterior Spinal Artery: This artery is formed by the midline union of paired branches of the vertebral arteries (Figs 5-4 and 5-5). It descends along the ventral surface of the cervical spinal cord, narrowing somewhat near T4.

B. Anterior Medial Spinal Artery: This is

Figure 5-1. Schematic illustration of the relationships between the spinal cord, spinal nerves, and vertebral column (lateral view), showing the termination of the dura (dura mater spinalis) and its continuation as the filum terminale externum. (Compare with Fig 4-5.)

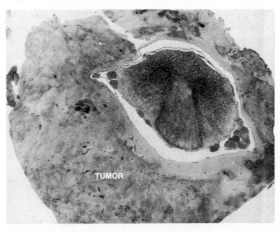

Figure 5-3. Epidural tumor in Hodgkin's disease, showing compression of the thoracic spinal cord (Weil stain). The illustration is positioned to conform with customary CT and MR imaging procedures.

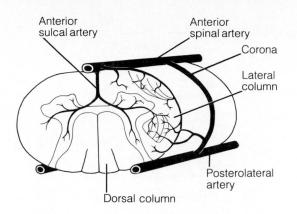

Figure 5-4. Cross section of the cervical spinal cord. The diagram shows the anterior and posterior spinal arteries with their branches and territories. There are numerous variations in the vascular supply.

the prolongation of the anterior spinal artery below T4.

C. Posterolateral Spinal Arteries: These arise from the vertebral arteries and course downward to the lower cervical and upper thoracic segments.

D. Radicular Arteries: Some (but not all) of the intercostal arteries from the aorta supply **segmental (radicular)** branches to the spinal cord, from T1 to L1; the largest of these branches, the **great ventral radicular artery,** also known as the **arteria radicularis magna,** or **artery of Adamkiewicz** (Fig 5-5), enters the spinal cord between segments T8 and L4. This artery usually arises on the left, and in most individuals, supplies most of the arterial blood supply for the lower half of the spinal cord. Although occlusion in this artery is rare, it results in major neurologic deficits (eg, paraplegia, loss of sensation in the legs, urinary incontinence). Some radicular arteries derived from the lumbar, iliolumbar, and lateral sacral arteries are present in the lumbosacral area. The largest such vessel appears to enter the intervertebral foramen at vertebra L2 to form the lowermost portion of the anterior spinal artery—the terminal artery— which runs along the filum terminale.

E. Posterior Spinal Arteries: These paired arteries are much smaller than the single large anterior spinal artery; they branch at various levels to form the posterolateral arterial plexus. The posterior spinal arteries supply the dorsal white columns and the posterior portion of the dorsal gray columns.

F. Sulcal Arteries: In each segment, the branches of the radicular arteries that enter the intervertebral foramens accompany the dorsal and

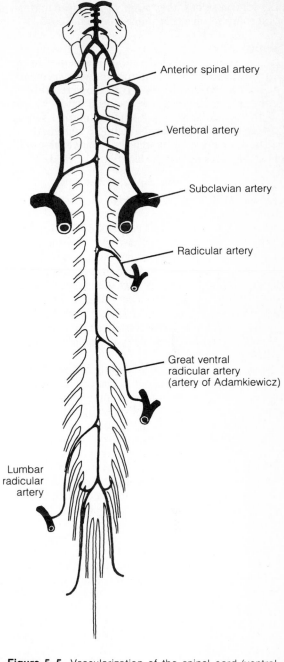

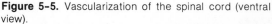

Figure 5-5. Vascularization of the spinal cord (ventral view).

ventral nerve roots. These branches unite directly with the posterior and anterior spinal arteries to form an irregular ring of arteries (an **arterial corona**) with vertical connections. Sulcal arteries branch from the coronal arteries at most levels. Anterior sulcal arteries (Fig 5-4) arise at various levels along the cervical and thoracic cord within the ventral sulcus; they supply the ventral and lateral columns on either side of the spinal cord.

Veins

An irregular external venous plexus lies in the epidural space; it communicates with segmental veins, basivertebral veins from the vertebral column, the basilar plexus in the head, and—by way of the pedicular veins—a smaller internal venous plexus that lies in the subarachnoid space. All venous drainage is ultimately into the venae cavae. Both plexuses extend the length of the cord.

THE VERTEBRAL COLUMN

The vertebral column consists of 33 vertebrae joined by ligaments and cartilage. The upper 24 vertebrae are separate and movable, but the lower 9 are fixed: 5 are fused to form the sacrum, and the last 4 are usually fused to form the coccyx. The vertebral column consists of 7 cervical (C1–7), 12 thoracic (T1–12), 5 lumbar (L1–5), 5 sacral (S1–5), and 4 coccygeal (Co1–4) vertebrae. In some individuals, vertebra L5 is partly or completely fused with the sacrum.

The vertebral column is slightly S-shaped when seen from the side (Fig 5–6). The cervical spine is ventrally convex, the thoracic spine ventrally concave, and the lumbar spine ventrally convex, with its curve ending at the lumbosacral angle. Ventral convexity is sometimes referred to as normal lordosis and dorsal convexity as normal kyphosis. The pelvic curve (sacrum plus coccyx) is concave downward and ventrally from the lumbosacral angle to the tip of the coccyx. The spinal cord in an adult is often slightly twisted along its long axis; this is called normal scoliosis.

Clinical Correlations

Abnormal curvatures of the spine can be caused by congenital malformations (eg, humpback) or by large intra-abdominal or intrathoracic masses. Abnormal angles may be caused by the collapse of one or more vertebral bodies as a result of trauma, infection, or tumors. Lumbar lordosis is more pronounced in late pregnancy. Thoracic kyphosis may be severe, especially in old age (this is often called dowager's hump).

Vertebrae

A typical vertebra (not C1, however) has a body and a vertebral (neural) arch that together surround the vertebral (spinal) canal (Fig 5–7). The neural arch is composed of a pedicle on each side supporting a lamina that extends posteriorly to the spinous process (spine). The pedicle has both superior and inferior notches that form the **intervertebral foramen.** Each vertebra has lateral **transverse**

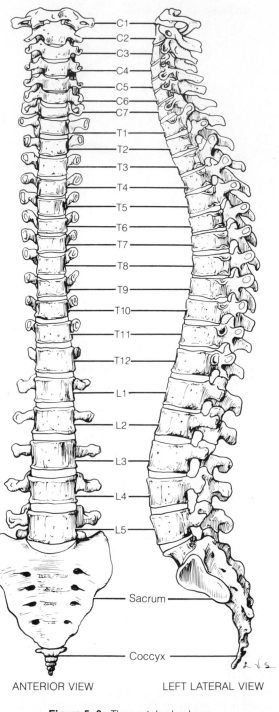

ANTERIOR VIEW   LEFT LATERAL VIEW

Figure 5–6. The vertebral column.

processes and superior and inferior **articular processes** with facets. The ventral portion of the neural arch is formed by the ventral body.

Articulation of a pair of vertebrae is body-to-body, with an intervening intervertebral disk, and at the superior and inferior articular facets on both

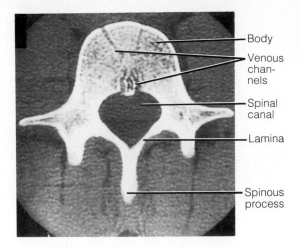

Body

Venous channels

Spinal canal

Lamina

Spinous process

Figure 5-7. CT image of a horizontal section at midlevel of vertebra L4.

sides. The intervertebral disks help absorb stress and strain transmitted to the vertebral column. They are thicker in the more mobile cervical and lumbar areas than in the thoracic region.

Each disk contains a core of primitive gelatinous large-celled tissue, the **nucleus pulposus,** surrounded by a thick **annulous fibrosus** (Fig 5–8). The disks are intimately attached to the hyaline cartilage that covers the superior and inferior surfaces of the vertebral bodies. The water content of

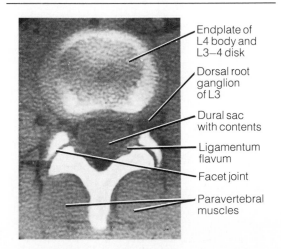

Endplate of L4 body and L3–4 disk

Dorsal root ganglion of L3

Dural sac with contents

Ligamentum flavum

Facet joint

Paravertebral muscles

Figure 5-8. CT image of a horizontal section through L4 at the level of the L3–4 intervertebral disk. (Reproduced, with permission, from deGroot J: *Correlative Neuroanatomy of Computed Tomography and Magnetic Resonance Imaging,* Lea & Febiger, 1984.)

the disks normally decreases with age resulting in a loss of height in older individuals.

Clinical Correlations

Spina bifida results from the failure of the vertebral canal to close normally because of a defect in vertebral development. There may be associated abnormalities that are caused by defective development of the spinal cord, brain stem, cerebrum, or cerebellum, there may also be other developmental defects such as meningoceles, meningomyeloceles, congenital tumors, or hydrocephalus. Since the bony spinal column closes by the twelfth week of intrauterine life, these defects must originate in early intrauterine life.

There are 2 main types of spina bifida: spina bifida occulta, in which there is a simple defect in the closure of the vertebra; and spina bifida with meningocele or meningomyelocele, where the defect is associated with saclike protrusions of the overlying meninges and skin, which may contain portions of the spinal cord or nerve roots. Simple failure of closure of one or more vertebral arches in the lumbosacral region is a common finding on routine examination of the spine by radiography or at autopsy.

Spina bifida occulta (Fig 5–9) is relatively common and is sometimes noticed as an incidental finding on roentgenographic examination of the vertebral column. The palpable bony defect, usually in the lumbar or sacral spine, is due to the failure of the laminas of the affected vertebrae to close. There may be associated abnormalities such as fat deposits, hypertrichosis (excessive hair) over the affected area, and dimpling of the overlying skin. Symptoms may be caused by intraspinal lipomas, adhesions, bony spicules, or maldevelopment of the spinal cord.

Meningocele is herniation of the meningeal membranes through the vertebral defect. It usually causes a soft, cystic, translucent tumor to appear low in the midline of the back.

In **meningomyelocele,** nerve roots and the spinal cord protrude through the vertebral defect and usually adhere to the inner wall of the meningeal sac. If the meningomyelocele is high in the vertebral column, the clinical picture may resemble that of complete or incomplete transection of the cord, or the symptoms of combined root and spinal cord defects may resemble those of syringomyelia.

Prophylactic repair of the sac and supportive closure of the tissues over the bony defect may be performed early in life. Excision of spinal sacs containing neural elements usually produces poor results. Closure of a sac, particularly a large one, may be followed by progressive hydrocephalus (see Chapter 10).

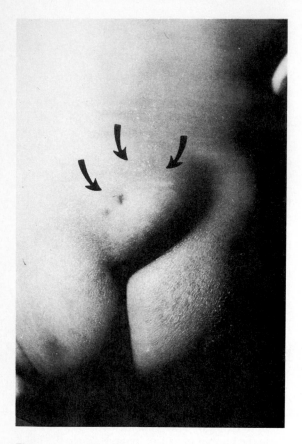

Figure 5-9. Spina bifida occulta. The arrows point to a swelling above the buttocks.

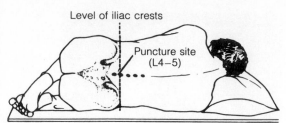

Figure 5-10. Decubitus position for lumbar puncture. (Reproduced, with permission, from Krupp MA et al: *Physician's Handbook*, 21st ed. Lange, 1985.)

Contraindications

There are few contraindications to lumbar puncture. When there is increased cranial pressure—especially when a tumor lies in the posterior fossa—spinal puncture should be done carefully or not at all, since life-threatening herniation of the cerebellum and medullary compression may follow the removal of cerebrospinal fluid.

Technique

Lumbar puncture is usually performed with the patient in the lateral decubitus position with legs drawn up (Fig 5-10); in this position, the manometric pressure of cerebrospinal fluid is normally 70–200 mm of water (average is 125 mm). If the puncture is done with the patient sitting upright (Fig 5–11), the fluid in the manometer normally rises to about the level of the midcervical spine. Inadvertent coughing, sneezing, or straining usually causes a prompt rise in pressure from the conges-

LUMBAR PUNCTURE

Location

Since the spinal cord in adults ends at the level of L1–2, a spinal (lumbar) puncture can be performed below that level—and above the sacrum—without injuring the cord.

Indications

Lumbar puncture is indicated when there is a need for chemical analysis or cytologic examination of the cerebrosinal fluid; injection of a contrast medium for radiologic examination; injection of therapeutic agents, eg, for treatment of myelitis or meningitis; or injection of anesthetics. The availability of new neuroradiologic techniques (CT scanning and MR imaging) has reduced the need for lumbar puncture.

Selective sacral anesthesia (as used in obstetrics) can be achieved by injecting anesthetic into the epidural space within the sacral canal (see Fig 5–11, below).

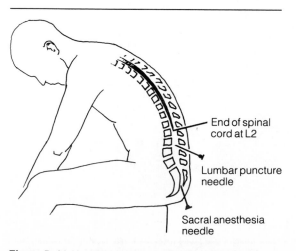

Figure 5–11. Lumbar puncture site with the patient in sitting position. The approach to the sacral hiatus for saddle-block anesthesia is also indicated.

tion of the spinal veins and the resultant increased pressure on the contents of the subarachnoid and epidural spaces. The pressure subsequently falls to its previous level.

After the initial pressure has been determined, 3–4 samples of 2–3 mL each are withdrawn into sterile tubes for laboratory examination. Routine examination usually includes cell counts and measurement of total protein. Cultures and special tests, such as those for sugar and chlorides, are done when indicated. The pressure is also routinely measured after the fluid is removed. In cases of spinal subarachnoid block above the puncture site, the pressure will be normal initially but will fall precipitously *after* the removal of 7–10 mL of fluid.

Other sites that reach the subarachnoid space are in the cisterna magna above the atlas, or in the C1–2 space. While the latter is easily done with radiographic guidance, cisternal puncture carries a risk of injury to the brain stem.

Complications

Despite hydration of the patient before and after lumbar puncture, severe headache may follow. The headache may be caused by the loss of fluid or leakage of fluid through the puncture site; it is characteristically relieved by lying down and exacerbated upon raising the head. Injection of the patient's own blood in the epidural space at the puncture site (blood patch) may give partial or complete relief. Serious complications, such as infection, epidural hematoma, uncal herniation, or cerebellar tonsil prolapse, are very rare.

Queckenstedt's Test

Queckenstedt's test can be used to demonstrate a block in the spinal fluid compartment. The test involves compressing the jugular veins during lumbar puncture. This normally produces a prompt rise in cerebrospinal fluid pressure that lasts as long as the compression is maintained, then promptly returns to its earlier level. A moderate rise in pressure occurs when one jugular vein is compressed, and a further rise occurs when the second jugular vein is compressed. If the cerebrospinal fluid pressure fails to rise and fall promptly, it is presumed that there is a block in the system between the site of the puncture and that of the jugular vein compression. The pressure can fail to rise on compression of one jugular because of thrombosis of the lateral sinus on the same side. The absence of a rise in pressure—or a slow rise and slow fall—upon compression of both veins implies a complete or partial block in the spinal subarachnoid compartment.

Queckenstedt's test is contraindicated if intracranial bleeding or an intracranial tumor is present or suspected; the test may abruptly precipitate

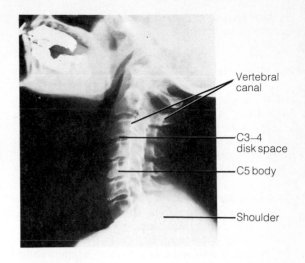

Figure 5-12. Roentgenograms through the neck (lateral view).

Vertebral canal

C3–4 disk space

C5 body

Shoulder

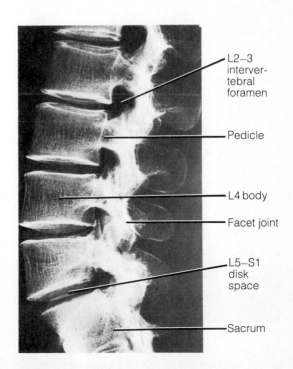

Figure 5-13. Roentgenogram of lumbar vertebrae (left lateral view). (Compare to Fig 5–6, right side.)

L2–3 intervertebral foramen

Pedicle

L4 body

Facet joint

L5–S1 disk space

Sacrum

further bleeding or cause herniation of the cerebellar tonsils, with medullary compression.

IMAGING OF THE SPINE & SPINAL CORD

The imaging methods that have been developed, particularly in this century, have great value in determining the precise site and extent of the involvement of pathologic processes in the spine and neighboring structures. (The methods themselves are discussed in detail in Chapter 22).

Roentgenography

Because roentgenograms (plain films) demonstrate the presence of calcium, various projections (anteroposterior, lateral, oblique) of the affected area show the skeletal components of the spine and foramens (Figs 5-12 and 5-13). Fractures or erosions of the vertebral column's bony elements are often easily seen, but the films provide little or no information about the spinal cord or other soft tissues. Because of this, roentgenograms are seldom used now (except in emergencies) to determine the location of fractures and foreign objects, eg, missile wounds.

Myelography

Roentgenography after injection of a radiopaque fluid into the subarachnoid shows the contours of the vertebral canal and the size of the spinal cord and roots. The contrast medium is usually injected via lumbar puncture but can be injected via a C1-2 puncture or a cisternal puncture (above the posterior arch of C1). Myelograms can show the defect caused by an extradural mass (eg, a herniated disk; see Fig 5-14), an intradural extramedullary mass (eg, tumor; see Fig 5-15) within the subarachnoid space, or an enlargement of the cord (intramedullary mass) and roots.

Computed Tomography

Information about the position, shape, and size of all the elements of the spine, cord, roots, ligaments, and surrounding soft tissue can be obtained by a series of thin (0.15–1 cm) transverse (axial) CT images, or scans, with or without contrast medium

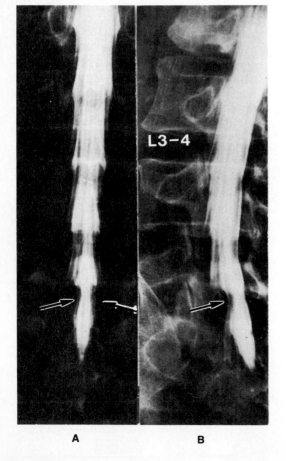

A   **B**

Figure 5-14. Myelograms of an extradural defect representing a herniated L4-5 disk. *A:* anteroposterior view. *B:* oblique view. Note amputation of L5 nerve, best seen in B.

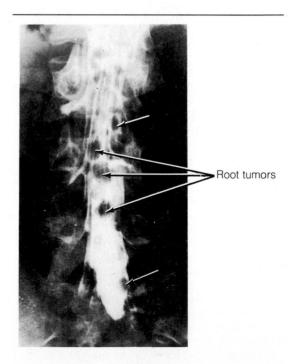

Figure 5-15. Myelogram (anteroposterior view) showing multiple root tumors (arrows) of the cauda equina in a patient with neurofibromatosis (von Recklinghausen's disease).

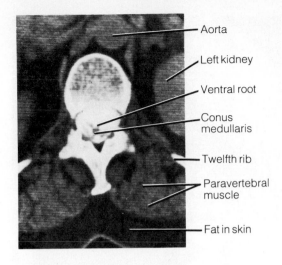

Aorta

Left kidney

Ventral root

Conus medullaris

Twelfth rib

Paravertebral muscle

Fat in skin

Figure 5–16. CT image of a horizontal section at the level of vertebra T12 in a 3-year-old child. The subarachnoid space was injected with contrast medium.

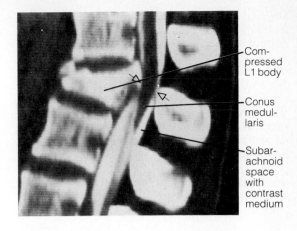

Compressed L1 body

Conus medullaris

Subarachnoid space with contrast medium

Figure 5–17. Reformatted CT image of midsagittal section of the lumbar spine of a patient who fell from a third-floor window. There is a compression fracture in the body of L1, and the lower cord is compressed between bony elements of L1 (arrows). The subarachnoid space was injected with contrast medium. (Reproduced, with permission, from Federle MP, Brant-Zawadski M [editors]. *Computed Tomography in the Evaluation of Trauma.* Williams & Wilkins, 1982.)

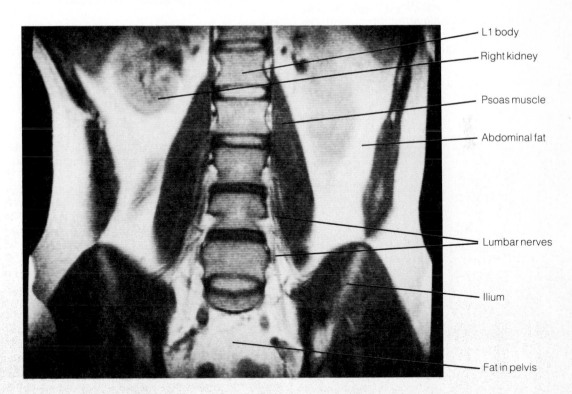

L1 body

Right kidney

Psoas muscle

Abdominal fat

Lumbar nerves

Ilium

Fat in pelvis

Figure 5–18. MR image of a coronal section through the body and (curved) lumbar spine. (Reproduced, with permission, from deGroot J: *Correlative Neuroanatomy of Computed Tomography and Magnetic Resonance Imaging.* Lea & Febiger, 1984.)

injected into the subarachnoid space (Figs 5–7 and 5–16). A series of transverse images can be reformed in other planes (sagittal, coronal, or oblique) to provide additional information (Fig 5–17).

Magnetic Resonance Imaging

MR imaging (MRI) can be used in any plane. It has been used, especially with sagittal images, to demonstrate the anatomy (Fig 5–18) or pathology of the spinal cord and surrounding spaces and structures (Figs 5–19, 5–20, and 5–21). Since the calcium of bone does not yield an MR signal, MR imaging is especially useful in showing suspected lesions of the soft tissues in and around the vertebral column (Figs 5–19 and 5–22).

CASE 4

A 49-year-old dock worker was reasonably healthy until he had an accident at work. A heavy piece of equipment fell high on his back, knocking him down—but not unconscious. He was unable to move his arms and legs and complained of vague shooting pains in both arms and some tingling in his right side below the axilla.

He was transported to the emergency room, where the following neurologic abnormalities were recorded: flaccid left hemiplegia, right triceps weakness, left extensor plantar response. Pain sensation was lost on the right side from the shoulder down, including the axilla and hand but not the thumb.

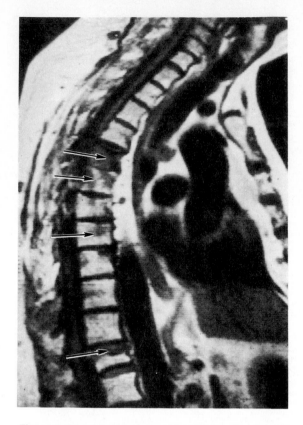

Figure 5–20. MR image of a midsagittal section through the lower neck and upper thorax of a patient with AIDS. Multiple masses are seen in the vertebral bodies at several levels (arrows): pathologic examination showed these to be malignant lymphomas.

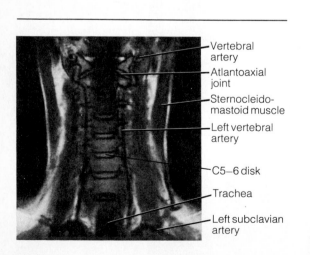

Vertebral artery

Atlantoaxial joint

Sternocleido-mastoid muscle

Left vertebral artery

C5–6 disk

Trachea

Left subclavian artery

Figure 5–19. MR image of a coronal section through the neck at the level of the cervical vertebrae. Because of the curvature of the neck, only 5 vertebral bodies are seen in this plane. (Reproduced, with permission, from Mills CM, de Groot J, Posin J: *Magnetic Resonance Imaging Atlas of the Head, Neck, and Spine.* Lea & Febiger, 1988.)

What is the tentative diagnosis? What neuroradiologic procedure would you request to localize the lesion?

The patient underwent back surgery to correct the problem. A few days postoperatively, he regained strength in his right arm and left leg, but the left arm continued to be weak. Pain sensation was not tested at this time.

Neurologic examination 3 weeks later disclosed fasciculations in the left deltoid; marked weakness in the left arm, more pronounced distally; mild spasticity of the left elbow; and minimal spasticity in the left knee on passive motion. Some deep tendon reflexes—all on the left side—were increased: biceps, triceps, quadriceps, and Achilles tendon. There was a left extensor plantar response. Position and vibration senses were intact, and pain sensation was absent on the right half of the body up to the level of the clavicle.

What is the sequence of pathologic events? Where is the lesion and which neural structures are

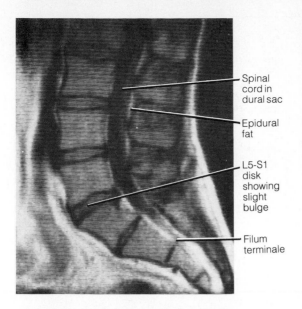

- Spinal cord in dural sac
- Epidural fat
- L5-S1 disk showing slight bulge
- Filum terminale

Figure 5–21. MR image of a midsagittal section through the lumbosacral vertebrae and dural sac. Note that the dural sac terminates at the level of S2. The epidural fat is clearly visible. The L5–S1 disk has degenerated and shows a slight posterior bulge.

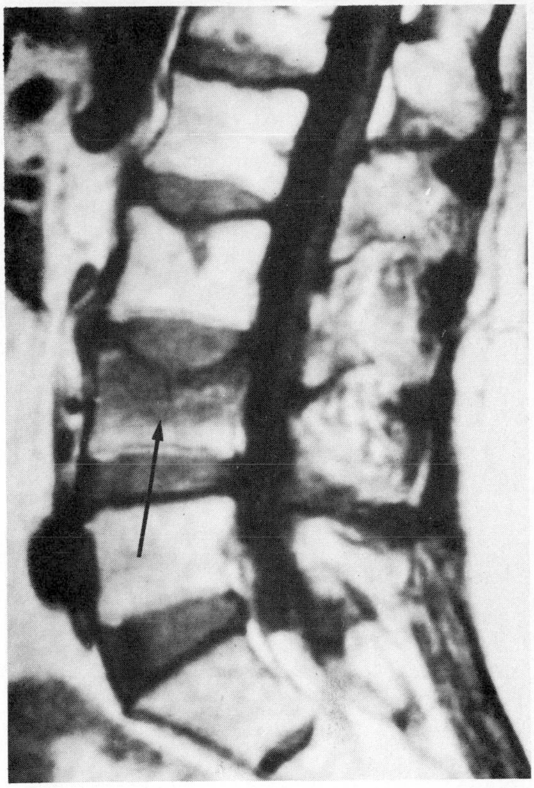

Figure 5–22. MR image of a midsagittal section through the lumbosacral spine. The mass visible in the body of L4 represents a metastasis of a colon carcinoma (arrow).

involved? Which syndrome is incompletely represented in this case? Which components of the complete syndrome are not present?

CASE 5

Two months before presentation, a 40-year-old camp counselor playing baseball sustained a minor injury, feeling a stab of pain to his lower back when he slid feet first into third base. Shortly after the incident, he noted dull pains in the same region in the mornings; these seemed to lessen during the day. Three weeks before presentation, he began to feel electric-shock-like pain shooting down the back of his right leg to his toes. The pain seemed to start in the right buttock and could be precipitated by coughing, sneezing, straining, or bending backward. The patient had also noted occasional tingling of his right calf and some spasms of the back and right leg muscles.

Neurologic examination showed no impairment of muscle strength, and there were normal deep tendon reflexes in the upper extremities. The Achilles tendon reflex was absent on the right and normal on the left, and there were flexor plantar responses on both sides. All sensory modalities were intact. There was marked spasm of the right paravertebral muscles and local tenderness on palpation of the spine at L5–S1 and at the sciatic nerve in the right buttock. Straight leg raising was limited to 30 degrees on the right but normal on the left. Radiographs of the lumbar spine were normal. The patient had a 12-day period of complete bed rest, but the symptoms persisted.

What is the most likely diagnosis?

Cases are discussed further in Chapter 25. Questions and answers pertaining to Section II (Chapters 4 and 5) are found in Appendix D).

REFERENCES

Crock HV, Yoshizawa H: *The Blood Supply of the Vertebral Column and Spinal Cord in Man*. Springer-Verlag, 1977.

Dorwart RH et al: Lumbosacral spine computed tomography. In: *Diagnostic Radiology*. Margulis AR, Gooding CA (editors). Univ of Calif Press, 1981.

Newton TH, Potts DG (editors): *Computed Tomography of the Spine and Spinal Cord*. Clavadel Press, 1983.

Norman D, Kjos BO: MR of the spine. In: *Magnetic Resonance Imaging of the Central Nervous System*. Raven, 1987.

Rothman RH, Simeone FA: *The Spine*. Saunders, 1975.

Section III.
Anatomy of the Brain

The Brain Stem & Cerebellum   6

DEVELOPMENT OF THE BRAIN & CRANIAL NERVES

The lower part of the cranial portion of the neural tube (neuraxis) gives rise to the brain stem. The tube undergoes local enlargement and shows 2 permanent flexures: the **cephalic flexure** at the upper end, and the varying **cervical flexure** at the lower end. The primitive central canal widens into a 4-sided pyramidal shape with a rhomboid floor; this becomes the fourth ventricle, which extends over the pons and the medulla. The curved central canal in the rostral brain stem becomes the **cerebral aqueduct.** The fourth ventricle and the cerebral aqueduct contain cerebrospinal fluid and are lined by ependyma. The roof of the rostral fourth ventricle undergoes intense cellular proliferation, and this lip produces the neurons and glia that will populate both the cerebellum and the **inferior olivary nucleus.**

The quadrigeminal plate, the midbrain tegmentum, and the cerebral peduncles develop from the **mesencephalon** (midbrain; Fig 6–1), and the cerebral aqueduct courses through it.

The **rhombencephalon** (Fig 6–1A) gives rise to the metencephalon and the myelencephalon. The **metencephalon** forms the cerebellum and pons; it contains part of the fourth ventricle. The **myelencephalon** forms the medulla oblongata; the lower part of the fourth ventricle lies within this portion of the brain stem.

As in the spinal cord, the embryonic brain stem has a central gray core with an **alar plate** (consisting mostly of sensory components) and a **basal plate** (mostly motor components). The gray columns are not continuous in the brain stem, however, and the development of the fourth ventricle causes wide lateral displacement of the alar plate in the lower brain stem. The basal plate takes the shape of a hinge (Fig 6–2). The process is reversed at the other end, resulting in the rhomboid shape of the floor of the fourth ventricle. In addition, long tracts, short neuronal connections, and nuclei become apposed to the brain stem. The cranial nerves, like the spinal nerves, take their origin from the basal plate cells (motor nerves) or from synapses in the alar plate cell groups (sensory nerves). Unlike spinal nerves, however, most cranial nerves emerge as one or more bundles of fibers from the basal or basilateral aspect of the brain stem (Figs 6–1 and 6–3). In addition, not all cranial nerves are mixed; ie, some have only sensory components and others have only motor components (see Chapter 7).

ORGANIZATION OF THE BRAIN STEM

Main Divisions & External Landmarks

Three major external divisions of the brain stem are recognizable: the medulla (medulla oblongata, or myelencephalon), a transition to the spinal cord; the pons (metencephalon together with the cerebellum); and the midbrain (mesencephalon) (Figs 6–3 and 6–4). The 3 internal longitudinal divisions of the brain stem are the **tectum** (mainly in the midbrain), **tegmentum,** and **basis** (Fig 6–4). The main external structures, seen from the dorsal aspect, are shown in Fig 6–5. The superior portion of the rhomboid fossa (which forms the floor of the fourth ventricle) extends over the pons, while the inferior portion covers the open portion of the medulla. The closed medulla forms the transition to the spinal cord.

Three pairs of cerebellar peduncles (inferior, middle, and superior) form connections with the cerebellum. The dorsal aspect of the midbrain shows 4 hillocks: the 2 superior and the 2 inferior colliculi, together called the **corpora quadrigemina.**

Internal Structural Components

Although the brain stem is a relatively small structure, it contains much that is essential for nor-

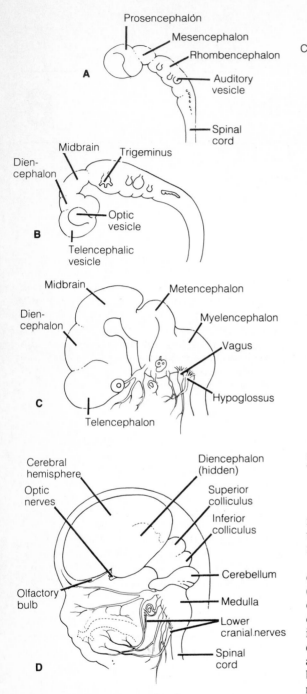

Figure 6-1. Four stages in early development of brain and cranial nerves (times are approximate). *A:* 3 1/2 weeks, *B:* 4 1/2 weeks, *C:* 7 weeks, *D:* 11 weeks.

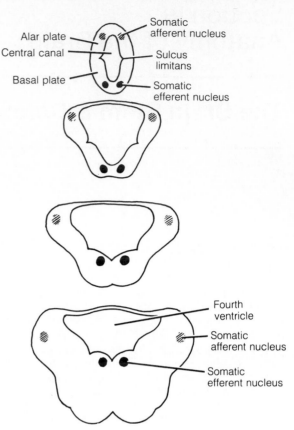

Figure 6-2. Schematic illustration of the widening of the central cavity in the lower brain stem during development.

mal brain function—indeed for normal body function. Internal structural components include the following:

A. Descending and Ascending Tracts: All descending tracts that terminate in the spinal cord (see Chapter 4) pass through the brain stem; in addition, several descending fiber systems terminate or originate in the brain stem. Similarly, all ascending tracts that reach the brain stem or the cerebral cortex pass through part or all of this region; other ascending tracts originate in the brain stem. The brain stem is therefore an important conduit or relay station for many longitudinal pathways, both descending and ascending (Table 6-1).

B. Cranial Nerve Nuclei: Almost all the cranial nerve nuclei are located in the brain stem (the exceptions are the first 2 nuclei, which are evaginations of the brain itself). Portions of the cranial nerves also pass through the brain stem.

C. Cerebellar Peduncles: The pathways to and from the cerebellum pass through 3 pairs of cerebellar peduncles (parts of the brain stem).

D. Descending Autonomic System Path-

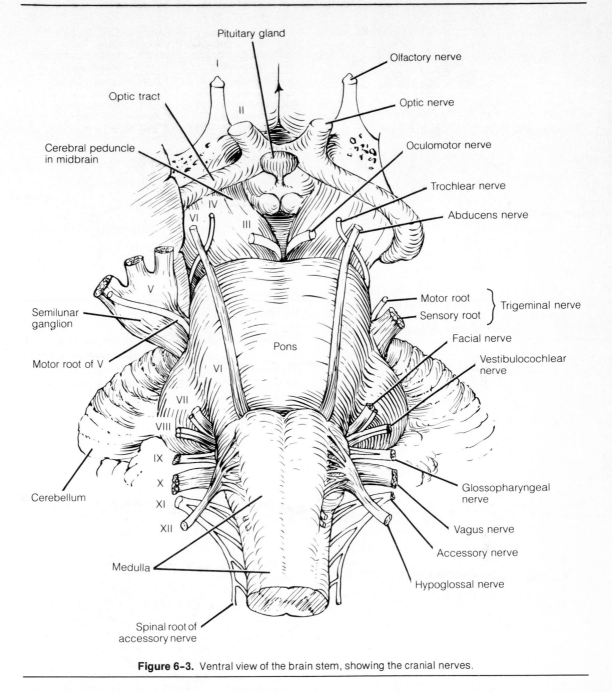

Figure 6-3. Ventral view of the brain stem, showing the cranial nerves.

ways: These paths to the spinal cord pass through the brain stem (see also Chapter 19).

E. Reticular Formation: Several of these areas in the tegmentum of the brain stem are vitally involved in the control of respiration, cardiovascular system functions, and states of consciousness, sleep, and alertness (see also Chapter 17).

F. Monoaminergic Pathways: These paths can be divided into 3 systems: the **serotoninergic** pathways from the raphe nuclei (see also Chapter 3); the **noradrenergic** pathways in the lateral reticular formation and the extensive efferents from the locus ceruleus; and the **dopaminergic** pathway from the basal midbrain to the basal ganglia, and others.

G. Cerebrospinal Fluid Pathway: This passes through the brain stem and reaches the subarachnoid space through openings in the fourth ventricle (see also Chapter 10).

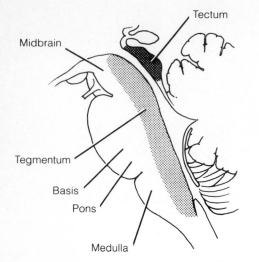

Figure 6-4. Drawing of the divisions of the brain stem in a midsagittal plane. The major internal longitudinal divisions are the tectum, tegmentum, and basis. The major external divisions are the midbrain, pons, and medulla.

Table 6-1. Major ascending and descending pathways in the brain stem.

Ascending	Descending
Medial lemniscus	Corticospinal tract
Spinothalamic tract	Corticonuclear tract
Trigeminal lemniscus	Corticopontine fibers
Lateral lemniscus	Rubrospinal tract
Reticular system fibers	Tectospinal tract
Medial longitudinal fasci-culus	Medial longitudinal fasci-culus
Inferior cerebellar pe-duncle	Vestibulospinal tract
Superior cerebellar pe-duncle	Reticulospinal tract
Secondary vestibulary fi-bers	Central tegmental tract
Secondary gustatory fi-bers	Descending tract of nerve V

CRANIAL NERVE NUCLEI IN THE BRAIN STEM

The functional composition of the lower 10 cranial nerves can best be analyzed by referring to the development of their nuclei (Fig 6–6). The nerves are usually referred to by name or by roman numeral (Table 6–2).

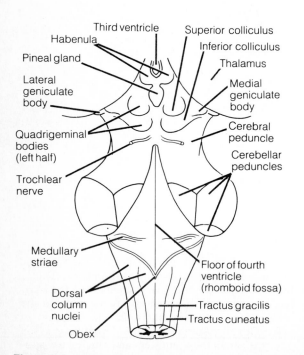

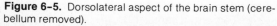

Figure 6-5. Dorsolateral aspect of the brain stem (cerebellum removed).

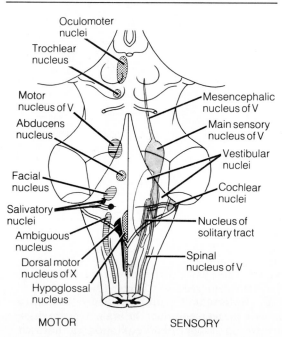

Figure 6-6. Cranial nerve nuclei. Dorsal view of the human brain stem with the positions of the cranial nerve nuclei projected upon the surface. Motor nuclei are on the left; sensory nuclei are on the right.

Table 6-2. Cranial nerves and nuclei in the brain stem.

Name	Nerve	Nuclei
Oculomotor	III	Oculomotor, Edinger-Westphal
Trochlear	IV	Trochlear
Trigeminal	V	Main sensory, spinal (descending), mesencephalic, motor (masticatory)
Abducens	VI	Abducens
Facial	VII	Facial, superior salivatory, gustatory (solitary)*
Vestibulocochlear	VIII	Cochlear (2 nuclei), vestibular (4 nuclei)
Glossopharyngeus	IX	Ambiguous,† inferior salivatory, solitary*
Vagus	X	Dorsal motor, ambiguous,† solitary*
Accessory	XI	Spinal accessory (C1–C5), ambiguous†
Hypoglossal	XII	Hypoglossal

*The solitary nucleus is shared by nerves VII, IX, and X.
†The ambiguous nucleus is shared by nerves IX, X, and XI.

Motor Components

Three types of basal plate derivatives can be found in the brain stem.

General somatic efferent (SE or GSE) components innervate striated muscles that are derived from somites and are involved with movements of the tongue and eyeballs: the hypoglossal nucleus of XII, oculomotor nucleus of III, trochlear nucleus of IV, and abducens nucleus of VI.

Branchial efferent (BE) components, sometimes referred to as **special visceral efferents (SVE),** innervate muscles that are derived from the branchial arches and are involved in chewing, making facial expressions, swallowing, producing vocal sounds, and turning the head: the masticatory nucleus of V; facial nucleus of VII; ambiguous nucleus of IX, X, and XI; and spinal accessory nucleus of XI located in the cord.

General visceral efferent (VE or GVE) components are parasympathetic preganglionic components that provide autonomic innervation of smooth muscles and the glands in the head, neck, and torso: the Edinger–Westphal nucleus of III, superior salivatory nucleus of VII, inferior salivatory nucleus of IX, and dorsal motor nucleus of X.

Sensory Components

Two types of alar-plate derivatives can be distinguished in the brain stem and are comparable to similar cell groups in the spinal cord.

General somatic afferent (SA or GSA) components receive and relay sensory stimuli from the skin and mucosa of most of the head: main sensory, descending, and mesencephalic nuclei of V.

General visceral afferent (VA or GVA) components relay sensory stimuli from the viscera and more specialized taste stimuli from the tongue and epiglottis: solitary nucleus for visceral input from IX and X and gustatory nucleus for special visceral taste fibers from VII, IX, and X.

Six **special sensory (SS) nuclei** can also be distinguished: the 4 vestibular and 2 cochlear nuclei that receive stimuli via vestibulocochlear nerve VIII. These nuclei are derived from the primitive auditory placode in the rhombencephalon.

Differences between Typical Spinal & Cranial Nerves

It is apparent that the simple and regular pattern of functional fiber components in spinal nerves is not found in cranial nerves. A single cranial nerve may contain one or more functional components; conversely, a single nucleus may contribute to the formation of one or more cranial nerves. Although some are solely efferent, most are mixed, and some contain many visceral components.

MEDULLA

The medulla (medulla oblongata, myelencephalon) can be divided into a caudal (closed; Fig 6–7B) portion and a rostral (open; Fig 6–7C) portion, based on the absence or presence of the lower fourth ventricle.

Ascending Tracts

In the closed medulla, the relay nuclei of the dorsal column pathway (nucleus gracilis and nucleus cuneatus) give rise to a crossed fiber bundle, the **medial lemniscus.** The lower part of the body is found in the ventral portion of the lemniscus and the upper part of the body in the dorsal. The **spinothalamic tract** (which crossed at spinal cord levels) continues upward throughout the medulla, as do the **spinoreticular tract** and the **ventral spinocerebellar pathway.** The **dorsal spinocerebellar tract** and the **cuneocerebellar tract** continue into the inferior cerebellar peduncle.

Descending Tracts

The **corticospinal tract** in the pyramid begins to cross at the transition between medulla and spinal cord; this decussation takes place over several millimeters. Some fibers from the corticospinal tract, which originate in the sensory cerebral cortex, end in the dorsal column nuclei and may modify their function. Because the fibers in the pyramid are corticospinal fibers only, a lesion here will not result in a typical upper-motor-neuron dysfunction. The **descending spinal tract of V** has its cell bodies, representing all 3 divisions of this tract, in the trigeminal ganglion. The fibers of the tract convey

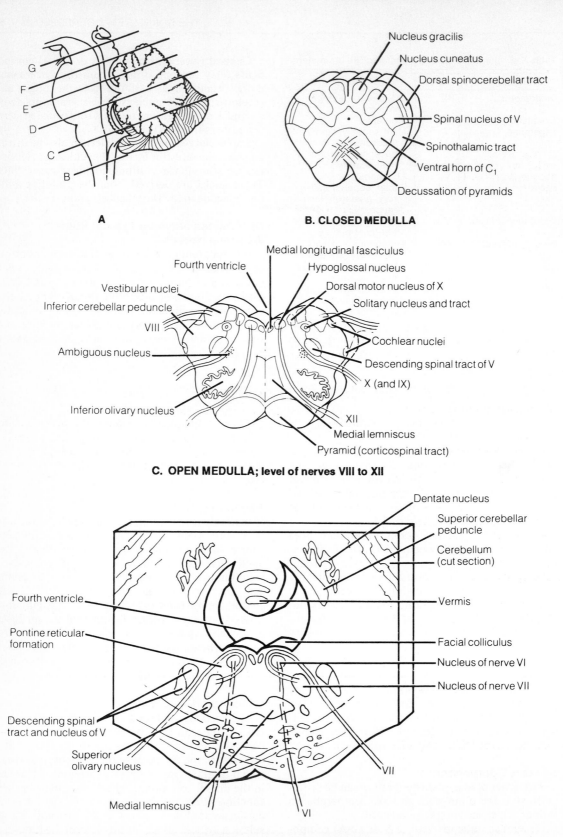

A: Key to levels of sections.

B. CLOSED MEDULLA

Nucleus gracilis
Nucleus cuneatus
Dorsal spinocerebellar tract
Spinal nucleus of V
Spinothalamic tract
Ventral horn of C_1
Decussation of pyramids

C. OPEN MEDULLA; level of nerves VIII to XII

Medial longitudinal fasciculus
Fourth ventricle
Hypoglossal nucleus
Vestibular nuclei
Dorsal motor nucleus of X
Inferior cerebellar peduncle
Solitary nucleus and tract
VIII
Ambiguous nucleus
Cochlear nuclei
Descending spinal tract of V
X (and IX)
Inferior olivary nucleus
XII
Medial lemniscus
Pyramid (corticospinal tract)

D. LOWER PONS; level of nerves VI and VII

Dentate nucleus
Superior cerebellar peduncle
Cerebellum (cut section)
Fourth ventricle
Vermis
Pontine reticular formation
Facial colliculus
Nucleus of nerve VI
Nucleus of nerve VII
Descending spinal tract and nucleus of V
Superior olivary nucleus
VII
Medial lemniscus
VI

Figure 6–7. *A:* Key to levels of sections. *B–G:* Schematic transverse sections through the brain stem.

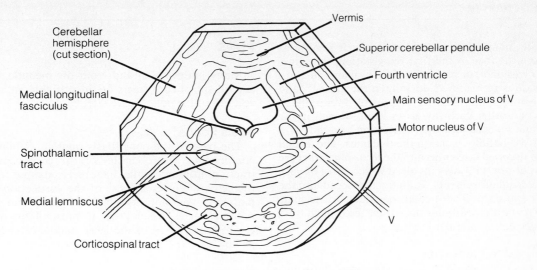

E. MIDDLE PONS; level of nerve V

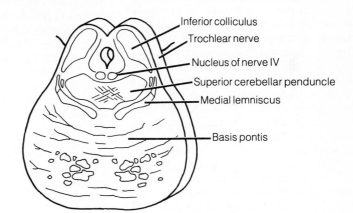

F. PONS/MIDBRAIN; level of nerve VI

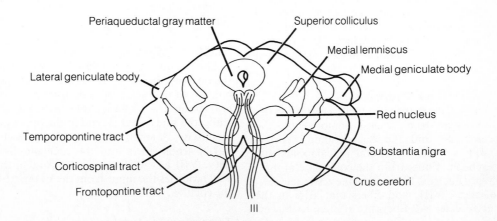

G. UPPER MIDBRAIN; level of nerve III

Figure 6-7. Continued.

pain, temperature, and crude touch sensations from the face to the first relay station, the spinal nucleus of V, or pars caudalis. The mandibular division is represented dorsally in the nucleus, and the ophthalmic division is represented ventrally. A second-order pathway arises from the cells in the spinal nucleus and then crosses and ascends in a diffuse bundle to end in the thalamus. The **medial longitudinal fasciculus** and the **tectospinal tract** are important pathways involved with control of gaze and head movements. Both tracts descend into the cervical cord. The medial longitudinal fasciculus arises in the vestibular nuclei, the tectospinal tract in the contralateral midbrain.

Cranial Nerve Nuclei

The hypoglossal nucleus, the dorsal motor nucleus of the vagus, and the solitary tract and nucleus are found in the medulla, grouped around the central canal; in the open medulla (Fig 6–7C), these nuclei lie below the fourth ventricle. The **hypoglossal nucleus,** which is homologous to the anterior horn nucleus in the cord, sends its fibers ventrally between the pyramid and inferior olivary nucleus to exit as nerve XII. This nerve innervates all the tongue muscles. The **dorsal motor nucleus of X** is a preganglionic parasympathetic nucleus that sends its fibers laterally into nerves IX and X. The branchial efferent component of the vagus arises from the ill-defined **nucleus ambiguous.**

The **solitary tract** is composed of visceral afferent fibers from nerves IX and X; it surrounds and ends in the **solitary nucleus.** Secondary fibers ascend in the brain stem to the thalamus. A rostral extension of the solitary nucleus, referred to as the **gustatory nucleus,** receives input from all 3 nerves that have a taste function: VII, IX and X.

The 4 **vestibular nuclei**—superior, inferior (or spinal), medial, and lateral—are found under the floor of the fourth ventricle, partly in the open medulla and partly in the pons. The ventral and dorsal **cochlear nuclei** are relay nuclei for fibers that arise in the spiral ganglion of the cochlea. The pathways of the vestibular and cochlear nuclei are discussed in Chapters 15 and 16.

Inferior Cerebellar Peduncle

The inferior cerebellar peduncle is formed in the open medulla from several components: the cuneocerebellar and the dorsal spinocerebellar tracts, fibers from the lateral reticular nucleus, olivocerebellar fibers from the contralateral inferior olivary nucleus, fibers from the vestibular division of nerve VIII, and fibers that arise in the vestibular nuclei. All fibers are afferent to the cerebellum.

PONS

Many pathways to and from the medulla and several spinal cord tracts are identifiable in cross sections of the pons (Figs 6–7D, E).

Basis Pontis

The base of the pons (basis pontis) contains 3 components: fiber bundles of the corticospinal tracts, **pontine nuclei** that have received input from the cerebral cortex by way of the corticopontine pathway, and pontocerebellar fibers from the pontine nuclei, which cross to most of the neocerebellum by way of the large middle cerebellar peduncle.

Tegmentum

The tegmentum of the pons is more complex than the base. The lower pons contains the nucleus of nerve VI (abducens nucleus) and the nuclei of nerve VII (the facial, superior salivatory, and gustatory nuclei). The branchial motor component of the facial nerve loops medially around the nucleus of nerve VI. The upper half of the pons harbors the main sensory nuclei of nerve V (Figs 6–7E and 6–8). The medial lemniscus assumes a different position (lower body, medial; upper body, lateral), and the spinothalamic tract courses even more laterally.

The **central tegmental tract** (from thalamus to inferior olivary nucleus), the **tectospinal tract** (from midbrain to cervical cord), and the **medial longitudinal fasciculus** are additional components of the pontine tegmentum.

Middle Cerebellar Peduncle

The middle cerebellar peduncle is the largest of the 3 cerebellar peduncles on each side of the brain stem. It contains numerous fibers that arise from the contralateral basis of the pons and end in the cerebellar hemisphere.

Auditory Pathways

The auditory system from the cochlear nuclei in the pontomedullary junction (see also Chapter 15) consists of fibers that ascend ipsilaterally in the lateral lemniscus. It also includes crossing fibers (the trapezoid body) that ascend in the opposite lateral lemniscus. A small **superior olivary nucleus** (Fig 6–7D) sends fibers into the cochlear division of nerve VIII as the olivocochlear bundle; this pathway modifies the input from the organ of Corti in the cochlea.

Trigeminal System

The 3 divisions of the **trigeminal nerve** (nerve V; Figs 6–7D, E, and Fig 6–8) all project to the brain stem: Fine touch function is relayed by the **main**

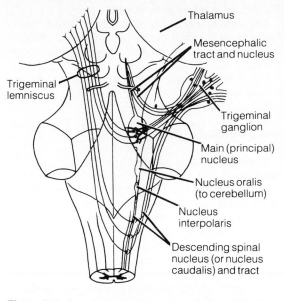

Figure 6-8. Schematic drawing of the trigeminal system.

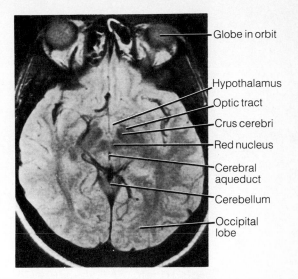

Figure 6-9. Magnetic resonance image of a horizontal section through the head at the level of the midbrain. Note that the position of the midbrain is reversed from that in Fig 6-7G.

sensory nucleus; pain and temperature are relayed into the **descending spinal tract of V;** and proprioceptive fibers form a **mesencephalic tract and nucleus** in the midbrain. Some first-order nuclei of this system are found within the brain stem, rather than in the trigeminal ganglion itself. The second-order neurons from the main sensory nucleus cross and ascend to the thalamus. The descending spinal tract of V sends fibers to the pars caudalis (the spinal nucleus in the medulla), the pars interpolaris (a link between trigeminal afferent components and the cerebellum), and the pars oralis. The **masticatory nucleus,** which is medial to the main sensory nucleus, sends branchial efferent fibers into the mandibular division of nerve V to innervate most of the muscles of mastication and the tensor tympani of the middle ear.

MIDBRAIN

The midbrain forms a transition (and fiber conduit) to the cerebrum (Figs 1-2, 1-3, and 6-10).

Basis

The base of the midbrain contains the **crus cerebri,** a massive fiber bundle that includes corticospinal, corticobulbar, and corticopontine pathways (Figs 6-7G and 6-9). The base also contains the **substantia nigra.** The substantia (whose cells contain neuromelanin) receives afferent fibers from the cerebral cortex and the striatum; it sends dopaminergic efferent fibers to the striatum (see Chapter 20).

The **corticobulbar fibers** from the motor cortex to interneurons of the efferent nuclei of cranial nerves are homologous with the corticospinal fibers (Fig 6-10). The corticobulbar fibers to the lower portion of the facial nucleus and the hypoglossal nucleus are crossed (from the opposite cerebral cortex). All other corticobulbar projections are bilaterally crossed (from both cortices). These cranial nerves are homologous with the spinal (motor) nerves, or lower motor neurons (LMN).

Tegmentum

The tegmentum of the midbrain contains all the ascending tracts from the spinal cord or lower brain stem and many of the descending systems. A large and richly vascularized **red nucleus** receives crossed efferent fibers from the cerebellum and sends fibers to the thalamus and the contralateral spinal cord via the rubrospinal tract. The red nucleus is an important component of motor coordination.

Two contiguous somatic efferent nuclear groups lie in the upper tegmentum: the **trochlear nucleus** (which forms contralateral nerve IV) and the **oculomotor nuclei** (which have efferent fibers in nerve III). Each eye muscle innervated by the oculomotor nerve has its own subgroup of innervating cells; the subgroup for the superior rectus muscle is contralateral. The preganglionic parasympathetic system destined for the eye (a synapse in the ciliary

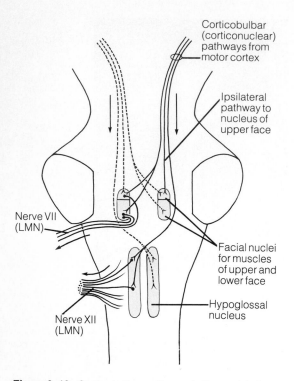

Figure 6-10. Corticobulbar pathways to the nuclei of cranial nerves VII and XII.

ganglion) has its origin in or near the Edinger-Westphal nucleus.

Tectum

The tectum, or roof, of the midbrain is formed by 2 pairs of colliculi and the **corpora quadrigemina.** The **superior colliculi** contain neurons that serve ocular reflexes; the **inferior colliculi** are involved in auditory reflexes and in determining the side on which a sound originates. The inferior colliculi receive input from both ears, and they project to the medial geniculate nucleus of the thalamus by way of the **inferior quadrigeminal brachium.** The **superior quadrigeminal brachium** links the lateral geniculate nucleus and the superior colliculus. The colliculi contribute to the formation of the crossed tectospinal tracts, which are involved in blinking and head-turning reflexes following sudden sounds or visual images.

Periaqueductal Gray Matter

The periaqueductal gray matter contains descending autonomic tracts as well as endorphin-producing cells that suppress pain. This region is the target for brain-stimulating implants used in patients suffering from chronic pain (see Chapter 13).

Superior Cerebellar Peduncle

The superior cerebellar peduncle contains efferent fibers from the dentate nucleus of the cerebellum to the opposite red nucleus (the dentato-rubro-thalamic system) and the ventral spinocerebellar tracts. The cerebellar fibers decussate just below the red nuclei.

VASCULARIZATION

The vessels that supply the brain stem are branches of the vertebrobasilar system (Fig 6–11; see also Chapter 11). Those classified as **circumferential vessels** are the posterior inferior cerebellar artery, the anterior inferior cerebellar artery, the superior cerebellar artery, the posterior cerebral artery, and the pontine artery. Each of these vessels sends small branches (a few or many) into the underlying brain stem structures along its course. Other vessels are classified as **median (paramedian) perforators,** since they penetrate the brain stem from the basilar artery. The small medullary and spinal branches of the vertebral artery make up a third group of vessels.

Lesions of the Brain Stem

The brain stem is an anatomically compact, functionally diverse, and clinically important structure. Even a single relatively small lesion nearly always damages several nuclei, reflex centers, tracts,

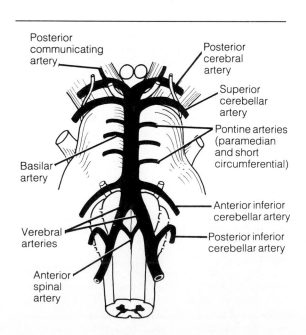

Figure 6-11. Principal arteries of the brain stem (ventral view).

or pathways. Such lesions are often vascular in nature (eg, hemorrhage, occlusive ischemia), but tumors, trauma, and degenerative or demyelinating processes can also injure the brain stem. The following are typical syndromes caused by intrinsic (intra-axial) lesions of the brain stem.

Medial (basal) medullary syndrome usually involves the pyramid, part or all of the medial lemniscus, and nerve XII. If it is unilateral, it is also known as **alternating hypoglossal hemiplegia** (Fig 6–12); the term refers to the finding that the cranial-nerve weakness is on the same side as the lesion, while the body paralysis is on the opposite side. Lesions can also result in bilateral defects. The area involved is supplied by the anterior spinal artery or by medial branches of the vertebral artery.

Lateral medullary, or **Wallenberg's, syndrome** (Fig 6–12) involves some (or all) of the following structures in the open medulla on the dorsolateral side: inferior cerebellar peduncle, vestibular nuclei, fibers or nuclei of nerve IX or X, spinal nucleus and tract of V, spinothalamic tract, and sympathetic pathways. (Involvement of the sympathetic pathways may lead to Horner's syndrome). The affected area is supplied by branches of the vertebral artery or the posterior inferior cerebellar artery.

Basal pontine syndromes (Fig 6–13) can involve both the corticospinal tract and a cranial nerve (VI, VII, or V) in the affected region, depending on the extent and level of the lesion. The syndrome is called **alternating abducens (VI),** facial (V), or tri-

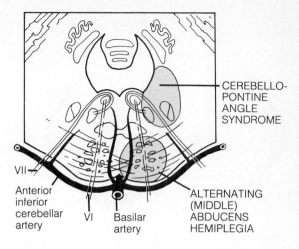

Figure 6–13. Clinical syndromes associated with pontine lesions (compare with Fig 6–7D).

geminal hemiplegia (V). If the lesion is large, it may include the medial lemniscus. The vascular supply comes from the perforators, or pontine branches, of the anterior inferior cerebellar artery.

Dorsal pons syndrome affects nerve VI or VII or their respective nuclei, with or without involvement of the medial lemniscus, spinothalamic tract, or lateral lemniscus. The "lateral gaze center" is often involved (see also Chapter 14). At a more rostral level, nerve V and its nuclei may no longer be functioning. The affected area is supplied by various perforators (pontine branches) of the circumferential arteries.

Peduncular syndrome, also called **alternating oculomotor hemiplegia** and **Weber's syndrome** in the basal midbrain (Fig 6–14), involves nerve III and portions of the cerebral peduncle. The arterial supply is by the posterior perforators and branches of the posterior cerebral artery.

Benedikt's syndrome (Fig 6–14) situated in the tegmentum of the midbrain, may damage the medial lemniscus, the red nucleus, and nerve III and its nucleus and associated tracts. This area is supplied by perforators and branches of circumferential arteries.

Vertical gaze palsy (an inability to move the eyes up or down), also called **Parinaud's syndrome** (Fig 6–14), is caused by compression of the tectum and adjacent areas (eg, by a tumor of the pineal gland).

Lesions near the Brain Stem

Space-occupying processes (eg, tumors, aneurysms, brain herniation) in the area surrounding the brain stem can affect the brain stem indirectly. The following disorders are typically caused by extrinsic (extra-axial) lesions.

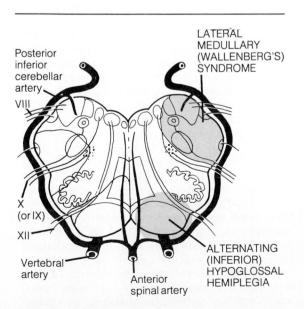

Figure 6–12. Clinical syndromes associated with medullary lesions (compare with Fig 6–7C).

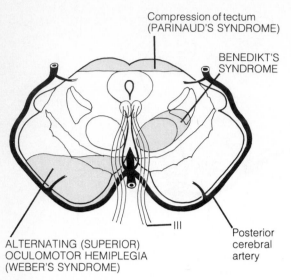

Figure 6-14. Clinical syndromes associated with midbrain lesions (compare with Fig 6-7G).

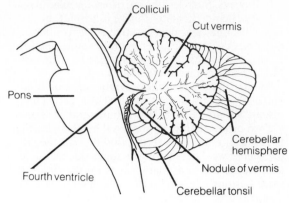

Figure 6-15. Midsagittal section through the cerebellum.

Cerebellopontine angle syndrome may involve nerve VIII or VII or deeper structures. It is most often caused by a tumor that begins by affecting the Schwann cells of a cranial nerve in that region, eg, a tumor at nerve VIII (Fig 6-3).

A tumor in the **pineal region** may compress the upper quadrigeminal plate and cause vertical gaze palsy, loss of pupillary reflexes, and other ocular manifestations. There may be accompanying obstructive hydrocephalus.

Other tumors near the brain stem include medulloblastoma, ependymoma of the fourth ventricle, glioma, meningioma, and congenital cysts. **Medulloblastoma,** a cerebellar tumor (usually of the vermis) that occurs in childhood, may fill the fourth ventricle and block the cerebrospinal fluid pathway. Although compression of the brain stem is rare, the tumor has a tendency to seed to the subarachnoid space of the spinal cord and the brain.

Aneurysms, local dilations of a vessel, (usually an artery), are rare in the region of the brain stem (see Chapter 11).

CEREBELLUM

Divisions

The cerebellum is divided into 2 hemispheres; they are connected by the **vermis,** which can be further subdivided (Fig 6-15). The phylogenetically old **archicerebellum** consists of the flocculus, the nodulus (nodule of the vermis), and interconnections **(flocculonodular system);** it is concerned with equilibrium and connects with the vestibular system (Fig 6-16). The **paleocerebellum** consists of the anterior portions of the hemispheres and the anterior and posterior vermis and is involved with propulsive, stereotyped movements such as swimming and walking (Fig 6-17). The remainder of the cerebellum is considered the **neocerebellum** and is concerned with the coordination of fine movement.

Functions

The cerebellum has 2 main functions: coordinating skilled voluntary movements by influencing muscle activity and controlling equilibrium and muscle tone through connections with the vestibular system and the spinal cord and its gamma motor neurons. There is a somatotropic organization of body parts within the cerebellar cortex (Fig 6-18). In addition, the cerebellum receives collateral input from the sensory and special sensory systems. Recent work suggests that the cerebellum is also involved in the mechanism of memory.

Peduncles

Three pairs of peduncles, located above and around the fourth ventricle, attach the cerebellum to the brain stem and contain pathways to and from the brain stem (see Figs 6-5 and 6-16 and Table 6-3). The inferior cerebellar peduncle contains many fiber systems from the spinal cord and lower brain stem as well as connections with the vestibular nuclei and nerve. The middle cerebellar peduncle consists of fibers from the contralateral pontine nuclei, which receive input from many areas of the cerebral cortex. The superior cerebellar peduncle, composed mostly of efferent fibers, sends impulses to both the thalamus and spinal cord, with relays in the red nuclei (see also Chapter 12).

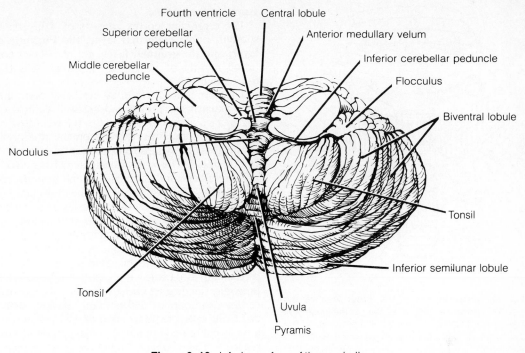

Figure 6–16. Inferior surface of the cerebellum.

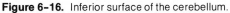

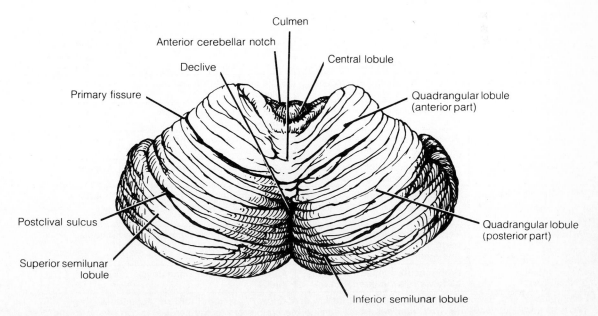

Figure 6–17. Superior surface of the cerebellum.

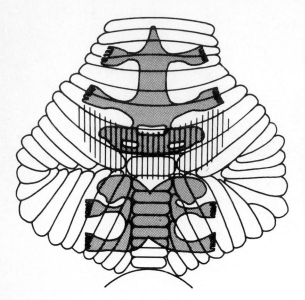

Figure 6-18. Cerebellar homunculi. Proprioceptive and tactile stimuli are projected as shown in the upper (inverted) homunculus and the lower (split) homunculus. The striped area represents the region from which evoked responses to auditory and visual stimuli are observed. (Redrawn and reproduced, with permission, from Snider R: The Cerebellum. *Sci Am* 1958;**199:**84.)

Cortical Layers

The cerebellar cortex consists of 3 layers: the subpial, outer **molecular layer,** the **Purkinje cell layer;** and the **granular layer,** an inner layer composed mainly of very small granular cells (Figs 6-19 and 6-20).

The fiber connections of the cerebellar cortex have been extensively studied and are well defined (Fig 6-21). Two axon types project to the cerebellar cortex. The climbing fibers extend from the inferior olivary nucleus and synapse onto the dendritic tree of the Purkinje cells. The mossy fibers extend from all other afferent fibers and terminate in the granule cells. These cells send their axons into the molecular layer to become parallel fibers that synapse on the Purkinje cell dendrites. All afferent fibers (both mossy and climbing) send collateral branches to the deep cerebellar nuclei (fastigial, globose, emboliform, and dentate). The Purkinje cell axons (of one-half of the cerebellum) also project to the deep cerebellar nuclei, especially the dentate nucleus. Because the cerebellar cortex also contains the inhibitory **basket, stellate,** and **Golgi cells,** the final output of the Purkinje cell is a finely calibrated impulse that may inhibit its target nucleus. The efferent output of the cerebellum (through the superior cerebellar peduncle) is a balance between the excitatory effects of afferent axon collaterals and the GABA-inhibitory effects of Purkinje cells (Table 6-4).

Cerebellum & Brain Stem in Whole-Head Sections

Magnetic resonance imaging shows the cerebellum and its relationship with the brain stem, cra-

Table 6-3. Functions and major terminations of the principal afferent systems to the cerebellum.*†

Afferent Tracts	Transmits	Distribution	Peduncle of Entry into Cerebellum
Dorsal spinocerebellar	Proprioceptive and exteroceptive impulses from body	Folia I–VI, pyramis and paramedian lobule	Inferior
Ventral spinocerebellar	Proprioceptive and exteroceptive impulses from body	Folia I–VI, pyramis and paramedian lobule	Superior
Cuneocerebellar	Proprioceptive impulses, especially from head and neck	Folia I–VI, pyramis and paramedian lobule	Inferior
Tectocerebellar	Auditory and visual impulses via inferior and superior colliculi	Folium, tuber, ansiform lobule	Superior
Vestibulocerebellar	Vestibular impulses from labyrinths, directly and via vestibular nuclei	Principally flocculonodular lobe	Inferior
Pontocerebellar	Impulses from motor and other parts of cerebral cortex via pontine nuclei	All cerebellar cortex except flocculonodular lobe	Middle
Olivocerebellar	Proprioceptive input from whole body via relay in inferior olive	All cerebellar cortex and deep nuclei	Inferior

*Reproduced, with permission, from Ganong WF: *Review of Medical Physiology,* 13th ed. Appleton & Lange, 1987.
†Several other pathways transmit impulses from nuclei in the brain stem to the cerebellar cortex and to the deep nuclei.

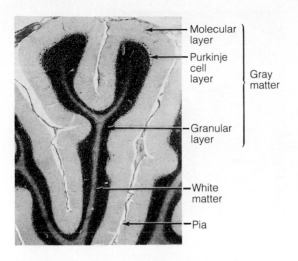

Figure 6–19. Photomicrograph of a portion of the cerebellum. Each lobule contains a core of white matter and 3 layers—granular, Purkinje, and molecular—of gray matter. H&E stain, × 28. (Reproduced, with permission, from Junqueira LC, Carneiro J, Kelley RO: *Basic Histology,* 6th ed. Appleton & Lange, 1989.)

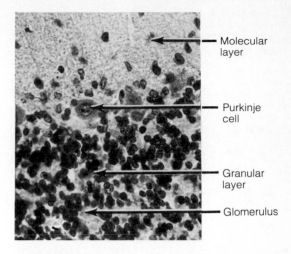

Figure 6–20. Photomicrograph of cerebellar cortex. This staining procedure does not reveal the unusually large dendritic arborization of the Purkinje cell. H&E stain, × 250. (Reproduced, with permission, from Junqueira LC, Carneiro J, Kelley RO: *Basic Histology,* 6th ed. Appleton & Lange, 1989.)

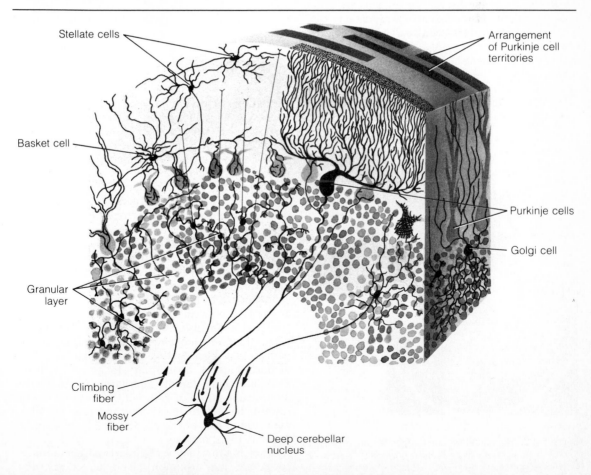

Figure 6–21. Schematic diagram of the cerebellar cortex.

Table 6-4. Excitatory and inhibitory effects.

Excitation	Inhibition
Mossy fibers → granular cell	Basket cell → Purkinje cell body
Olive → climbing	Stellate cell → Purkinje cell dendrite
Climbing → Purkinje cell	Golgi cell → granular cell
Granular cell → Purkinje cell	Purkinje cell → roof nuclei (including dentate)
Granular cell → Golgi cell	Purkinje cell → lat. vestib. nuclei
Granular cell → basket cell	Purkinje cell → Purkinje cells
Granular cell → stellate cell	Purkinje cell → Golgi cells

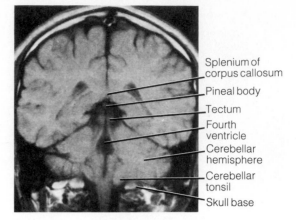

Figure 6-23. MR image of a coronal section through the head at the level of the fourth ventricle.

nial nerves, skull, and vessels (Figs 6–22 and 6–23). These images are increasingly useful in determining the location, nature (solid or cystic), and extent of cerebellar lesions (see the discussion of Chiari malformation, below).

Clinical Correlations

Signs of cerebellar disorders in humans are usually the result of a lesion that affects more than one region of the cerebellum (see also Chapter 12). The most characteristic signs of a cerebellar disorder are **hypotonia** (diminished muscle tone) and **ataxia** (loss of the coordinated muscular contractions required for the production of smooth movements). In general, unilateral lesions of the cerebellum lead to motor disabilities ipsilateral to the side of the lesion. Note that alcohol intoxication can mimic cerebellar ataxia.

Some lesions are confined to a particular subdivision of the cerebellum. For example, lesions of the **vestibulocerebellum** (involving the flocculus, nodulus, and caudal vermis) cause disturbances of equilibrium, characterized by unsteady walking and swaying when standing. **Nystagmus** (rhythmic oscillations of the eyeballs) may also be present. Because such lesions often involve midline structures, they can cause bilateral signs. Lesions of the **paleocerebellum** and **neocerebellum** usually involve portions of a cerebellar hemisphere and result in clumsy movements of the extremities (ataxia) on the same side as the cerebellar lesion. With these lesions it is difficult to determine the predominant involvement of one or the other of these portions of the cerebellum.

Several types of **asynergy** (loss of coordination) can be demonstrated in patients with cerebellar lesions: There can be the decomposition of movement into its component parts; **dysmetria,** which is characterized by the inability to place an extremity at a precise point in space (eg, touch the finger to the nose); or **intention tremor,** a tremor that arises when voluntary movements are attempted. The patient may also exhibit **adiadochokinesis (dysdiadochokinesis),** an inability to make, or difficulty in making, rapidly alternating or successive movements; ataxia of gait, with a tendency to fall toward the side of the lesion; and **rebound phenomenon,** a loss of the normal checks of agonist and antagonist muscles.

Fig 6–24 shows a type of **Chiari malformation,** a congenital malformation characterized by displacement of the lower cerebellum into the spinal

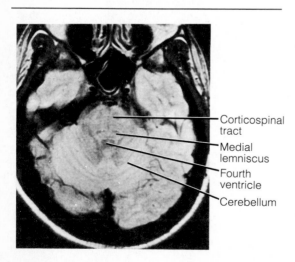

Figure 6-22. Horizontal section through the head at the level of the lower pons. Note that the position of the pons is reversed from that of Fig 6–7D, to conform with customary CT and MR procedures.

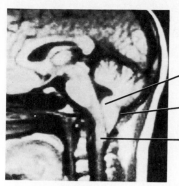

Figure 6–24. MR image of a midsagittal section showing Chiari malformation (compare with Fig 1–4).

canal. This malformation is also associated with deformation of the brain stem. It can produce obstructive hydrocephalus by blocking the cerebrospinal fluid pathway from the fourth ventricle to the subarachnoid space (see Chapter 10).

CASE 6

A 60-year-old technician had a sudden onset of double vision and dizziness. Three weeks later (one day prior to admission), she noted a sudden drooping of her right eyelid.

Neurologic examination showed unequal pupils (right smaller than left, both responding to light and accommodation), ptosis of the right eyelid, mild enophthalmos and decreased sweating on the right side of the face, and nystagmus on left lateral gaze. The corneal reflex was diminished on the right but normal on the left. Although pain sensation was decreased on the right side of the face, touch sensation was normal; there was minor right peripheral facial weakness. The uvula deviated to the left, and mild hoarseness was noted. Muscle strength was intact, but the patient could not execute a right finger-to-nose test or make rapid alternating movements. There was an intention tremor, and further examination revealed ataxia in the right lower extremity. Reflexes were all normal.

Pain sensation was decreased on the left side of the body; senses of touch, vibration and position were intact.

What is the differential diagnosis? What is the most likely diagnosis?

CASE 7

A 27-year-old graduate student was admitted with a chief complaint of having double vision for 2 weeks. Earlier, he had noticed persistent tingling of all the fingers on his left hand. More recently, he felt as though ants were crawling on the left side of his face and the left half of his tongue. He also thought that both legs had become weaker recently.

Neurologic examination showed a scotoma in the upper field of the left eye, weakness of the left medial rectus muscle, coarse horizontal nystagmus on left lateral gaze, and mild weakness of the left central facial muscles. All other muscles had normal strength. The deep tendon reflexes were normal on the right and livelier on the left, and there was a left extensor plantar response. The sensory system was unremarkable.

The patient was discharged a few days later, seemingly improved after corticosteroid treatment. He was readmitted 3 weeks later, however, because he noted difficulty in walking and his speech had become thickened. Neurologic examination showed the following additional findings: wide-based ataxic gait, minor slurring of speech, bilateral tremor in the finger-to-nose test, and disorganization of rapid alternating movements. A CT scan was within normal limits. Lumbar puncture showed 56 mg protein, with a relatively increased level of gamma globulins. All other cerebrospinal fluid findings were normal. Treatment with high doses of corticosteroids seemed to improve the neurological deficits, and the patient was discharged.

What is the differential diagnosis at this point?

Two months later, the patient's symptoms recurred, and he was admitted to a nursing home. He gradually became quadriplegic, and his visual and brain stem problems increased.

What is the diagnosis?

Cases are discussed further in Chapter 24.

REFERENCES

Chan-Palay V: *Cerebellar Dentate Nucleus: Organization, Cytology and Transmitters.* Springer-Verlag, 1977.

DeArmand SJ: *Structure of the Human Brain: A Photographic Atlas,* 3rd ed. Oxford Univ Press, 1989.

Llinas RR: The cortex of the cerebellum. *Sci Am* 1975;**232**:56.

Montemurro DG, Bruni JE: *The Human Brain in Dissection.* Saunders, 1981.

Moruzzi G: Active processes in the brain during sleep. *Harvey Lect* 1963;**58**:233.

Riley HA: *An Atlas of the Basal Ganglia, Brain Stem and Spinal Cord.* Williams & Wilkins, 1943.

Scheibel ME, Scheibel AB: Anatomical basis of attention: Mechanisms in vertebrate brains. Pages 577–602 in: *The Neurosciences.* Quarton GC, Melnechuck T, Schmitt FO (editors). Rockefeller Univ Press, 1967.

Cranial Nerves & Pathways

7

ORIGIN OF CRANIAL NERVE FIBERS

The 12 pairs of cranial nerves are usually referred to by either name or roman numeral (see Fig 7–1 and Table 7–1). Note that the olfactory peduncle (see Chapter 18) and the optic nerve (see Chapter 14) are not true nerves but fiber tracts of the brain, while nerve XI (the spinal accessory nerve) is derived, in part, from the upper cervical segments of the spinal cord. The remaining 9 pairs relate to the brain stem.

The superficial origin of a cranial nerve is the area of the brain where the nerve emerges or enters. Cranial nerve fibers with motor (efferent) functions arise from collections of cells (motor nuclei) that lie deep within the brain stem; they are homologous to the anterior horn cells of the spinal cord. Cranial nerve fibers with sensory (afferent) functions have their cells of origin (first-order nuclei) outside the brain stem, usually in ganglia that are homologous to the dorsal root ganglia of the spinal nerves. Second-order sensory nuclei lie within the brain stem (see Chapter 6 and Fig 6–6).

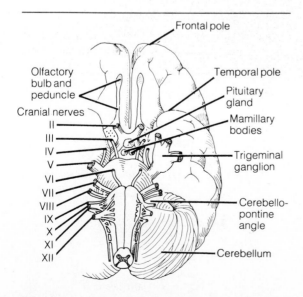

Figure 7-1. Ventral view of the brain stem with cranial nerves.

FUNCTIONAL COMPONENTS OF THE CRANIAL NERVES

A cranial nerve can have one or more functions (as shown in Table 7–1). The functional components are conveyed from or to the brain stem by 6 types of nerve fibers:

(1) **Somatic efferent fibers,** also called general somatic efferent fibers, they innervate striated muscles that are derived from somites and are involved in eye (nerves III, IV, and VI) and tongue (nerve XII) movements.

(2) **Branchial efferent fibers,** also known as special visceral efferent fibers, are special somatic efferent components. They innervate muscles that are derived from the branchial (gill) arches and are involved in chewing (nerve V), making facial expressions (nerve VII), swallowing (nerves IX and X), producing vocal sounds (nerve X), and turning the head (nerve XI).

(3) **Visceral efferent fibers** are also called general visceral efferent fibers (preganglionic parasympathetic components of the cranial division); they course through nerves III (smooth muscles of the inner eye), VII (salivatory and lacrimal glands), IX (the parotid gland), and X (the muscles of the heart, lung, and bowel that are involved in movement and secretion; see also Chapter 19).

(4) **Visceral afferent fibers,** also called general

Table 7-1. Composition of cranial nerves.

Nerve	Functional Component	Nerve	Functional Component
I	SS	VII	BE, VE, VA (taste), (SA)*
II	SS	VIII	SS
III	SE, BE	IX	BE, VE, VA, (SA)*
IV	SE	X	BE, VE, VA, (SA)*
V	SA, BE	XI	BE
VI	SE	XII	SE

Efferent (motor)	Afferent (sensory)
SE—somatic; general SE	VA—visceral; general VA, special VA
BE—branchial; special VE	SA—somatic; general SA
VE—visceral; general VE	SS—special sensory

*Most nerves with SE components have a few SA fibers for proprioception.

visceral afferent fibers, convey sensation from the alimentary tract, heart, vessels, and lungs by way of nerves IX and X. A specialized visceral afferent component is involved with the sense of taste; fibers carrying gustatory impulses are present in cranial nerves VII, IX, and X.

(5) **Somatic afferent fibers,** often called general somatic afferent fibers, convey sensation from the skin and the mucous membranes of the head. They are found mainly in the trigeminal nerve (V). A small number of afferent fibers travel with the facial (VII), glossopharyngeal (IX), and vagus (X) nerves; these fibers terminate on trigeminal nuclei in the brain stem.

(6) **Special sensory fibers** are found in nerves I (involved in smell), II (vision), and VIII (hearing and equilibrium).

Differences between Cranial & Spinal Nerves

Unlike the spinal nerves, cranial nerves are not found at regular intervals. They differ in other aspects as well: The spinal nerves, for example, contain neither branchial efferent nor special sensory components. Some cranial nerves contain motor components only (most motor nerves have a few proprioceptive fibers), and some contain large visceral components. Other cranial nerves are completely or mostly sensory, and still others are mixed, with both types of components. The mixed cranial nerves enter and exit at the same point on the brain stem; this point is ventral or ventrolateral except for nerve IV, which exits from the dorsal surface (Fig 7–1).

Ganglia Related to Cranial Nerves

The 2 types of ganglia related to cranial nerves are those without synapses, which are found in afferent (somatic or visceral) components and are homologous to dorsal root ganglia; and ganglia with synapses, which are found in efferent visceral (autonomic) components (Table 7–2).

The named ganglia of the cranial **parasympathetic division** of the autonomic nervous system are the **ciliary ganglion** (nerve III), the **pterygopalatine** and **submandibular ganglia** (VIII), **optic ganglion** (IX), and **intramural ganglion** (X). The first 4 of these ganglia have a close association with branches of V; the trigeminal branches may course through the autonomic ganglia. Of the ganglia for the taste components of nerves VII, IX, and X, only the **geniculate ganglion** (VII) is specifically named.

The chain of **sympathetic division** ganglia lies in the neck region and consists of 3 **cervical ganglia:** inferior, middle, and superior. Postganglionic fibers then form a sympathetic plexus to supply structures in the head via the **carotid plexus.**

Table 7–2. Ganglia related to cranial nerves.

Ganglion	Nerve	Functional Type	Synapse
Ciliary	III	VE (para-sympathetic)	+
Ptertgopalatine	VII	VE (para-sympathetic)	+
Submandibular	VII	VE (para-sympathetic)	+
Otic	IX	VE (para-sympathetic)	+
Intramural (in viscus)	X	VE (para-sympathetic)	+
Semilunar	V	SA	−
Geniculate	VII	VA (taste)	−
Inferior and superior	IX	SA, VA (taste)	−
Inferior and superior	X	SA, VA (taste)	−
Spiral	VIII (cochlear)	SS	−
Vestibular	VIII (vestibular)	SS	−

ANATOMIC RELATIONSHIPS OF THE CRANIAL NERVES

Cranial Nerve I: Olfactory Nerve

The true olfactory nerves are short connections between the olfactory mucosa within the nose, and the olfactory bulb within the cranial cavity (see Fig 7–2 and Chapter 18). There are 9–15 of these nerves on each side of the brain.

Cranial Nerve II: Optic Nerve

The optic nerve arises from the ganglion cells in

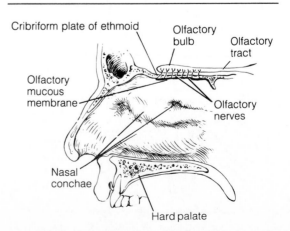

Cribriform plate of ethmoid — Olfactory bulb — Olfactory tract

Olfactory mucous membrane — Olfactory nerves

Nasal conchae

Hard palate

Figure 7–2. Lateral view of the olfactory bulb, tract, mucous membrane, and nerves.

the retina and then passes through the optic papilla to the orbit, where it is contained within meningeal sheaths. The nerve changes its name to optic tract when the fibers have passed through the optic chiasm (Figs 6–3 and 7–3; see also Chapter 14).

Cranial Nerve III: Oculomotor Nerve

The oculomotor nerve leaves the brain on the medial side of the cerebral peduncle, behind the posterior cerebral artery and in front of the superior cerebellar artery. It then passes anteriorly, parallel to the internal carotid artery in the lateral wall of the cavernous sinus, leaving the cranial cavity by way of the superior orbital fissure. The somatic efferent portion of the nerve innervates the **levator palpebrae superioris muscle;** the **superior, medial,** and **inferior rectus muscles;** and the **inferior oblique muscle** (Fig 7–4). The visceral efferent portion innervates 2 smooth intraocular muscles: the **ciliary** and the **constrictor pupillae.**

Cranial Nerve IV: Trochlear Nerve

The small trochlear nerve is the only crossed cranial nerve. It originates in the lower midbrain and emerges contralaterally on the dorsal surface of the brain stem. The nerve then curves ventrally between the posterior cerebral and superior cerebellar arteries (lateral to the oculomotor nerve). It continues anteriorly in the lateral wall of the cavernous sinus and enters the orbit via the superior orbital fissure. It innervates the superior oblique muscle (Fig 7–4). *Note:* Because nerves III, IV, and VI are generally grouped together for discussion, nerve V is discussed after nerve VI.

Cranial Nerve VI: Abducens Nerve

A. Anatomy: The abducens nerve emerges

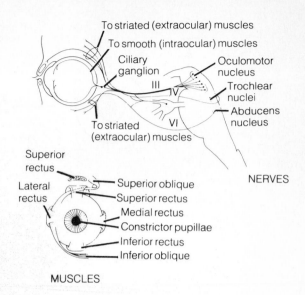

Figure 7–4. The oculomotor, trochlear, and abducens nerves; ocular muscles.

from the pontomedullary fissure, passes through the cavernous sinus close to the internal carotid, and exits from the cranial cavity via the superior orbital fissure. Its long intracranial course makes it vulnerable to pathologic processes in the posterior and middle cranial fossae. The nerve innervates the lateral rectus muscle (Fig 7–4).

A few sensory (proprioceptive) fibers from the muscles of the eye are present in nerves III, IV, and VI and in some other nerves that innervate striated muscles. The central termination of these fibers is in the mesencephalic nucleus of V (see below).

B. Action of the External Eye Muscles: The actions of eye muscles operating singly and in tandem are shown in Tables 7–3 and 7–4 (see Fig 7–5). The levator palpebrae superioris muscle has no action on the eyeball but lifts the upper eyelid when contracted. Closing the eyelids is performed

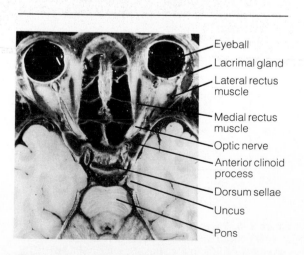

Figure 7–3. Horizontal section through the head at the level of the orbits.

Table 7–3. Functions of the ocular muscles.*

Muscle	Primary Action	Secondary Action
Lateral rectus	Abduction	None
Medial rectus	Abduction	None
Superior rectus	Elevation	Adduction, intorsion
Inferior rectus	Depression	Adduction, extorsion
Superior oblique	Depression	Intorsion, abduction
Inferior oblique	Elevation	Extorsion, abduction

*Reproduced, with permission, from Vaughan D, Asbury T: *General Ophthalmology,* 11th ed. Appleton & Lange, 1986.

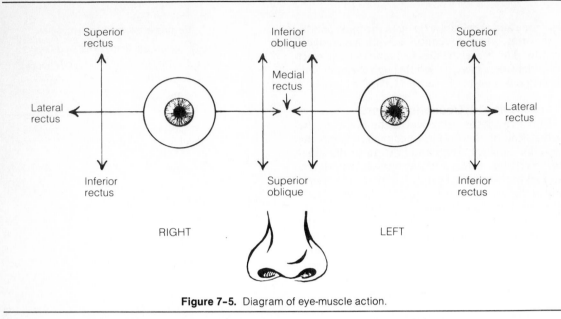

Figure 7-5. Diagram of eye-muscle action.

by contraction of the orbicular muscle of the eye; this muscle is innervated by nerve VII.

C. Control of Ocular-Muscle Movements: The oculomotor system is normally precise (Fig 7-6). It can aid vision by accurately fixating on an object of interest without head movements or by aligning the most acute portion of each retina at the point of interest. When the eyes scan the environment, they do so in short, rapid movements called **saccades.** When a target moves, a different form of ocular movement—smooth pursuit—is used to keep the image in sharp focus. This compensatory function is achieved by the **vestibulo-ocular reflex** (see Chapter 16).

The 6 individual muscles that move one eye normally act together with the muscles of the other eye

Table 7-4. Yoke muscle combinations.*

Cardinal Direction of Gaze	Yoke Muscles
Eyes up, right	Right superior rectus and left inferior oblique
Eyes right	Right lateral rectus and left medial rectus
Eyes down, right	Right inferior rectus and left superior oblique
Eyes down, left	Right superior oblique and left inferior rectus
Eyes left	Right medial rectus and left lateral rectus
Eyes up, left	Right inferior oblique and left superior rectus

*Reproduced, with permission, from Vaughan D, Asbury T: *General Ophthalmology,* 11th ed. Appleton & Lange, 1986.

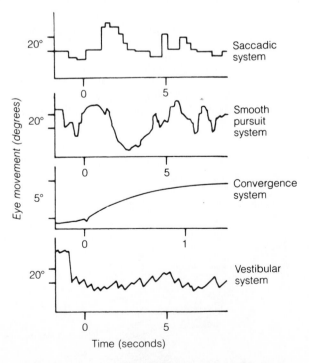

Figure 7-6. Types of eye-movement control. (Modified and reproduced, with permission, from Robinson DA: Eye movement control in primates. *Science* 1968;**161:**1219. (Copyright 1968 by the American Association for the Advancement of Science.)

in controlled movement. Both eyes move to follow an object in space, but they move by simultaneously contracting and relaxing different muscles; this is called a **conjugate gaze** movement. Fixating on a single point is called **vergence,** which requires a different set of muscles, including the intraocular muscles. Each of the extraocular muscles is brought into play in conjugate gaze movements or vergence.

1. Gaze and vergence centers–Conjugate gaze and vergence are controlled from 3 areas in the brain stem. There are 2 lateral gaze centers in the paramedian pontine reticular formation near the left and right abducens nuclei and a vergence center in the pretectum just above the superior colliculi. Each of these 3 areas can be activated during head movement by the vestibular system via the medial longitudinal fasciculus (see Chapter 16). In addition, regions in the contralateral frontal lobe (the eye field area) influence the lateral gaze centers, while regions in the occipital lobe influence the vergence center (Fig 7–7).

2. Control of pupillary size–The diameter of the pupil is affected by parasympathetic efferent fibers in the oculomotor nerve and sympathetic fibers from the superior cervical ganglion (Fig 7–8). **Constriction (miosis)** of the pupil is caused by the stimulation of parasympathetic fibers, whereas **dilation (mydriasis)** is caused by sympathetic activation. The size of both pupils is normally affected simultaneously by one or more of such causes as emotion, pain, drugs, and changes in light intensity and accommodation.

3. Reflexes–The **pupillary light reflex** is a constriction of both eyes in response to a bright light. Even if the light hits only one eye, both pupils usually constrict; this is a **consensual response.** The pathways for the reflex (Fig 7–9) include optic nerve fibers (or their collaterals) to the pretectum, a nuclear area between thalamus and midbrain. Short fibers go from the pretectum to both Edinger-Westphal nuclei by way of the posterior commissure and to both ciliary ganglia by way of the oculomotor nerves. Postganglionic parasympathetic fibers to the constrictor muscles are activated, and the sympathetic nerves of the dilator muscle are inhibited. The interaction between these components of the autonomic nervous system can be used to localize a lesion in the reflex pathways.

The **accommodation reflex** involves pathways from the visual cortex in the occipital lobe to the pretectum. From here, fibers to all nuclei of nerves III, IV, and VI cause vergence of the extraocular

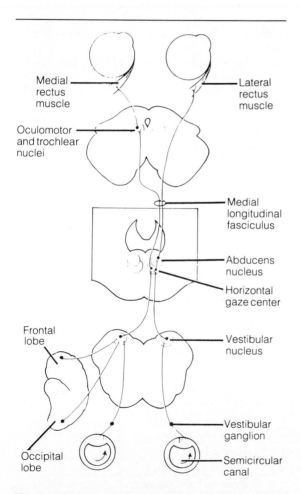

Medial rectus muscle

Lateral rectus muscle

Oculomotor and trochlear nuclei

Medial longitudinal fasciculus

Abducens nucleus

Horizontal gaze center

Frontal lobe

Vestibular nucleus

Occipital lobe

Vestibular ganglion

Semicircular canal

Figure 7-7. Conjugate right gaze. The impulses for voluntary conjugate movements in right lateral gaze are initiated in the left frontal lobe. Involuntary conjugate movements in right lateral gaze are initiated in the occipital lobes.

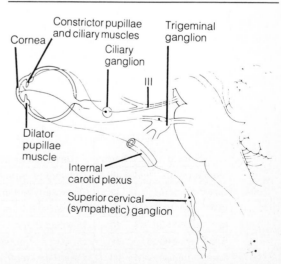

Cornea

Constrictor pupillae and ciliary muscles

Ciliary ganglion

Trigeminal ganglion

III

Dilator pupillae muscle

Internal carotid plexus

Superior cervical (sympathetic) ganglion

Figure 7-8. Innervation of the eye.

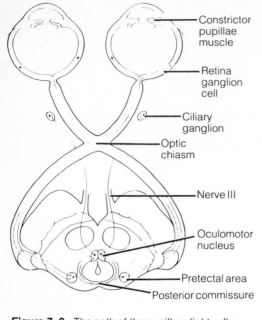

Figure 7-9. The path of the pupillary light reflex.

Labels in figure:
- Constrictor pupillae muscle
- Retina ganglion cell
- Ciliary ganglion
- Optic chiasm
- Nerve III
- Oculomotor nucleus
- Pretectal area
- Posterior commissure

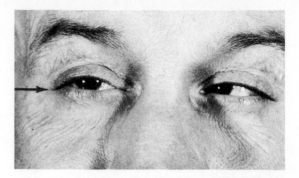

Figure 7-10. Right abducens paralysis. Right eye fails to abduct on lateral gaze.

muscles as well as parasympathetic activation of the constrictor and ciliary muscles within each eye.

D. Clinical correlations for Nerves III, IV, and VI:

1. Symptoms and signs-Clinical findings include strabismus, diplopia, and ptosis. **Strabismus (squint)** is the deviation of one or both eyes. In internal strabismus, the visual axes cross each other; in external strabismus, the visual axes diverge from each other. **Diplopia (double vision)** is a subjective phenomenon reported to be present when the patient is—usually—looking with both eyes; it is caused by misalignment of the visual axes. **Ptosis (lid drop)** is caused by weakness or paralysis of the levator palpebrae superioris muscle; it is sometimes seen in patients with myasthenia gravis.

2. Classification of ophthalmoplegias-Le-

sions that cause ophthalmoplegia (paralysis) of nerves III, IV, and V may be acute, chronic, or progressive; they may also be central or peripheral (Table 7-5).

a. Oculomotor (nerve III) paralysis. External ophthalmoplegia is characterized by divergent strabismus, diplopia, and ptosis. Internal ophthalmoplegia is characterized by dilated pupils and loss of light and accommodation reflexes. There may be paralysis of individual muscles of nerve III, as shown in Table 7-5.

b. Trochlear (nerve IV) paralysis. This rare condition is characterized by slight convergent strabismus and diplopia on looking downward. The patient cannot look downward and inward and hence has difficulty in descending stairs. The head is tilted as a compensatory adjustment; this may be the first indication of a trochlear lesion.

c. Abducens (nerve VI) paralysis. This eye palsy is the most common, owing to the long course of nerve VI. Features of abducens paralysis include convergent strabismus and diplopia (Fig 7-10).

Cranial Nerve V: Trigeminal Nerve

A. Anatomy: The trigeminal nerve, shown in

Table 7-5. Paralyses of individual eye muscles.*

Muscle	Nerve	Deviation of Eyeball	Diplopia Present When Looking*	Direction of Image
Medial rectus	III	Outward (external squint)	Toward nose	Vertical
Superior rectus	III	Downward and inward	Upward and outward	Oblique
Inferior rectus	III	Upward and inward	Downward and outward	Oblique
Inferior oblique	III	Downward and outward	Upward and inward	Oblique
Superior oblique	IV	Upward and outward	Downward and inward	Oblique
Lateral rectus	VI	Inward (internal squint)	Toward temple	Vertical

*Diplopia is noted only when the affected eye attempts these movements.

Fig 7–11, contains a large sensory root, which carries sensation from the skin and mucosa of most of the head, and a smaller motor root, which innervates most of the chewing muscles and the tensor tympani muscle of the middle ear. The efferent fibers of the nerve (the minor portion) originate in the motor nucleus in the pons; this cell group receives bilateral input from the corticobulbar tracts and reflex connections from the spinal tract of nerve V. The sensory root (the main portion of the nerve) arises from cells in the semilunar ganglion (also known as the gasserian or trigeminal ganglion) in a pocket of dura (Meckel's cave) lateral to the cavernous sinus. It passes posteriorly between the superior petrosal sinus in the tentorium and the skull base and enters the pons. Fibers of the **ophthalmic division** enter the cranial cavity through the superior orbital fissure. Fibers of the **maxillary division** pass through the foramen rotundum. Sensory fibers of the **mandibular division,** joined by

the motor fibers involved in mastication, course through the foramen ovale. Touch pathways pass from the nerve's main sensory nucleus to the thalamus and higher centers through its dorsal secondary tract. Pain and temperature pathways pass from the spinal tract and nucleus to the thalamus via the ventral secondary tract. The reflex connections pass to the cerebellum and the motor nuclei of cranial nerves V, VII, and IX. The sensory distribution of the divisions of the face is shown in Fig 7–12.

B. Clinical Correlations: Symptoms and signs of nerve V involvement include loss of sensation of one or more sensory modalities of the nerve; impaired hearing from paralysis of the tensor tympani muscle; paralysis of the muscles of mastication, with deviation of the mandible to the affected side; loss of reflexes (cornea, jaw jerk, sneeze); trismus (lockjaw); and, in some disorders, tonic spasm of the muscles of mastication.

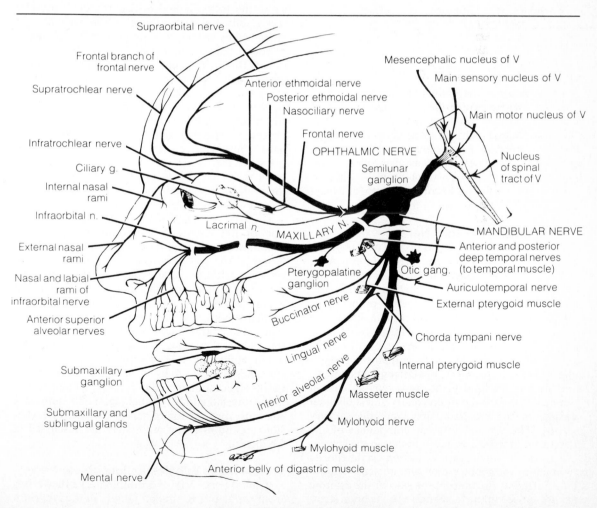

Figure 7–11. The trigeminal nerve.

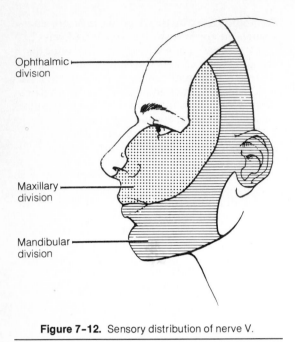

Ophthalmic
division

Maxillary
division

Mandibular
division

Figure 7–12. Sensory distribution of nerve V.

Tic douloureux (trigeminal neuralgia) is characterized by severe pain in the distribution of one or more branches of the trigeminal nerve. Excruciating paroxysmal pain of short duration can be caused by pressure from a small vessel on the root entry zone of the nerve. It may also follow irritation of the trigger zone, a point on the lip, face, or tongue that is sensitive to cold, pressure, or a blast of air. Involvement is usually unilateral.

Cranial Nerve VII: Facial Nerve
A. Anatomy: The facial nerve consists of the **facial nerve proper** and the **nervus intermedius.** Both parts pass through the internal auditory meatus, where the geniculate ganglion for the taste component lies. The facial nerve proper exits through the stylomastoid foramen; it innervates the muscles of facial expression, the platysma muscle, and the stapedius muscle in the inner ear. The nervus intermedius sends parasympathetic preganglionic fibers to the **pterygopalatine ganglion** to innervate the lacrimal gland and, via the chorda tympani nerve, to the submaxillary and sublingual ganglia in the mouth to innervate the salivary glands. The visceral afferent component of the nervus intermedius, with cell bodies in the geniculate ganglion, carries taste sensation via the chorda tympani to the solitary tract and nucleus. The somatic afferent fibers from the skin of the external ear are carried in the facial nerve to the brain stem. These fibers connect there to the trigeminal nuclei and are, in fact, part of the trigeminal sensory system.

The superior salivatory nucleus receives cortical impulses from the nucleus of the solitary tract via the dorsal longitudinal fasciculus and reflex connections.

The taste fibers are connected with the cerebral cortex through the medial lemnisci and thalamus and with the salivatory nucleus and motor nucleus of VII by reflex neurons. The cortical taste area is located in the inferior central (face) region; it extends onto the opercular surface of the parietal lobe and adjacent insular cortex.

B. Clinical Correlations: The facial nucleus receives crossed and uncrossed fibers by way of the corticobulbar (corticonuclear) tract (see Fig 6–10). The facial muscles below the forehead receive contralateral cortical innervation (crossed corticobulbar fibers only). Therefore, a lesion rostral to the facial nucleus—a central facial lesion—results in paralysis of the contralateral facial muscles except the frontalis and orbicularis oculi muscles. Because the frontalis and orbicularis oculi muscles receive bilateral cortical innervation, they are not paralyzed by lesions involving one motor cortex or its corticobulbar pathways. The complete destruction of the facial nucleus itself or its branchial efferent fibers (facial nerve proper) paralyzes all ipsilateral face muscles; this is equivalent to a peripheral facial lesion. Chilling of the face, middle ear infections, or less commonly encountered disorders can cause **peripheral facial paralysis (Bell's palsy).** Seventy-five percent of all facial nerve lesions are forms of palsy, and the condition can occur at any age. When an attempt is made to close the eyelids, the eyeball on the affected side may turn upward (Bell's phenomenon; see Fig 7–14).

The symptoms and signs depend upon the location of the lesion. A lesion in or outside the stylomastoid foramen results in a flaccid paralysis (lower motor neuron type) of all the muscles of facial expression in the affected side; this can occur from a stab wound or from swelling of the parotid gland (eg, as seen in mumps). A lesion in the facial canal involving the chorda tympani nerve results in reduced salivation and loss of taste sensation from the ipsilateral anterior two-thirds of the tongue. A lesion higher up in the canal can paralyze the stapedius muscle. A lesion in the middle ear involves all components of nerve VII, while a tumor in the internal auditory canal (eg, a Schwannoma) can cause dysfunction of nerves VII and VIII. (Lesions in and near the brain stem are discussed in Chapter 6).

Cranial Nerve VIII: Vestibulocochlear Nerve
Cranial nerve VIII is a double nerve that arises from spiral and vestibular ganglia in the labyrinth of the inner ear (Fig 7–15). It passes into the cranial

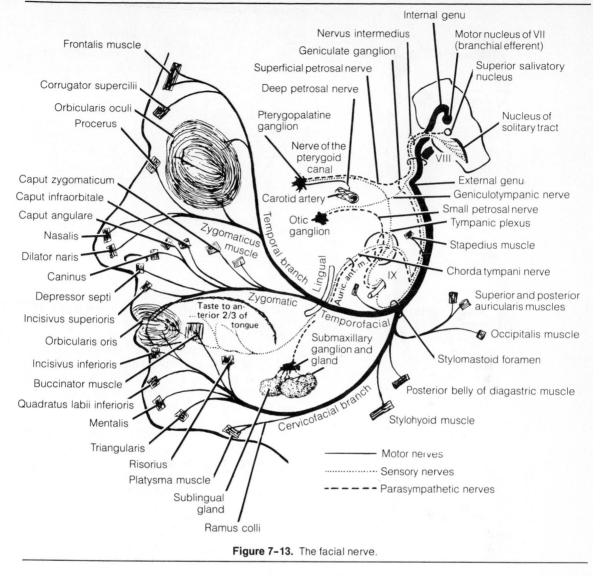

Figure 7–13. The facial nerve.

cavity via the internal acoustic meatus and enters the brain stem behind the posterior edge of the middle cerebellar peduncle in the pontocerebellar angle. The cochlear nerve is concerned with hearing (audition); the vestibular nerve is part of the system of equilibrium (position sense). The functional anatomy of the auditory system (and its clinical correlations) is discussed in Chapter 15; the vestibular system and its clinical correlations are discussed in Chapter 16.

Cranial Nerve IX: Glossopharyngeal Nerve

A. Anatomy: Cranial nerve IX contains several types of fibers (Fig 7–16). Branchial efferent fibers from the **ambiguous nucleus** pass to the stylopharyngeus muscle.

Visceral efferent (parasympathetic pregangli-

onic) fibers from the **inferior salivatory nucleus** pass through the tympanic plexus and lesser petrosal nerve to the **otic ganglion,** from which the postganglionic fibers pass to the **parotid gland.** The inferior salivatory nucleus receives cortical impulses via the dorsal longitudinal fasciculus and reflexes from the nucleus of the solitary tract.

Visceral afferent fibers arise from unipolar cells in the **inferior** (formerly **petrosal**) **ganglia.** Centrally, they terminate in the solitary tract and its nucleus. Peripherally, they supply general sensation to the pharynx, soft palate, posterior third of the tongue, fauces, tonsils, auditory tube, and tympanic cavity. Through the sinus nerve, they supply special receptors in the **carotid body** and **carotid sinus** that are concerned with reflex control of respiration, blood pressure, and heart rate. Spe-

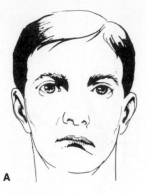

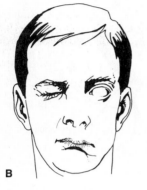

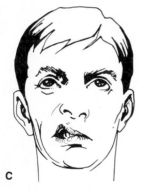

Figure 7–14. Bell's palsy. *A:* In repose. *B:* Patient after being asked to close his eyes. *C:* Patient after being asked to show his teeth.

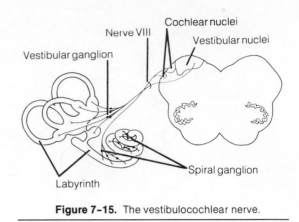

Figure 7–15. The vestibulocochlear nerve.

cial visceral afferents supply the taste buds of the posterior third of the tongue and carry impulses via the **superior ganglia** to the gustatory nucleus of the brain stem. A few somatic afferent fibers enter by way of the glossopharyngeal nerve and end in the trigeminal nuclei. The tongue receives its sensory innervation through multiple pathways: 3 cranial

nerves contain taste fibers, and the general sensory afferent fibers are mediated by nerve V (Fig 7–17); the pathway for taste sensation is shown in Fig 7–18.

B. Clinical Correlations: The glossopharyngeal nerve is rarely involved alone (eg, by neuralgia); it is generally involved with the vagus and accessory nerves. The **pharyngeal (gag) reflex** depends on nerve IX for its sensory component, while nerve X innervates the motor component. Stroking the affected side of the pharynx does not produce gagging if the nerve is injured. The **carotid sinus reflex** depends on nerve IX for its sensory component. Pressure over the sinus normally produces slowing of the heart rate and a fall in blood pressure.

Cranial Nerve X: Vagus Nerve

A. Anatomy: Branchial efferent fibers from the ambiguous nucleus contribute rootlets to the vagus nerve and the cranial component of the accessory nerve (XI). Those of the vagus nerve pass to the muscles of the soft palate and pharynx (Fig 7–19). Those of the accessory nerve join the vagus outside the skull and pass, via the recurrent laryngeal nerve, to the intrinsic muscles of the larynx.

Visceral efferent fibers from the **dorsal motor nucleus** of the vagus course to the thoracic and abdominal viscera. Their postganglionic fibers arise in the terminal ganglia within or near the viscera. They inhibit heart rate and adrenal secretion and stimulate gastrointestinal peristalsis and gastric, hepatic, and pancreatic glandular activity (see Chapter 19).

Somatic afferent fibers of unipolar cells in the **superior** (formerly **jugular) ganglion** send peripheral branches via the auricular branch of nerve X to the external auditory meatus and part of the earlobe. They also send peripheral branches via the recurrent meningeal branch to the dura of the pos-

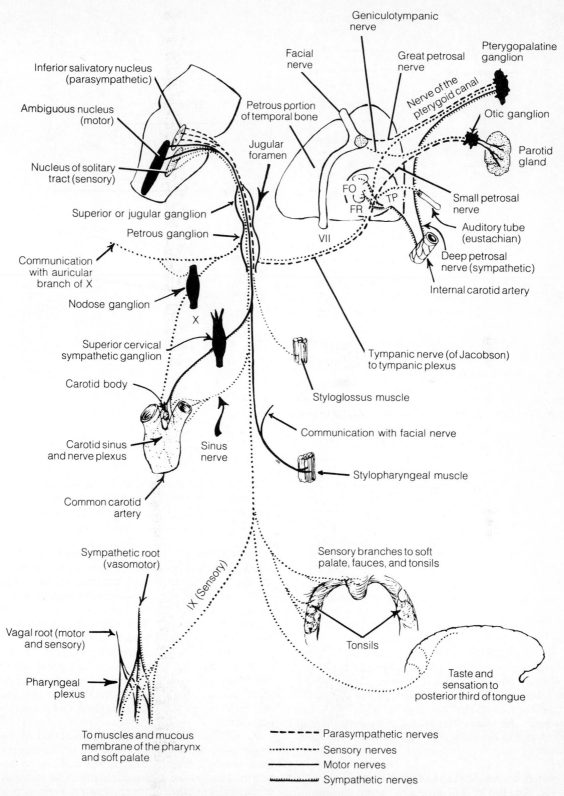

Inferior salivatory nucleus (parasympathetic)

Ambiguous nucleus (motor)

Nucleus of solitary tract (sensory)

Geniculotympanic nerve

Facial nerve

Great petrosal nerve

Pterygopalatine ganglion

Petrous portion of temporal bone

Nerve of the Pterygoid canal

Otic ganglion

Parotid gland

Jugular foramen

Superior or jugular ganglion

Petrous ganglion

FO

FR

TP

VII

Small petrosal nerve

Auditory tube (eustachian)

Deep petrosal nerve (sympathetic)

Internal carotid artery

Communication with auricular branch of X

Nodose ganglion

X

Superior cervical sympathetic ganglion

Carotid body

Carotid sinus and nerve plexus

Sinus nerve

Common carotid artery

Tympanic nerve (of Jacobson) to tympanic plexus

Styloglossus muscle

Communication with facial nerve

Stylopharyngeal muscle

Sympathetic root (vasomotor)

IX (Sensory)

Sensory branches to soft palate, fauces, and tonsils

Vagal root (motor and sensory)

Pharyngeal plexus

Tonsils

Taste and sensation to posterior third of tongue

To muscles and mucous membrane of the pharynx and soft palate

– – – – – Parasympathetic nerves

· · · · · · · Sensory nerves

———— Motor nerves

Sympathetic nerves

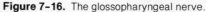

Figure 7–16. The glossopharyngeal nerve.

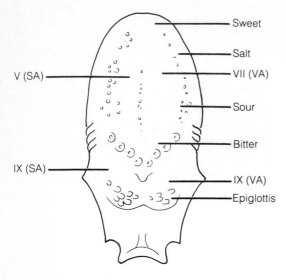

Figure 7-17. Sensory innervation of the tongue.

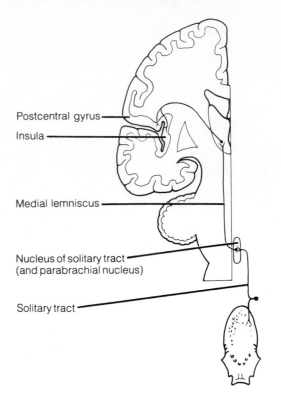

Figure 7-18. Diagram of taste pathways.

terior fossa. Central branches pass with nerve X to the brain stem and end in the spinal tract of the trigeminal nerve and its nucleus.

Visceral afferent fibers of unipolar cells in the **inferior** (formerly **nodose) ganglion** send peripheral branches to the pharynx, larynx, trachea, esophagus, and the thoracic and abdominal viscera. They also send a few special afferent fibers to taste buds in the epiglottic region. Central branches run to the solitary tract and terminate in its nucleus. The visceral afferent fibers of the vagus nerve carry the sensations of abdominal distention and nausea and the impulses concerned with regulating the depth of respiration and controlling blood pressure. A few special visceral afferent fibers for taste from the epiglottis pass via the inferior ganglion to the gustatory nucleus of the brain stem.

The ambiguous nucleus receives cortical connections from the corticobulbar tract and reflex connections from the extrapyramidal and tectobulbar tracts and the nucleus of the solitary tract.

B. Clinical Correlations: Lesions of the vagus nerve may be intramedullary or peripheral. Vagus nerve lesions near the skull base often involve the glossopharyngeal and accessory nerves and sometimes the hypoglossal nerve as well (Fig 7–20). Lesions in the vagus branches can cause unilateral weakness of the palate and shortening of the vocal cords.

Cranial Nerve XI: Accessory Nerve

A. Anatomy: The accessory nerve consists of 2 separate components: the cranial component and the spinal component (Fig 7–21).

In the cranial component, branchial efferent fibers (from the ambiguous nucleus to the intrinsic muscles of the larynx) join the accessory nerve inside the skull, but are part of the vagus outside the skull.

In the spinal component, the branchial efferent fibers from the lateral part of the anterior horns of the first 5 or 6 cervical cord segments ascend as the spinal root of the accessory nerve through the foramen magnum and leave the cranial cavity through the jugular foramen. These fibers supply the sternocleidomastoid muscle and partly supply the trapezius muscle. The central connections of the spinal component are those of the typical lower motor neuron: voluntary impulses via the corticospinal tracts, postural impulses via the basal ganglia, and reflexes via the vestibulospinal and tectospinal tracts.

B. Clinical Correlations: Interruption of the spinal component leads to paralysis of the sternocleidomastoid muscle, causing the inability to rotate the head to the contralateral side, and paralysis of the upper portion of the trapezius muscle, which is characterized by a winglike scapula and the inability to shrug the ipsilateral shoulder.

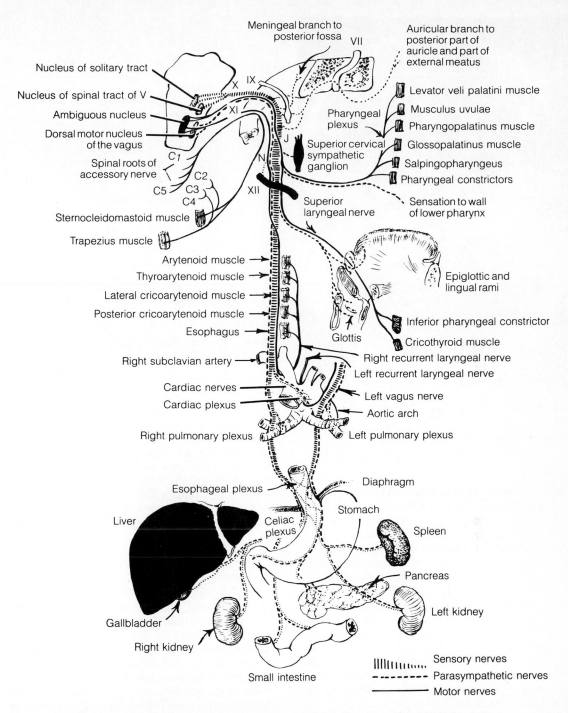

Meningeal branch to posterior fossa VII

Auricular branch to posterior part of auricle and part of external meatus

Nucleus of solitary tract

Nucleus of spinal tract of V

Ambiguous nucleus

Dorsal motor nucleus of the vagus

Spinal roots of accessory nerve

Sternocleidomastoid muscle

Trapezius muscle

Arytenoid muscle

Thyroarytenoid muscle

Lateral cricoarytenoid muscle

Posterior cricoarytenoid muscle

Esophagus

Right subclavian artery

Cardiac nerves

Cardiac plexus

Right pulmonary plexus

Esophageal plexus

Liver

Gallbladder

Right kidney

Small intestine

X IX

XI

C1

C2
C3
C4
C5

XII

Pharyngeal plexus

Superior cervical sympathetic ganglion

J

N

Levator veli palatini muscle

Musculus uvulae

Pharyngopalatinus muscle

Glossopalatinus muscle

Salpingopharyngeus

Pharyngeal constrictors

Sensation to wall of lower pharynx

Superior laryngeal nerve

Epiglottic and lingual rami

Inferior pharyngeal constrictor

Cricothyroid muscle

Glottis

Right recurrent laryngeal nerve

Left recurrent laryngeal nerve

Left vagus nerve

Aortic arch

Left pulmonary plexus

Diaphragm

Stomach

Celiac plexus

Spleen

Pancreas

Left kidney

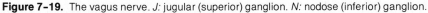

|||||||||||...... Sensory nerves

--------- Parasympathetic nerves

————— Motor nerves

Figure 7–19. The vagus nerve. *J:* jugular (superior) ganglion. *N:* nodose (inferior) ganglion.

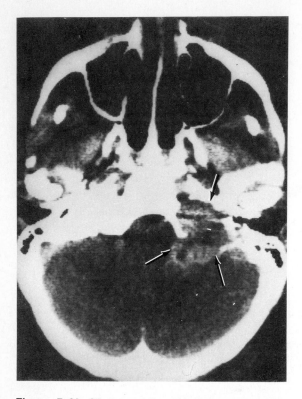

Figure 7–20. CT image through horizontal section through the head at the level of the posterior fossa. A large mass (arrows) has eroded the left jugular foramen.

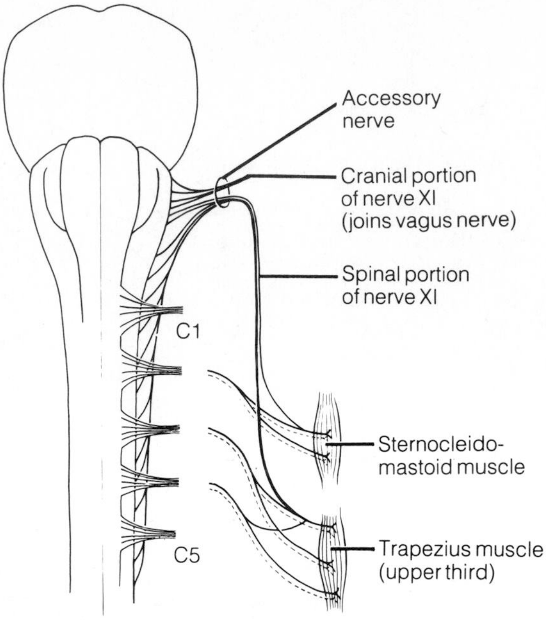

Figure 7–21. Schematic illustration of the accessory nerve, viewed from below.

Labels in Figure 7-21:
Accessory nerve
Cranial portion of nerve XI (joins vagus nerve)
Spinal portion of nerve XI
C1
Sternocleido-mastoid muscle
C5
Trapezius muscle (upper third)

Cranial Nerve XII: Hypoglossal Nerve

A. Anatomy: Somatic efferent fibers from the **hypoglossal nucleus** in the ventromedian portion of the gray matter of the medulla emerge between the pyramid and the olive to form the hypoglossal nerve (Fig 7–22). The nerve leaves the skull through the hypoglossal canal and passes to the muscles of the tongue. A few proprioceptive fibers from the tongue course in the hypoglossal nerve and end in the trigeminal nuclei of the brain stem. The hypoglossal nerve distributes motor branches to the geniohyoid and infrahyoid muscles with fibers derived from communicating branches of the first cervical nerve. A sensory recurrent meningeal branch of the nerve XII innervates the dura of the posterior fossa of the skull.

Central connections of the hypoglossal nucleus include the corticobulbar (corticonuclear) motor system (with crossed fibers, as shown in Fig 6–10), as well as reflex neurons from the sensory nuclei of the trigeminal nerve and the nucleus of the solitary tract (not shown).

B. Clinical Correlations: Peripheral lesions that affect the hypoglossal nerve usually come from mechanical causes (Fig 7–23). Nuclear and supranuclear lesions can have many causes (eg, tumors, bleeding, demyelination).

Lesions of the medulla produce characteristic symptoms that are related to the involvement of the nuclei of the last 4 cranial nerves that lie within the medulla and the motor and sensory pathways through it. Extramedullary lesions of the posterior fossa may involve the roots of the last 4 cranial nerves between their emergence from the medulla and their exit from the skull.

CASE 8

A 24-year-old medical student noticed while shaving one morning that he was unable to move the left side of his face. He worried that a serious problem, possibly a stroke, might have occurred. He had suffered from influenzalike symptoms the day before this sudden attack.

Neurologic examination showed that the patient could not wrinkle his forehead on the left side; neither could he show his teeth or purse his lips on that side. Taste sensation was abnormal in the left anterior two-thirds of the tongue, and he had trouble closing his left eye. A test to determine tear secretion showed that secretion on the right side was normal, but the left lacrimal gland produced little fluid. Loud noises caused discomfort in the patient, who was in good health otherwise, and there were no additional signs or symptoms.

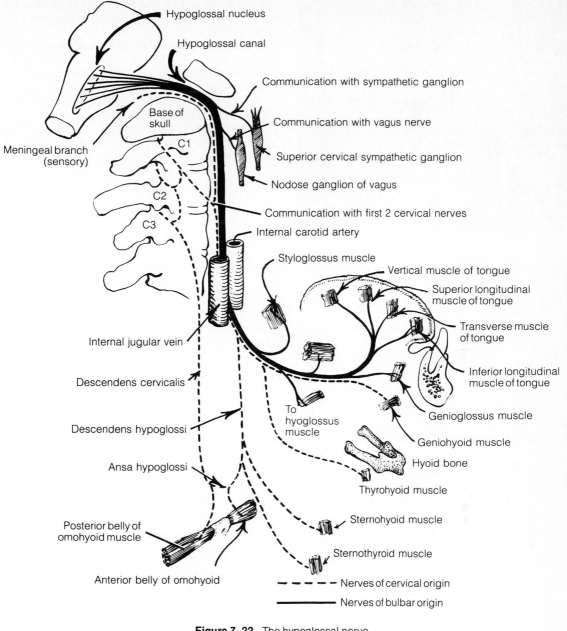

Figure 7–22. The hypoglossal nerve.

What is the differential diagnosis? What is the most likely diagnosis?

CASE 9

A 56-year-old mailman complained of attacks of severe stabbing pains in the right side of the face.

These pain attacks had started to appear about 6 months earlier and had lately seemed to come more often. The pain would occur several times a day, lasting only a few seconds. He was unable to shave, since touching his right cheek would trigger an excruciating pain (he now had a full beard). On windy days the attacks seemed to occur more frequently. Sometimes drinking or eating would trig-

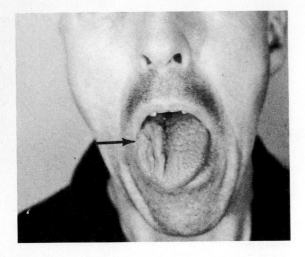

Figure 7-23. Right hypoglossal paralysis. Atrophy of the right side of the tongue and deviation of the tongue to the right occurred 2 months (after surgical section the right hypoglossal nerve.)

ger the pain, and he had lost weight recently. He had seen a dentist who had not found any tooth-related problems.

The neurologic examination was almost entirely normal; however, when testing his face for touch and pain sensibility, a pain attack was set off each time his right cheek was touched.

What is the most likely diagnosis? Would a radiologic examination be useful?

Cases are discussed further in Chapter 24. Tests designed to determine the function of cranial nerves are described in Appendix A.

REFERENCES

Bannister R: *Brain's Clinical Neurology,* 6th ed. Oxford Univ Press, 1984.

Bender MB: Brain control of conjugate horizontal and vertical eye movements. *Brain* 1980;**103:**23.

Samii M, Jannetta PJ, (editors): *The Cranial Nerves.* Springer-Verlag, 1981.

Diencephalon

8

The diencephalon, which is part of the cerebrum, includes the thalamus and its geniculate bodies, the hypothalamus, the subthalamus, and the epithalamus (Fig 8-1). The third ventricle lies between the halves of the diencephalon. A small groove on the lateral wall of the slim third ventricle—the hypothalamic sulcus—separates the thalamus and epithalamus dorsally and the hypothalamus and subthalamus inferiorly. The development of the diencephalon is mentioned briefly in Chapter 9 (Figs 9-1, 9-3, and 9-4).

THALAMUS

Landmarks

Each half of the brain contains a thalamus (**dorsal thalamus**), a large, ovoid, gray mass of nuclei. Its broad posterior end, the **pulvinar,** extends over the medial and lateral **geniculate bodies** (Fig 8-2). The narrower rostral end of the thalamus contains the **anterior thalamic tubercle.** In many individuals there is a short **interthalamic adhesion (massa intermedia)** between the thalami, across the narrow third ventricle (see Fig 8-1); this adhesion has no functional significance.

White Matter

The **thalamic radiations** are the fiber bundles that emerge from the lateral surface of the thalamus and terminate in the cerebral cortex. The **external medullary lamina** is a layer of myelinated fibers on the lateral surface of the thalamus close to the internal capsule. The **internal medullary lamina** (Fig 8-3) is a vertical sheet of white matter that bifurcates in its anterior portion and thus divides the gray matter of the thalamus into lateral, medial, and anterior portions.

Thalamic Nuclei

There are 5 groups of thalamic nuclei, each with specific fiber connections (Figs 8-3, 8-4, and 8-5).

A. Anterior Nuclear Group: This group forms the anterior tubercle of the thalamus and is bordered by the limbs of the internal lamina. It receives fibers from the mamillary bodies via the mamillothalamic tract and projects to the cingulate cortex of the cerebrum.

B. Nuclei of the Midline: These groups of cells are located just beneath the lining of the third ventricle and in the interthalamic adhesion. They connect with the hypothalamus and central periaqueductal gray matter. The **centromedian nucleus** connects with the cerebellum and corpus striatum.

C. Medial Nuclei: These include most of the gray substance medial to the internal medullary lamina: the **intralaminar nuclei** as well as the **dorsomedial nucleus,** which projects to the frontal cortex.

D. Lateral Nuclear Mass: This constitutes a large part of the thalamus anterior to the pulvinar between the internal and external medullary laminas. The mass includes a **reticular nucleus** between the external medullary lamina and the internal capsule; an **anteroventral nucleus (ventralis anterior [VA]),** which connects with the corpus striatum; a **lateroventral nucleus (ventralis lateralis [VL]),** which projects to the cerebral motor cortex; a **dorsolateral nucleus,** which projects to the parietal lobe cortex; and a **posteroventral (ventralis basalis)** group, which ends in the postcentral gyrus and receives fibers from the medial lemniscus and the spinothalamic and trigeminal tracts. The posteroventral group is divided into the **posterolateral (PVL) nucleus,** which relays sensory input from the body, and the **posteromedial (PVM) nucleus,** which relays sensory input from the face. The posteroventral nuclei project information via the internal capsule to the sensory cortex of the cerebral hemisphere (see Chapter 9).

E. Posterior Nuclei: These include the pulvinar nucleus, the medial geniculate nucleus, and the

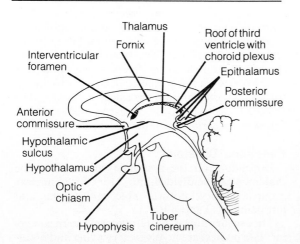

Figure 8-1. Midsagittal section through the diencephalon.

Thalamus

Fornix

Roof of third ventricle with choroid plexus

Interventricular foramen

Epithalamus

Posterior commissure

Anterior commissure

Hypothalamic sulcus

Hypothalamus

Optic chiasm

Tuber cinereum

Hypophysis

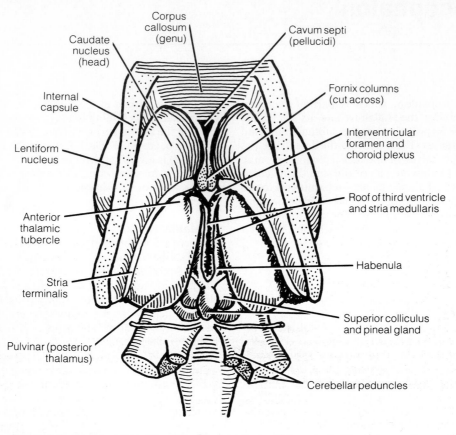

Figure 8-2. Dorsal aspect of the diencephalon after partial removal of the corpus callosum.

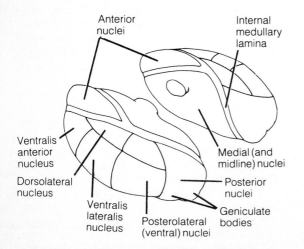

Figure 8-3. Diagrams of the thalamus. Oblique lateral and medial views. (Modified, after Netter.)

lateral geniculate nucleus. The **pulvinar nucleus** is a large posterior nuclear group that connects with the parietal and temporal lobe cortices. The **medial geniculate nucleus,** which lies lateral to the midbrain under the pulvinar, receives acoustic fibers from the lateral lemniscus and inferior colliculus. It projects fibers via the acoustic radiation to the temporal lobe cortex. The **lateral geniculate nucleus** receives most of the fibers of the optic tract and projects via the geniculocalcarine radiation to the visual cortex around the calcarine fissure. The geniculate nuclei or bodies appear as oval elevations below the posterior end of the thalamus (Fig 8–2).

Functional Divisions

Depending on the anatomic connections, the thalamus can be divided into 5 functional nuclear groups: sensory, motor, limbic, multimodal, and intralaminar (Table 8–1).

The **sensory nuclei** (posteroventral group and geniculate bodies) are involved in relaying and modifying sensory signals from the body, face, retina, cochlea, and taste receptors (see also Chapter 13). The thalamus (rather than the sensory cortex) is

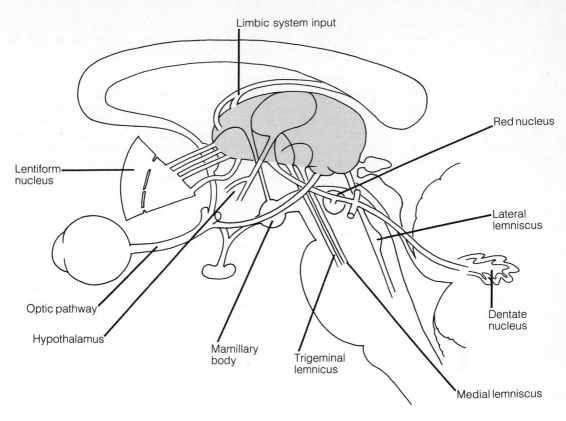

Limbic system input

Red nucleus

Lentiform
nucleus

Lateral
lemniscus

Optic pathway

Hypothalamus

Dentate
nucleus

Mamillary
body

Trigeminal
lemnicus

Medial lemniscus

Figure 8-4. Schematic lateral view of the thalamus with afferent fiber systems. (Modified, after JH LaVail.)

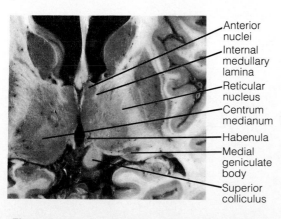

Anterior
nuclei

Internal
medullary
lamina

Reticular
nucleus

Centrum
medianum

Habenula

Medial
geniculate
body

Superior
colliculus

Figure 8-5. Horizontal section through the thalamus.

Table 8-1. Functional divisions of thalamic nuclei.

Type	Nucleus
Sensory	Lateral geniculate Medial geniculate Ventral posterior (posteroventral); medial part Ventral posterior (posteroventral); lateral part
Motor	Ventral anterior Ventral lateral
Limbic	Anterior Dorsomedial
Multimodal	Pulvinar Lateral posterior (postero lateral) Lateral dorsal (dorsolateral)
Intralaminar	Reticular Centrum medianum Intralaminar

thought to be the crucial structure for the perception of some types of sensation, especially pain, and the sensory cortex may function to give finer detail to the sensation.

The thalamic motor nuclei (ventralis anterior and lateralis) convey motor information from the cerebellum and globus pallidus to the precentral motor cortex. The nuclei have also been called motor relay nuclei on the basis of these connections (see also Chapter 12).

There are 3 anterior **limbic nuclei** interposed between the mamillary nuclei of the hypothalamus (see below) and the cingulate gyrus of the cerebral cortex. The dorsomedial nucleus receives input from the olfactory cortex and amygdala regions, and projects reciprocally to the prefrontal cortex and the hypothalamus (see also Chapter 18).

The **multimodal nuclei** (pulvinar, posterolateral and dorsolateral) have connections with the association areas in the parietal lobe (see Chapter 9). Other diencephalic regions may contribute to these connections.

Other, nonspecific thalamic nuclei include the intralaminar and reticular nuclei and the centrum medianum; the projections of these nuclei are not known in detail. Interaction with cortical motor areas, the caudate nucleus, the putamen, and the cerebellum have been demonstrated.

Clinical Correlations

Thalamic syndrome is characterized by immediate hemianesthesia, with the threshold of sensitivity to pinprick, heat, and cold rising later. When a sensation is felt, sometimes referred to as thalamic hyperpathia, it is disagreeable and unpleasant. The syndrome usually appears during recovery from a thalamic infarct.

HYPOTHALAMUS

Landmarks

The hypothalamus lies below and in front of the thalamus; it forms the floor and lower walls of the third ventricle (Fig 8-1). External landmarks of the hypothalamus are the **optic chiasm;** the **tuber cinereum,** with its infundibulum extending to the posterior lobe of the hypophysis; and the **mamillary bodies** lying between the cerebral peduncles (Fig 8-6).

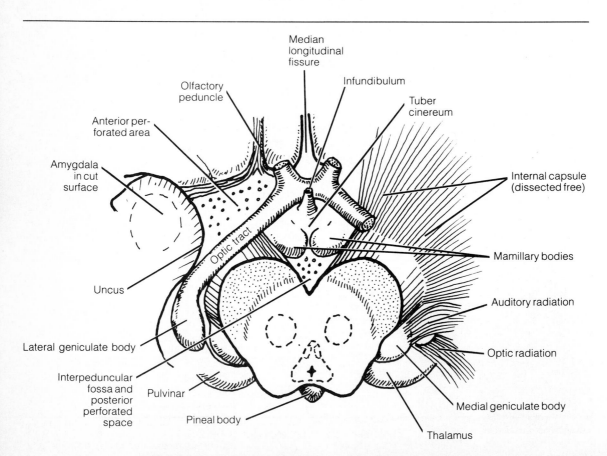

Figure 8-6. Diencephalon from below, with adjacent structures.

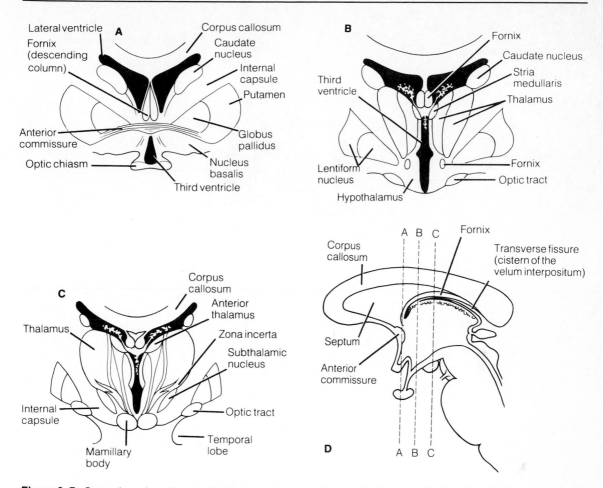

Figure 8–7. Coronal sections through the diencephalon and adjacent structures. *A:* Section through the optic chiasm and the anterior commissure. *B:* Section through the tuber cinereum and the anterior portion of the thalamus. *C:* Section through the mamillary bodies and middle thalamus. *D:* Key to the section levels.

The hypothalamus can be divided into an anterior portion, the chiasmatic region, including the lamina terminalis; the central hypothalamus, including the tuber cinereum and the infundibulum; and the posterior portion, the mamillary area (Fig 8–7).

The right and left sides of the hypothalamus can each be further divided into a medial hypothalamic area that contains many nuclei and a lateral hypothalamic area that contains fiber systems (eg, the medial forebrain bundle) and diffuse lateral nuclei.

Hypothalamic Nuclei

Each half of the medial hypothalamus can be divided into 3 parts (Fig 8–8): the **supraoptic portion,** which is farthest anterior and contains the **supraoptic suprachiasmatic,** and **paraventricular nuclei;** the **tuberal** portion, which lies immediately behind the supraoptic portion and contains the **ventromedial, dorsomedial,** and **arcuate nuclei** in addition to

the median eminence; and the **mamillary** portion. This last part is farthest posterior and contains the **posterior nucleus** and several **mamillary nuclei.** There is also the **preoptic area,** a region that lies anterior to the hypothalamus, between the optic chiasm and the anterior commissure.

Fiber Connections

Afferent connections to the hypothalamus include part of the medial forebrain bundle, which sends fibers to the hypothalamus from nuclei in the **parolfactory area** and **corpus striatum;** thalamohypothalamic fibers from the medial and midline thalamic nuclei; and the fornix, which brings fibers from the hippocampus to the mamillary bodies. These connections also include the **stria terminalis,** which brings fibers from the **amygdala; pallidohypothalamic fibers,** which lead from the **lentiform nucleus** to the **ventromedial hypothalamic nucleus;** and the inferior mamillary pe-

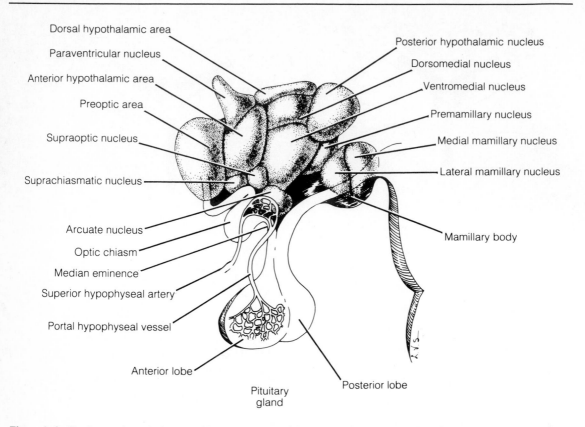

Figure 8-8. The human hypothalamus, with a superimposed diagrammatic representation of the portal-hypophyseal vessels. (Reproduced, with permission, from Ganong WF: *Review of Medical Physiology,* 14th ed. Appleton & Lange, 1989.)

duncle, which sends fibers from the tegmentum of the midbrain. These and other connections are shown in Table 8-2.

Efferent tracts from the hypothalamus include the **hypothalamohypophyseal tract,** which runs from the supraoptic and paraventricular nuclei to the **neurohypophysis;** the **mamillotegmental tract** (part of the medial forebrain bundle) going to the tegmentum; and the **mamillothalamic tract (tract of Vicq d'Azyr),** from the mamillary nuclei to the anterior thalamic nuclei. There are also the **periventricular system,** including the dorsal fasciculus to the lower brain levels; the **tuberohypophyseal tract,** which goes from the tuberal portion of the hypothalamus to the posterior pituitary; and fibers from the septal region, by way of the fornix, to the hippocampus (see Chapter 18).

Functions

Although the hypothalamus is small (it weighs 4 gm—about 0.3% of the total brain weight), the hypothalamic region has important regulatory functions, as outlined in Table 8-3).

A. Eating: A tonically active feeding center in the lateral hypothalamus evokes eating behavior. A satiety center in the ventromedial nucleus stops hunger and inhibits the feeding center when a high blood glucose level is reached after food intake. Damage to the feeding center leads to anorexia (loss of appetite) and severe loss of body weight; lesions of the satiety center lead to hyperphagia (overeating) and obesity.

B. Autonomic Function: Although anatomically discrete centers have not been identified, the posterolateral and dorsomedial areas of the hypothalamus function as a sympathetic (catecholamine) activating region, while an anterior area functions as a parasympathetic activating region. The evidence for this is derived from studying the effects of lesions in humans and animals (see also Chapter 19).

C. Body Temperature: When some regions of the hypothalamus are appropriately stimulated, they evoke autonomic responses that result in loss, conservation, or production of body heat (Table 8-4). A fall in body temperature, for example, causes vasoconstriction, which conserves heat, and shivering, which produces heat. A rise in body temperature results in sweating and cutaneous vasodi-

Table 8-2. Principal pathways to and from the hypothalamus.*

Tract	Type†	Description
Medial forebrain bundle	A, E	Connects limbic lobe and midbrain via lateral hypothalamus, where fibers enter and leave it; includes direct amygdalohypothalamic fibers, which are sometimes referred to as a separate pathway.
Fornix	A, E	Connects hippocampus to hypothalamus; mostly mamillary bodies.
Stria terminalis	A	Connects amygdala to hypothalamus, especially ventromedial region.
Mamillary peduncle	A	Diverges from sensory pathways in midbrain to enter hypothalamus; may be the pathway by which sensory stimuli enter.
Ventral noradrenergic bundle	A	Axons of noradrenergic neurons projecting from nucleus of solitary tract and other hindbrain nuclei to paraventricular nuclei and other parts of hypothalamus.
Dorsal noradrenergic bundle	A	Axons of noradrenergic neurons projecting from locus ceruleus to dorsal hypothalamus.
Serotoinergic neurons	A	Axons of serotonin-secreting neurons projecting from raphe nuclei to hypothalamus.
Adrenergic neurons	A	Axons of epinephrine-secreting neurons from medulla to ventral hypothalamus.
Retinohypothalamic fibers	A	Optic nerve fibers to suprachiasmatic nuclei from optic chiasm.
Periventricular system (including dorsal longitudinal fasciculus of Schütz)	A, E	Interconnects hypothalamus and midbrain; efferent projections to spinal cord, afferent from sensory pathways.
Mamillothalmic tract of Vicq d'Azyr	E	Connects mamillary nuclei to anterior thalamic nuclei.
Mamillotegmental tract	E	Connects hypothalamus with reticular portions of midbrain.
Hypothalamohypophyseal tract (supraopticohypophyseal and paraventriculohypophyseal tracts)	E	Axons of neurons in supraoptic and paraventricular nuclei; end in pituitary stalk and posterior pituitary.

*Modified with permission, from Ganong WF: *Review of Medical Physiology,* 13th ed. Appleton & Lange, 1987.
†A = principally afferent; E = principally efferent.

lation. Normally, the hypothalamic set-point, or thermostat, lies just below 37°C of body temperature. A higher temperature, or fever, is the result of a change in the set-point, eg, by pyrogens in the blood.

D. Water Balance: Hypothalamic influence on vasopressin secretion by the posterior pituitary is activated by osmoreceptors that are stimulated by any increase in blood osmolarity. Pain, stress, and emotional states also stimulate vasopressin secretion. Lack of secretion caused by hypothalamic or pituitary lesions, for example, can result in polyuria (increased urine excretion) and polydipsia (increased thirst).

E. Anterior Pituitary Function: The hypothalamus exerts a direct influence on secretions of the anterior pituitary and an indirect influence on secretions of other endocrine glands by releasing or inhibiting hormones carried by the pituitary portal vessels (Fig 8-9). It thus regulates many endocrine functions, including reproduction, sexual behavior, thyroid and adrenal cortex secretions, and growth.

F. Circadian rhythm: Many body functions (eg, temperature, corticosteroid levels, oxygen consumption) are cyclically influenced by light-intensity changes that have a circadian (day-to-day) rhythm. A retinosuprachiasmatic pathway reacts to changes in light intensity. The suprachiasmatic nucleus itself functions as an independent clock with a period of about 25 hours per cycle; lesions in this nucleus cause the loss of all circadian cycles.

G. Expression of Emotion: The hypothalamus is involved in the expression of rage, fear, aversion, sexual behavior, and pleasure. Patterns of expression and behavior are subject to limbic system influence and, in part, to changes in visceral system function (see Chapters 18 and 19).

Clinical Correlations

Several clinical problems related to dysfunction of the hypothalamus have been discussed in the previous paragraphs (Table 8-5). Lesions in the hypothalamus are most often caused by tumors that arise from either the hypothalamus itself (eg, glioma, hamartoma, germinoma) or adjacent structures (eg, pituitary adenoma, craniopharyngioma, thalamic glioma). Somnolence or even coma may

Table 8-3. Principal hypothalamic regulatory mechanisms.*

Function	Afferents From	Integrating Areas
Temperature regulation	Cutaneous cold receptors; temperature-sensitive cells in hypothalamus	Anterior hypothalamus (response to heat) posterior hypothalamus (response to cold)
Neuroendocrine control of Catecholamines	Emotional stimuli, probably via limbic system	Dorsomedial and posterior hypothalamus
Vasopressin	Osmoreceptors, volume receptors, others	Supraoptic and paraventricular nuclei
Oxytocin	Touch receptors in breast, uterus, genitalia	Supraoptic and paraventricular nuclei
Thyroid-stimulating hormone (thyrotropin, TSH) via thyrotropin-stimulating hormone (TRH)	Temperature receptors, perhaps others	Dorsomedial nuclei and neighboring areas
Adrenocorticotropic hormone (ACTH) and β-lipotropin (β-LPH) via corticortropin-releasing hormone (CRH)	Limbic system (emotional stimuli); reticular formation ("systemic" stimuli); hypothalamic or anterior pituitary cells sensitive to circulating blood cortisol level; suprachiasmatic nuclei (diurnal rhythm)	Paraventricular nuclei
Follicle-stimulating hormone (FSH) and luteinizing hormone (LH) via luteinizing-hormone–releasing hormone (LHRH)	Hypothalamic cells sensitive to estrogens; eyes, touch receptors in skin and genitalia of reflex ovulating species	Preoptic area, other areas
Prolactin via prolactin-inhibiting hormone (PIH) and prolactin-releasing hormone (PRH)	Touch receptors in breasts, other unknown receptors	Arcuate nucleus, other areas (hypothalamus inhibits secretion)
Growth hormone via somatostatin and growth-hormone–releasing hormone (GRH)	Unknown receptors	Periventricular nucleus, arcuate nucleus
"Appetitive" behavior Thirst	Osmoreceptors, subfornical organ	Lateral superior hypothalamus
Hunger	"Glucostat" cells sensitive to rate of glucose utilization	Ventromedial satiety center, lateral hunger center; also limbic components
Sexual behavior	Cells sensitive to circulating estrogen and androgen, others	Anterior ventral hypothalamus plus (in the male) piriform cortex
Defensive reactions Fear, rage	Sense organs and neocortex, paths unknown	In limbic system and hypothalamus
Control of various endocrine and activity rhythms	Retina via retinohypothalamic fibers	Suprachiasmatic nuclei

*Reproduced and modified with permission, from Ganong WF: *Review of Medical Physiology,* 14th ed. Appleton & Lange, 1989.

be the result of bilateral lesions of the lateral hypothalamus and its reticular formation components (see Chapter 17). Even relatively minor destruction in the hypothalamus can cause a considerable loss of function.

SUBTHALAMUS

Landmarks

The subthalamus is the zone of brain tissue that lies between the dorsal thalamus and the tegmentum of the midbrain. The hypothalamus lies medial and rostral to the subthalamus; the internal capsule lies lateral to it (Fig 8-7C). The **subthalamic nucleus,** or **body of Luys,** is a cylindrical mass of gray substance dorsolateral to the upper end of the substantia nigra; it extends posteriorly as far as the lateral aspect of the red nucleus.

Fiber Connections

The subthalamus receives fibers from the globus pallidus; these form part of the efferent descending path from the corpus striatum. Fibers from the

Table 8-4. Temperature-regulating mechanisms.*

Activated by cold:	Result
Shivering	
Hunger	Increased
Increased voluntary activity	heat
Increased secretion of norepinephrine and epinephrine	production
Cutaneous vasoconstriction	Decreased
Curling up	heat
Horripilation	loss
Activated by heat:	
Cutaneous vasodilation	Increased
Sweating	heat
Increased respiration	loss
Anorexia	Decreased
Apathy and inertia	heat production

*Reproduced, with permission, from Ganong WF: *Review of Medical Physiology,* 13th ed. Appleton & Lange, 1987.

Table 8-5. Symptoms and signs in 60 cases of hypothalamic disease.*

	Percentage of Cases
Endocrine and metabolic findings	
Precocious puberty	40
Hypogonadism	32
Diabetes insipidus	35
Obesity	25
Abnormalities of temperature regulation	22
Emaciation	18
Bulimia	8
Anorexia	7
Neurologic findings	
Eye signs	78
Pyramidal and sensory deficits	75
Headache	65
Extrapyramidal signs	62
Vomiting	40
Psychic disturbances, rage attacks, etc	35
Somnolence	30
Convulsions	15

*Data from Bauer HG: Endocrine and other clinical manifestations of hypothalamic disease. *J Clin Endocrinol* 1954;**14**:13. See also Kahana L et al: Endocrine manifestations of intracranial extrasellar lesions. *J Clin Endocrinol* 1962;**22**:304. Table reproduced, with permission, from Ganong WF: *Review of Medical Physiology,* 14th ed. Appleton & Lange, 1989.

globus pallidus also occupy the **fields of Forel,** which lie anterior to the red nucleus and contain cells that may be a rostral extension of reticular nuclei. The ventromedial portion is usually designated as field H, the dorsomedial portion as field H_1, and the ventrolateral portion as field H_2. The **fasciculus lenticularis** (field H_2) runs medially from the globus pallidus and is joined by the **ansa lenticularis,** which bends acutely in field H. The

thalamic fasciculus extends through field H_1 to the anterior ventral nucleus of the thalamus. The **zona incerta** is a thin zone of gray substance above the fasciculus lenticularis. The tracts and nuclear areas of the subthalamus are involved in several functional pathways for sensory, motor, and reticular function (see Chapters 12, 13, and 17).

Clinical Correlations

Lesions in the subthalamic nucleus usually result in hemiballismus, a motor disorder that affects one side of the body. (In rare cases, the lesions cause ballismus, affecting both sides.) Intermittent flailing of the affected extremities may lead to severe trauma or fractures; muscle-relaxant drugs may give temporary relief.

EPITHALAMUS

The epithalamus consists of the habenular trigones on each side of the third ventricle, the pineal body (pineal gland, or epiphysis cerebri), and the habenular commissure (Fig 8-1).

Habenular Trigone

The habenular trigone is a small triangular area in front of the superior colliculus. It contains the **habenular nuclei,** which receive fibers from the stria medullaris thalami and are joined via the

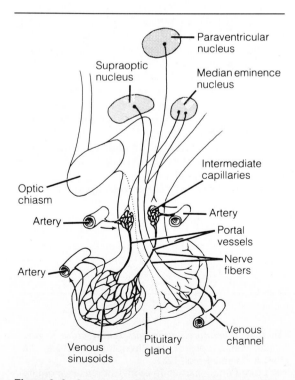

Figure 8-9. Schematic view of the pituitary portal system of vessels and neurohypophyseal pathways.

Paraventricular nucleus

Supraoptic nucleus

Median eminence nucleus

Optic chiasm

Artery

Artery

Intermediate capillaries

Artery

Portal vessels

Nerve fibers

Venous channel

Venous sinusoids

Pituitary gland

habenular commissure. The **habenulopeduncular tract** extends from the habenular nucleus to the interpeduncular nucleus in the midbrain. The function of these structures in humans is not known.

Pineal Body

The pineal body is a small mass that normally lies in the depression between the superior colliculi (Figs 8–1 and 8–10). Its base is attached by the pineal stalk. The ventral lamina of the stalk is continuous with the posterior commissure and the dorsal lamina with the habenular commissure. At their proximal ends, the laminas of the stalk are separated, forming the pineal recess of the third ventricle. The pineal body is said to secrete hormones that are absorbed into its blood vessels.

Clinical Correlations

A tumor in the pineal region may obstruct the cerebral aqueduct or cause inability to move the eyes in the vertical plane (Parinaud's syndrome). One type of tumor (germinoma) produces precocious sexual development, and interruption of the posterior commissure abolishes the consensual light reflex.

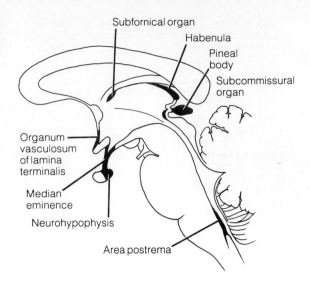

Figure 8–10. Location of the circumventricular organs. There is no blood-brain barrier in these organs (see Chapter 10).

CIRCUMVENTRICULAR ORGANS

Several small areas (Fig 8–10) in or near the wall of the third ventricle, the aqueduct, and the fourth ventricle may be of functional importance with regard to cerebrospinal fluid composition, hormone secretion into the ventricles, and the maintenance of normal cerebrospinal fluid pressure. Most of the research has been performed in experimental animals. The functions of the habenula, the pineal body, and the pituitary gland in humans have been discussed above.

CASE 10

A 21-year-old mailman was referred to neurology service for an evaluation of severe headaches, from which he said he had been suffering for 6 months. He reported that the pain was not constant but had become more pronounced during the past month, and he felt that his eyesight had deteriorated in the past few weeks. He also stated that he now often felt cold, even in warm weather.

Neurologic examination showed partial (incomplete) bitemporal hemianopia. There was no clear papilledema, but the disks had become flattened and slightly pale. The patient had indicated that he was sexually inactive; further examination showed underdeveloped testes and the absence of pubic and axillary hair.

What is the differential diagnosis? Which neuroradiologic procedures are needed? What is the most likely diagnosis?

Cases are discussed further in Chapter 24.

REFERENCES

Ganong WF: Brain mechanisms regulating the secretions of the pituitary gland. Pages 549–564 in: *The Neurosciences.* Schmitt FO, Worden FG (editors). MIT Press, 1974.

Ganten D, Pfaff D (editors): *Morphology of Hypothalamus and its Connections.* Springer Verlag, 1980.

Hensel H: *Thermoreception and Temperature Regulation.* Monographs of the Physiological Society. No 38. Academic Press, 1981.

Jones EG: Functional subdivisions and synaptic organization of the mammalian thalamus. *Int Rev Physiol* 1981;**25**:173.

Meijer JH, Rietveld WJ: Neurophysiology of the supra-chiasmatic circadian pacemaker in rodents. *Physiol Rev* 1989, Vol 89.

Morgan PJ, Panksepp J (editors): *Handbook of the Hypothalamus.* Marcel Dekker, 1979.

Purpura DP, Yahr MD (editors): *The Thalamus.* Columbia Univ Press, 1986.

Steriade M, Llinas RR: The functional states of the thalamus. *Physiol Rev* 1988, Vol 68.

Wurtman RJ, Axelrod J, Kelly DE: *The Pineal.* Academic Press, 1968.

9   Cerebral Hemispheres/Telencephalon

DEVELOPMENT

The **telencephalon (endbrain)** gives rise to left and right cerebral hemispheres, each with a lateral ventricle. Each full-grown hemisphere contains a cerebral cortex, subcortical white matter, and deep masses of gray matter, collectively called **basal ganglia** (lentiform and caudate nuclei; see Fig 9–1). The hemispheres undergo a pattern of extensive differential growth; in the later stages, they resemble an arch over the lateral fissure (Fig 9–2).

The derivatives of the neural tube, or **neuraxis,** include the spinal cord, the brain stem, and the diencephalon. The upper end of the neural tube just below the anterior commissure (see below) is the lamina terminalis. The cerebral hemispheres and the cerebellum, however, are not considered part of the neuraxis.

The basal ganglia arise from the base of the primitive telencephalic vesicles (Fig 9–3). The growing hemispheres gradually cover most of the diencephalon and the upper part of the brain stem. Fiber connections (commissures) between the hemispheres are formed first at the rostral portions as the anterior commissure, later extending posteriorly as the **corpus callosum** (Fig 9–4).

ANATOMY OF THE CEREBRAL HEMISPHERES

The 2 cerebral hemispheres make up the largest portion of the brain.

Main Sulci & Fissures

The surfaces of the cerebral hemispheres contain many fissures and sulci that separate the frontal, parietal, occipital, and temporal lobes from both each other and the insula (Figs 9–5 and 9–6). Fissures, which tend to be deeper than sulci, are visible earlier during development and separate important and often large functional areas. The portions of brain lying between the sulci are called **convolutions,** or **gyri.** Some gyri are relatively constant in location and contour, while others show considerable variation.

The **lateral cerebral fissure** separates the temporal lobe from the frontal and parietal lobes. This fissure resulted from the differential growth pattern of the adjacent cerebral hemisphere (Fig 9–2). The insula (Fig 9–7), a portion of cortex that did not grow much during development, lies deep

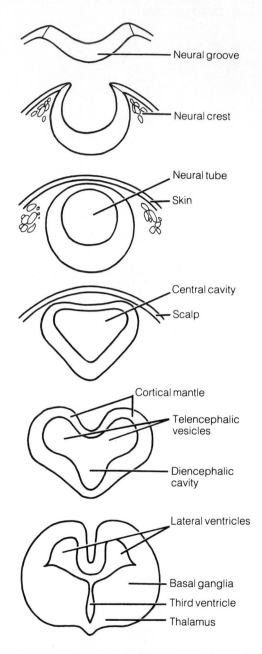

Figure 9-1. Cross sections showing early development from neural groove to cerebrum.

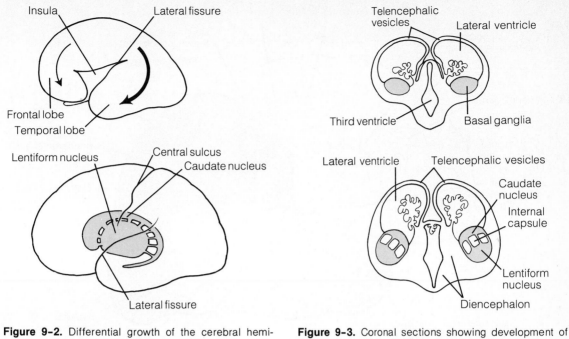

Figure 9-2. Differential growth of the cerebral hemisphere and deeper telencephalic structures.

Figure 9-3. Coronal sections showing development of the basal ganglia in the floor of the lateral ventricle.

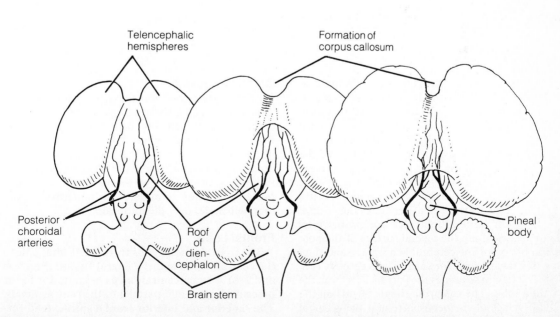

Figure 9-4. Dorsal view of developing cerebrum, showing formation of the corpus callosum, which covers the subarachnoid cistern and vessels over the diencephalon.

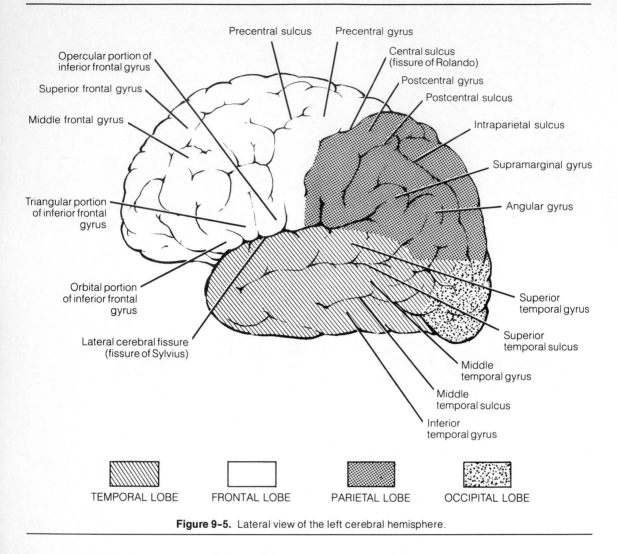

Precentral sulcus
Precentral gyrus
Central sulcus (fissure of Rolando)
Postcentral gyrus
Postcentral sulcus
Intraparietal sulcus
Supramarginal gyrus
Angular gyrus
Opercular portion of inferior frontal gyrus
Superior frontal gyrus
Middle frontal gyrus
Triangular portion of inferior frontal gyrus
Orbital portion of inferior frontal gyrus
Lateral cerebral fissure (fissure of Sylvius)
Superior temporal gyrus
Superior temporal sulcus
Middle temporal gyrus
Middle temporal sulcus
Inferior temporal gyrus

TEMPORAL LOBE   FRONTAL LOBE   PARIETAL LOBE   OCCIPITAL LOBE

Figure 9–5. Lateral view of the left cerebral hemisphere.

within the fissure. The **circular sulcus (circuminsular fissure)** surrounds the insula and separates it from the adjacent frontal, parietal, and temporal lobes. The hemispheres are separated by a deep median fissure, the **longitudinal cerebral fissure.** The **central sulcus** arises about the middle of the hemisphere, beginning near the longitudinal cerebral fissure and extending downward and forward to about 2.5 cm above the lateral cerebral fissure (Fig 9–5). The central sulcus separates the frontal lobe from the parietal lobe. The **parieto-occipital fissure** passes along the medial surface of the posterior portion of the cerebral hemisphere and then runs downward and forward as a deep cleft (Fig 9–6). The fissure separates the parietal lobe from the occipital lobe. The **calcarine fissure** begins on the medial surface of the hemisphere near the occipital pole and extends forward to an area slightly below the splenium of the corpus callosum (Fig 9–6).

Corpus Callosum

The corpus callosum (Figs 9–4 and 9–6) is a large myelinated bundle of fibers, the great white commissure that crosses the longitudinal cerebral fissure and interconnects large portions of the hemispheres. The body of the corpus callosum is arched; its anterior curved portion, the **genu,** continues anteroventrally as the rostrum. The thick posterior portion terminates in the curved splenium, which lies over the midbrain.

Frontal Lobe

The frontal lobe extends from the frontal pole to the central sulcus and the lateral fissure (Figs 9–5 and 9–6). The **precentral sulcus** lies anterior to the **precentral gyrus** and parallel to the central sulcus. The **superior** and **inferior frontal sulci** extend forward and downward from the precentral sulcus, dividing the lateral surface of the frontal lobe into 3

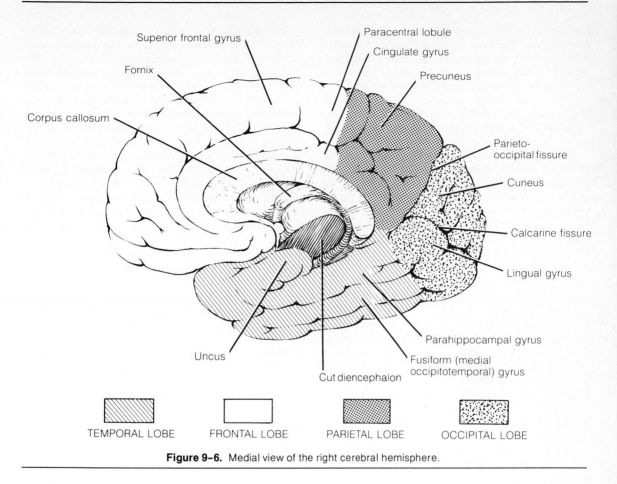

Figure 9–6. Medial view of the right cerebral hemisphere.

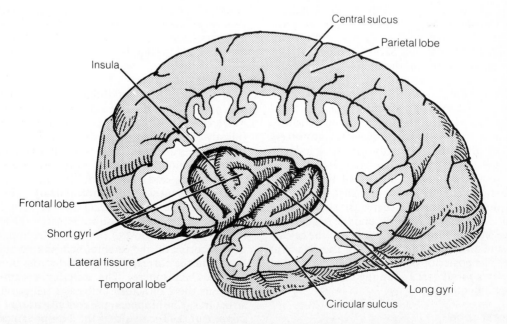

Figure 9–7. Dissection of the left hemisphere to show the insula.

parallel gyri: the **superior, middle,** and **inferior frontal gyri.** The inferior frontal gyrus is divided into 3 parts by the anterior horizontal and ascending rami of the lateral cerebral fissure. The orbital part lies rostral to the anterior horizontal ramus; the triangular, wedge-shaped portion lies between the anterior horizontal and anterior ascending rami; and the opercular part is between the ascending ramus and the precentral sulcus.

The **orbital sulci** and **gyri** are irregular in contour and location. The **olfactory sulcus** lies beneath the olfactory tract on the orbital surface; lying medial to it is the **straight gyrus (gyrus rectus).** The **cingulate gyrus** is the crescent-shaped, or arched, convolution on the medial surface between the cingulate sulcus and the corpus callosum. The **paracentral lobule** is the **quadrilateral gyrus** around the end of the central sulcus on the medial surface of the hemisphere and is the continuation of the precentral and postcentral gyri.

Parietal Lobe

The parietal lobe extends from the central sulcus to the parieto-occipital fissure; laterally, it extends to the level of the lateral cerebral fissure (Figs 9–5 and 9–6). The **postcentral sulcus** lies behind the postcentral gyrus. The **intraparietal sulcus** is a horizontal groove that sometimes unites with the postcentral sulcus. The **superior parietal lobule** lies above the horizontal portion of the intraparietal sulcus, and the **inferior parietal lobule** lies below it.

The **supramarginal gyrus** is the portion of the inferior parietal lobule that arches above the ascending end of the posterior ramus of the lateral cerebral fissure. The **angular gyrus** arches above the end of the superior temporal sulcus and becomes continuous with the middle temporal gyrus. The **precuneus** is the posterior portion of the medial surface between the parieto-occipital fissure and the ascending end of the cingulate sulcus.

Occipital Lobe

The pyramid-shaped occipital lobe (Figs 9–5 and 9–6) is situated behind the parieto-occipital fissure. The **lateral occipital sulcus** extends transversely along its lateral surface, dividing the occipital lobe into a superior and an inferior gyrus. The calcarine fissure divides the medial surface of the occipital lobe into the cuneus and the lingual gyrus. The wedge-shaped **cuneus** lies between the calcarine and parieto-occipital fissures, and the **lingual (lateral occipitotemporal) gyrus** is between the calcarine fissure and the posterior part of the collateral fissure. The posterior part of the **fusiform (medial occipitotemporal) gyrus** is on the basal surface of the occipital lobe.

Temporal Lobe

The temporal lobe (Figs 9–5 and 9–6) lies below the lateral cerebral fissure and extends back to the level of the parieto-occipital fissure on the medial surface of the hemisphere. The lateral surface of the temporal lobe is divided into the parallel **superior, middle,** and **inferior temporal gyri,** which are separated by the **superior** and **middle temporal sulci.** The **inferior temporal sulcus** extends along the lower surface of the temporal lobe from the temporal pole to the occipital lobe. The **transverse temporal gyrus** occupies the posterior part of the superior temporal surface. The **fusiform gyrus** is medial, and the inferior temporal gyrus lateral, to the inferior temporal sulcus on the basal aspect of the temporal lobe. The **hippocampal fissure** extends along the inferomedian aspect of the lobe from the area of the splenium of the corpus callosum to the uncus. The **parahippocampal gyrus** lies between the hippocampal fissure and the anterior part of the collateral fissure. Its anterior part, the most medial portion of the temporal lobe, curves in the form of a hook; it is known as the **uncus.**

Insula

The insula (Fig 9–7) is a sunken portion of the cerebral cortex. It lies deep within the lateral cerebral fissure and can be exposed by separating the upper and lower lips (**opercula**) of the lateral fissure. The deep circular sulcus bounds the insula. Several short gyri, formed by shallow sulci, occupy the anterior portion of the insula; a long gyrus occupies the posterior part.

Limbic System Components

The cortical components of the limbic system include the cingulate, parahippocampal, and subcallosal gyri as well as the hippocampal formation. The anatomy and function of these components are discussed in Chapter 18.

White Matter

The white matter of the adult cerebral hemisphere (Fig 9–8 and Table 9–1) contains myelinated nerve fibers of many sizes as well as neuroglia (mostly oligodendrocytes). The white center of the upper cerebral hemisphere, sometimes called the **centrum semiovale,** contains transverse fibers, projection fibers, and association fibers.

A. Transverse (Commissural) Fibers: Transverse fibers interconnect the 2 cerebral hemispheres. The **corpus callosum** comprises the largest bundle of fibers; most of these arise from parts of the neocortex of one cerebral hemisphere and terminate in the corresponding parts of the opposite cerebral hemisphere. The **anterior commissure** connects the 2 olfactory bulbs and temporal lobe structures. The **hippocampal commissure,** or **commissure of the fornix,** joins the 2 hippocampi; it is variable in size (see also Chapter 18).

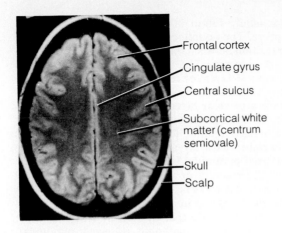

Frontal cortex
Cingulate gyrus
Central sulcus
Subcortical white matter (centrum semiovale)
Skull
Scalp

Figure 9-8. MR image of a horizontal section through the upper head.

B. Projection Fibers: These fibers connect the cerebral cortex with lower portions of the brain or the spinal cord. The **corticopetal (afferent) fibers** include the geniculocalcarine radiation from the lateral geniculate body to the calcarine cortex, the auditory radiation from the medial geniculate body to the auditory cortex, and thalamic radiations from the thalamic nuclei to specific cerebrocortical areas. **Corticofugal (efferent) fibers** proceed from the cerebral cortex to the thalamus, brain stem, or spinal cord.

C. Association Fibers: These fibers connect the various portions of a cerebral hemisphere (Fig 9-9). Short association fibers, or **U fibers,** connect adjacent gyri; those located in the deeper portions of the white matter are the intracortical fibers and those just beneath the cortex are called subcortical fibers. Long association fibers connect more widely separated areas. The **uncinate fasciculus** crosses the bottom of the lateral cerebral fissure and connects the inferior frontal lobe gyri with the anterior temporal lobe. The **cingulum,** a white

Table 9-1. Myelinated nerve fibers in the cerebral hemisphere.

Type of Fiber	Name	Function
Transverse (commisural)	Corpus callosum Anterior commissure Hippocampal commissure	Connect homologous areas of the 2 cerebral hemispheres
Projection	Corticopetal (afferent) fibers	Connect the thalamus to the cerebral cortex
	Corcitofugal (efferent) fibers	Connect the cerebral cortex to lower portions of the brain or the spinal cord
Association	Short association (U) fibers Long association fibers Uncinate fasciculus Arcuate fasciculus Longitudinal fasciculi (inferior and superior) Occipitofrontal fasciculus Cingululm	Connect gyri, lobes, or widely separated areas within each cerebral hemisphere

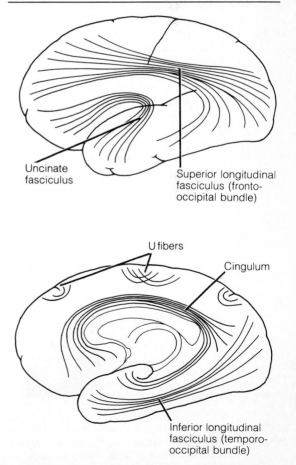

Uncinate fasciculus
Superior longitudinal fasciculus (fronto-occipital bundle)
U fibers
Cingulum
Inferior longitudinal fasciculus (temporo-occipital bundle)

Figure 9-9. Diagram of the major association systems.

band within the cingulate gyrus, connects the anterior perforated substance and the parahippocampal gyrus. The **arcuate fasciculus** sweeps around the insula and connects the superior and middle frontal convolutions with the temporal lobe and frontal pole. The **superior longitudinal fasciculus** connects portions of the frontal lobe with occipital and temporal areas. The **inferior longitudinal fasciculus,** which extends parallel to the lateral border of the inferior and posterior horns of the lateral ventricle, connects the temporal and occipital lobes. The **occipitofrontal fasciculus** extends backward from the frontal lobe, radiating into the temporal and occipital lobes.

MICROSCOPIC STRUCTURE OF THE CORTEX

A. Types of Cortices: The cortex of the cerebrum is considered to comprise 2 types: allocortex and isocortex. The **allocortex (archicortex)** is found predominantly in the limbic system cortex (see Chapter 18). The **isocortex (neocortex)** is more commonly found in most of the cerebral hemisphere. The **juxtallocortex (mesocortex)** forms the transition between the allocortex and isocortex.

B. Layers: The isocortex (Fig 9–10) consists of up to 6 layers of cells (the organization of these layers is referred to as **cytoarchitecture**). The outermost **molecular layer (I)** contains nonspecific afferent fibers that come from within the cortex or from the thalamus. The **external granular layer (II)** is a rather dense layer composed of small cells. The **external pyramidal layer (III)** contains pyramidal cells, frequently in row formation. The **internal granular layer (IV)** is usually a thin layer with cells similar to those in the external granular layer. These cells receive specific afferent fibers from the thalamus. The **ganglionic (internal pyramidal) layer (V)** contains, in most areas, pyramidal cells that are fewer in number but larger in size than those in the external pyramidal layer. These cells project to distal structures (eg, brain stem and spinal cord). The **fusiform (multiform) layer (VI)** consists of irregular fusiform cells whose axons enter the adjacent white matter.

C. Columns: Although the cortex is arranged in layers, its constituent groups of neurons with

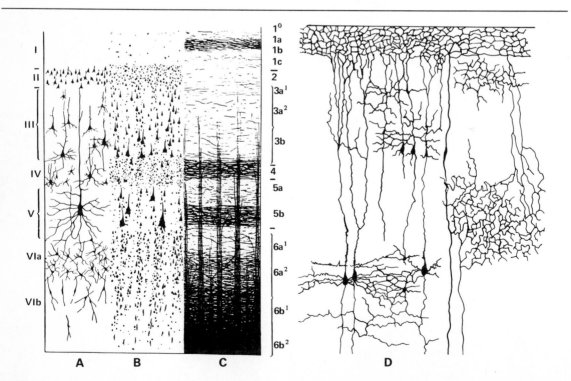

Figure 9–10. Diagram of the structure of the cerebral cortex. *A:* Golgi neuronal stain. *B:* Nissl cellular stain. *C:* Weigert myelin stain. *D:* Neuronal connections. Roman and Arabic numerals indicate the layers of the isocortex (neocortex); *4:* external line of Baillarger (line of Gennari in the occipital lobe); *5b:* internal line of Baillarger. (A, B, and C reproduced, with permission, from Ranson SW, Clark SL: *The Anatomy of the Nervous System,* 10th ed. Saunders, 1959. D reproduced, with permission, from Ganong WF: *Review of Medical Physiology,* 14th ed, Appleton & Lange, 1989.)

similar functions are interconnected in vertically oriented columns. It is the vast number of such local circuits that gives the brain its complex functions (see also the section on electroencephalograms in Chapter 23).

D. Myeloarchitecture: Myelinated fiber layers between the cortical layers give the appearance of white lines. The **line of Gennari** (Fig 9–10) in the striated area of the occipital lobe is prominent and visible to the naked eye; it forms the outer portion of the internal granular layer (IV). Elsewhere in the cortex, this line is thinner and is known as the **external line of Baillarger.** The **internal line of Baillarger** is formed at the inner aspect of the ganglionic layer (V).

E. Classification of Principal Areas: Division and classification of the cerebral cortex has been attempted by many investigators on the basis of cytoarchitecture. Inferences concerning its structure and function are drawn largely from observations on animals, especially primates. The most commonly employed system is **Brodmann's** classification system (Figs 9–11 and 9–12), which

uses numbers to label individual areas of the cortex that Brodmann believed differed from others. The areas have been used as a reference base for the localization of physiologic and pathologic processes. Ablation and stimulation, electrically and with various chemicals, has led to functional localizations. The principal areas and their functional correlations are shown in Figs 9–11, 9–12, and 9–13.

1. Frontal lobe-Area 4 is the primary motor area in the precentral gyrus. Area 6 is a part of the associated motor tract circuit, and area 8 is concerned with eye movements and pupillary changes. The remaining areas are frontal association areas.

2. Parietal lobe-Areas 3, 1, and 2 are the postcentral primary sensory areas. The remaining areas are sensory or multimodal association areas.

3. Occipital lobe-Area 17 is the striate—the principal visual—cortex. Areas 18 and 19 are visual association areas.

4. Temporal lobe-Area 41 is the primary auditory cortex; area 42 is the associative (secondary) auditory cortex. The remaining areas are multimodal association areas.

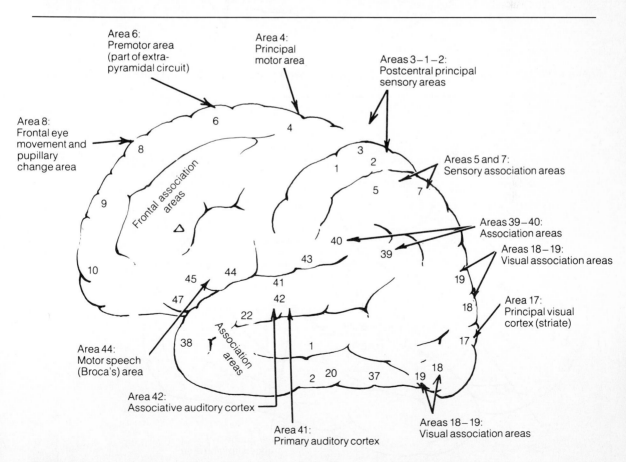

Figure 9–11. Lateral aspect of the cerebrum. The cortical areas are shown according to Brodmann, with functional localizations.

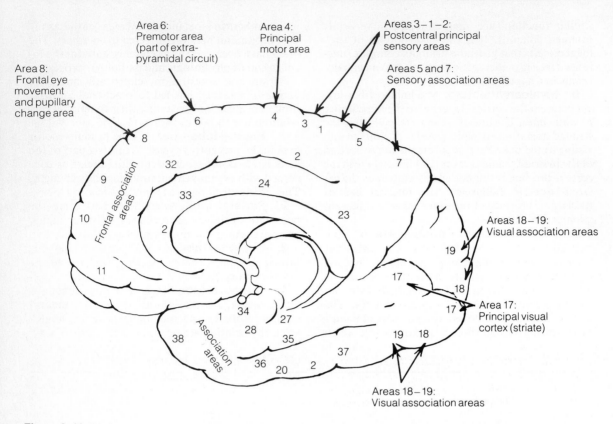

Area 8:
Frontal eye
movement
and pupillary
change area

Area 6:
Premotor area
(part of extra-
pyramidal circuit)

Area 4:
Principal
motor area

Areas 3–1–2:
Postcentral principal
sensory areas

Areas 5 and 7:
Sensory association areas

Frontal association areas

Association areas

Areas 18–19:
Visual association areas

Area 17:
Principal visual
cortex (striate)

Areas 18–19:
Visual association areas

Figure 9–12. Medial aspect of the cerebrum. The cortical areas are shown according to Brodmann, with functional localizations.

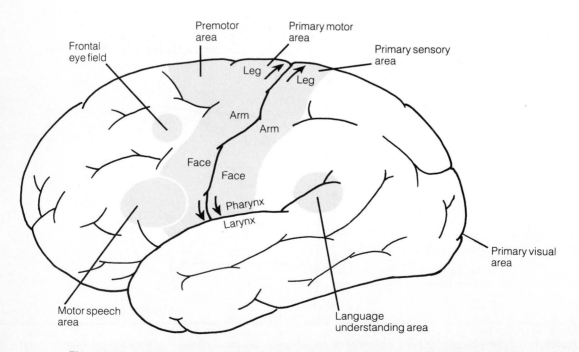

Frontal
eye field

Premotor
area

Primary motor
area

Primary sensory
area

Leg

Leg

Arm

Arm

Face

Face

Pharynx

Larynx

Primary visual
area

Motor speech
area

Language
understanding area

Figure 9–13. Lateral view of the left hemisphere, showing the functions of the cortical areas.

PHYSIOLOGY OF THE CORTEX

A. Primary Motor Projection Cortex: The functions of the **olfactory receptive cortex** and related areas are discussed in Chapter 18.

1. Location and function-The primary motor projection cortex (area 4; see Chapter 12) is located on the anterior wall of the central sulcus and the adjacent portion of the precentral gyrus, corresponding generally to the distribution of the giant pyramidal (Betz) cells. These cells control voluntary movements of skeletal muscle on the opposite side of the body, with the impulses traveling over their axons in the corticobulbar and corticospinal tracts to the nuclei of the cerebrospinal nerves. A somatotopic representation within the motor areas, mapped by electrical stimulation during brain surgery, appears in Fig 9–14. Secondary and tertiary areas of motor function can be mapped roughly around the primary motor cortex where stimulation produces gross movements. Contralateral conjugate deviation of the head and eyes occurs upon stimulation of the posterior part of the middle frontal gyrus (area 8).

2. Clinical correlations-Irritative lesions of the motor centers may cause convulsive seizures that begin as focal twitchings and spread to involve large muscle groups (jacksonian epilepsy). There may also be modification of consciousness and postconvulsive weakness or paralysis. Destructive lesions of the motor cortex (area 4) produce contralateral flaccid paresis, or paralysis, of affected

muscle groups. Spasticity is more apt to occur if area 6 is also ablated.

B. Primary Sensory Projection Cortex:

1. Location and function-The primary sensory projection cortex for sensation information received from the skin and mucosa of the body and face is located in the postcentral gyrus and is called the **somatesthetic area** (areas 3, 1, and 2; see Fig 9–15). From the thalamic radiations, this area receives fibers that convey touch and proprioceptive (muscle, joint, and tendon) sensations from the opposite side of the body (see also Chapter 13).

Experimental studies indicate that a relatively wide portion of the adjacent frontal and parietal lobes can be considered a secondary sensory cortex since this area also receives sensory stimuli. The primary **sensorimotor area** is therefore considered capable of functioning as both a motor and a sensory cortex, with the portion of the cortex anterior to the central sulcus predominantly motor and that behind it predominantly sensory.

The **cortical taste area** is located in the facial sensory area and extends onto the opercular surface of the lateral cerebral fissure (see Fig 7–18).

2. Clinical correlations-Irritative lesions of this area produce **paresthesias** (eg, numbness; abnormal sensations of ants crawling on the body, electric shock, or pins and needles) on the opposite

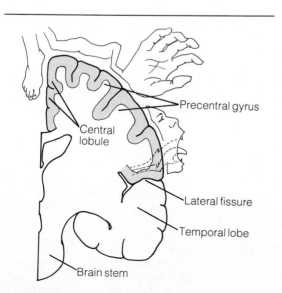

Figure 9–14. Motor homunculus, drawn on a coronal section through the precentral gyrus. The figure shows the location of cortical control of various body parts.

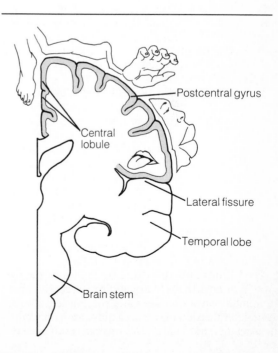

Figure 9–15. Sensory homunculus, drawn overlying a coronal section through the postcentral gyrus. The figure shows the location of the cortical representation of various body parts.

side of the body. Destructive lesions produce objective impairments in sensibility, such as an impaired ability to localize or measure the intensity of painful stimuli and impaired perception of various forms of cutaneous sensation. Complete anesthesia on a cortical basis is rare.

C. Primary Visual Receptive Cortex and Visual Association Cortex:

1. Location and function–The primary visual receptive (striate) cortex (area 17) is located in the occipital lobe. It lies in the cortex of the calcarine fissure and adjacent portions of the cuneus and the lingual gyrus.

In primates, an extensive posterior portion of the occipital pole is concerned primarily with macular vision; the more anterior parts of the calcarine cortex are concerned with peripheral vision. The visual cortex in the right occipital lobe receives impulses from the right half of each retina, while the left visual cortex (area 17) receives impulses from the left half of each retina. The upper portion of area 17 represents the upper half of each retina, while the lower portion represents the lower half. Visual association is a function of areas 18 and 19. Area 19 can receive stimuli from the entire cerebral cortex; area 18 receives stimuli mainly from area 17 (see also Chapter 14).

2. Clinical correlations–Irritative lesions of area 17 can produce such visual hallucinations as flashes of light, rainbows, brilliant stars, or bright lines. Destructive lesions can cause contralateral homonymous defects of the visual fields without destruction of macular vision. Injury to areas 18 and 19 can produce visual disorganization, with defective spatial orientation in the homonymous halves of the visual field.

D. Primary Auditory Receptive Cortex:

1. Location and function–The primary auditory receptive area (41; see also Chapter 15) is located in the transverse temporal gyrus, which lies in the superior temporal gyrus toward the lateral cerebral fissure. It receives the auditory radiation from the cochlea of each ear, and there is point-to-point projection of the cochlea upon the acoustic area (tonotopia). In humans, low tones are projected or represented in the frontolateral portion and high tones in the occipitomedial portion of area 41. Low tones are detected near the apex of the cochlea and high tones near the base.

2. Clinical correlations–Irritation of the region in or near the primary auditory receptive area in humans causes buzzing and roaring sensations. A unilateral lesion in this area may cause only mild hearing loss, but bilateral lesions can result in deafness.

BASAL GANGLIA

The traditional term *basal ganglia* refers to masses of gray matter deep within the cerebral hemispheres. The term is debatable, however, because these masses are nuclei rather than ganglia—and some of them are not basal. Anatomically, the basal ganglia include the **caudate nucleus** and the **putamen** (together called the **corpus striatum**), the **globus pallidus,** and other gray areas at the base of the forebrain. Together, the putamen and the globus pallidus form the **lentiform nucleus.** The caudate nucleus is separated from the lentiform nucleus and thalamus by a complex fiber system, the **internal capsule.** Functionally, these collections of neurons together with their fibrous connections and neurotransmitters form an associated motor system that includes nuclei in the subthalamus and midbrain (see Chapter 12).

Caudate Nucleus

The caudate nucleus, an elongated gray mass whose pear-shaped head is continuous with the putamen, lies adjacent to the inferior border of the anterior horn of the lateral ventricle. The slender end continues backward and downward as the tail; it enters the roof of the temporal horn of the lateral ventricle and tapers off at the level of the amygdala.

Lentiform Nucleus

The lentiform nucleus is situated between the insula and the internal capsule. The external medullary lamina divides the nucleus into 2 parts, the putamen and the globus pallidus. The putamen is the larger, convex gray mass lying lateral to and just beneath the insular cortex. The striped appearance of the corpus striatum is caused by the white fasciculi of the internal capsule that are situated between the gray putamen and the caudate nucleus. The globus pallidus is the smaller, triangular median zone whose numerous myelinated fibers make it appear lighter in color. A medullary lamina divides the globus pallidus into 2 portions.

Claustrum & External Capsule

The claustrum is a thin layer of gray substance situated just beneath the insular cortex and separated from the more median putamen by the thin lamina of white matter known as the external capsule.

Fiber Connections

Most portions of the basal ganglia are interconnected by 2-way fiber systems (Fig 9–16). The caudate nucleus sends many fibers to the putamen, which in turn sends short fibers to the globus pallidus. The putamen and globus pallidus receive some fibers from the substantia nigra, and the thal-

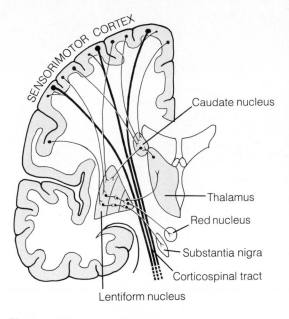

Figure 9-16. Connections between the basal ganglia, the thalamus, and the cortex.

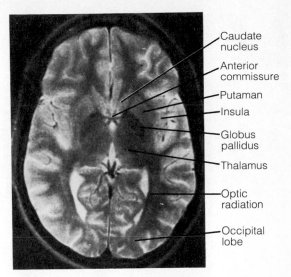

Figure 9-17. MR image of a horizontal section through the head.

amus sends fibers to the caudate nucleus. Efferent fibers from the corpus striatum leave via the globus pallidus. Some fibers pass through the internal capsule and form a bundle, the **fasciculus lenticularis,** on the medial side. Other fibers sweep the medial border of the internal capsule to form a loop, the **ansa lenticularis.** Both these sets of fibers have some terminals in the subthalamic and red nuclei; others continue upward to the thalamus via the fasciculus thalamicus.

Internal Capsule

The internal capsule is a broad band of myelinated fibers that separate the lentiform nucleus from the medial caudate nucleus and thalamus. It consists of an anterior limb, a posterior limb, a retrolenticular part, and a sublenticular part. The capsule is not one of the basal ganglia, but a related fiber bundle. In horizontal section, it presents a *V* appearance, with the **genu** (apex) pointing medially (Fig 9-17).

The anterior limb of the internal capsule separates the lentiform nucleus from the caudate nucleus. It contains thalamocortical and corticothalamic fibers that join the lateral thalamic nucleus and the frontal lobe cortex, frontopontine tracts from the frontal lobe to the pontine nuclei, and fibers from the caudate nucleus to the putamen.

The posterior limb of the internal capsule, located between the thalamus and the lentiform nucleus, contains the corticobulbar and corticospinal tracts, with the fibers to the arm in front of the fibers to the leg. Corticorubral fibers from the frontal lobe cortex to the red nucleus accompany the corticospinal tract. The posterior one-third of the limb contains fibers from the posterolateral nucleus of the thalamus to the postcentral gyrus. The retrolenticular part contains optic fibers from the geniculate body to the calcarine cortex and fibers from the occipital cortex to the pontine nuclei. The sublenticular part, which lies below the lentiform nucleus, contains parietotemporopontine fibers from the temporal and parietal lobe cortex to the pontine nuclei and auditory radiations from the medial geniculate body to the transverse temporal gyrus.

Lower horizontal sections through the head show the descending fibers of the internal capsule contained in the crus cerebri, the ventral part of the cerebral peduncle of the midbrain (Fig 9-18).

CASE 11

A 44-year-old woman gave a history of dizzy spells associated with disorientation and confusion. These spells had begun about a year previously and had become more frequent in the last several months. The patient had recently begun to complain of general headaches, and after she had what she described as "a fit," her husband insisted she see a doctor.

Neurologic examination showed apathy, impair-

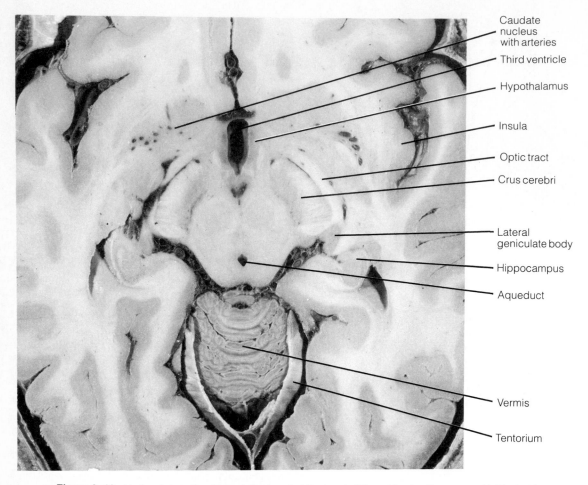

Caudate nucleus with arteries

Third ventricle

Hypothalamus

Insula

Optic tract

Crus cerebri

Lateral geniculate body

Hippocampus

Aqueduct

Vermis

Tentorium

Figure 9–18. Horizontal section through the head at the level of the midbrain. (Compare with Fig 6–9.)

ment of memory, possible left papilledema, facial asymmetry, lack of movement on the right side of the face, and general weakness but symmetric reflexes in the remainder of the body. An electroencephalogram showed a slow-wave focus in the left hemisphere, and a skull film showed a calcified mass in the left frontoparietal region.

What is the differential diagnosis based on the above findings?

A brain biopsy was performed and a diagnosis made. By the next day, the patient had become comatose with dilated fixed pupils, and she died soon afterward. At autopsy, findings included small hemorrhages in the brain stem and extensive pathologic changes in the forebrain.

What happened after the brain biopsy? What is the most likely diagnosis?

CASE 12

A 12-year-old girl began to have increasingly severe ear pain and fever. A few days later, her mother noticed a discharge from the left ear and took her to her family physician. The doctor prescribed antibiotics. One week later, the girl developed a severe, constant, left-frontal headache with swelling around the left eye. The following week, she developed left-sided facial weakness.

What is the differential diagnosis at this point?

The girl was then referred to a neurologist. At the time of admission, she was confused (almost delirious), and spoke unintelligibly, sometimes displayed silly behavior, and had a temperature of 100°F (37.8°C). Neurologic examination showed confusion of past and recent events, severe difficulty in naming objects, bilateral papilledema, normal extraocular movements, minor left peripheral facial paralysis, and decreased hearing ability on the left. The patient resisted neck flexion. An electroencephalogram showed slow-wave activity in the left hemisphere, especially in the fronto-temporal region.

Which diagnostic neuroradiologic procedure would be helpful? What is the most likely diagnosis?

Cases are discussed further in Chapter 24.

REFERENCES

Dray A: The physiology and pharmacology of mammalian basal ganglia. *Prog Neurobiol* 1980;**14**:221.

Ralston HJ: *Neuroanatomy: Clinical and Experimental.* Lea & Febiger, in press.

Romanes GJ: *Cunningham's Anatomy,* 18th ed. Oxford Univ Press, 1986.

Schmitt FO et al: *The Organization of the Cerebral Cortex.* MIT Press, 1981.

Warwick R, et al: *Gray's Anatomy,* 37th ed. Saunders, 1989.

Yahr MD (editor): *The Basal Ganglia.* Raven, 1976.

10 Ventricles & Coverings of the Brain

VENTRICULAR SYSTEM

Within the brain substance is a communicating system of 5 cavities that are lined with ependyma and filled with cerebrospinal fluid (CSF). These cavities are designated as the 2 lateral ventricles, the third ventricle (between the halves of the diencephalon), the cerebral aqueduct, and the fourth ventricle within the brain stem (Fig 10–1).

Lateral Ventricles

The irregularly shaped lateral ventricles are the largest of the ventricles; they include 2 central portions (body and atrium) and 3 extensions (horns).

The **choroid plexus** of the lateral ventricle is a fringelike vascular process of pia mater containing capillaries of the choroid arteries. It projects into the ventricular cavity and is covered by an epithelial layer of ependymal origin (Figs 10–2 and 10–3). The attachment of the plexus to the adjacent brain structures is known as the **tela choroidea.** The choroid plexus extends from the interventricular foramen, where it joins with the plexuses of the third ventricle and opposite lateral ventricle, to the end of the inferior horn (there is no choroid plexus in the anterior and posterior horns). The arteries to the plexus consist of the **anterior choroidal artery,** a branch of the internal carotid artery that enters the plexus at the inferior horn; and the lateral **posterior choroidal arteries,** which are branches of the posterior cerebral artery.

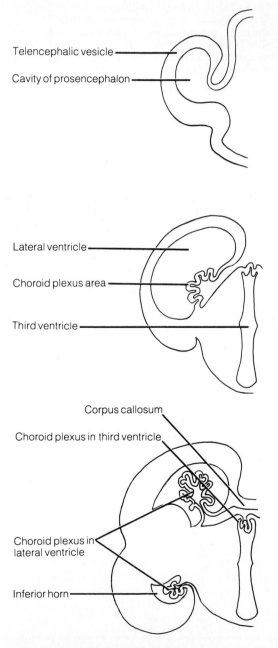

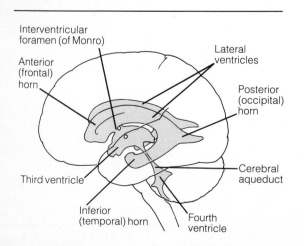

Figure 10–1. The ventricular system.

Figure 10–2. Three stages of development of the choroid plexus in the lateral ventricle (coronal sections).

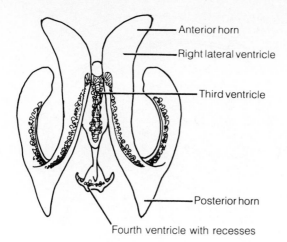

Figure 10–3. Dorsal view of the choroid plexus in the ventricular system. Note the absence of choroid in the aqueduct and the anterior and posterior horns.

The **anterior (frontal) horn** is in front of the interventricular foramen. Its roof and anterior border are formed by the corpus callosum; its vertical medial wall by the septum pellucidum; and the floor and lateral wall by the bulging head of the caudate nucleus. During development and early life, the septum contains the **cavum septi pellucidi** (erroneously called the fifth ventricle). This fluid-filled cavity (its posterior portion is called the **cavum vergae**) may persist; it sometimes extends to the splenium.

The central part, or body, of the lateral ventricle is the long, narrow portion that extends from the interventricular foramen to a point opposite the splenium of the corpus callosum. Its roof is formed by the corpus callosum and its medial wall by the posterior portion of the septum pellucidum. The floor contains (from medial to lateral side) the fornix, the choroid plexus, the lateral part of the dorsal surface of the thalamus, the stria terminalis, the vena terminalis, and the caudate nucleus. The **atrium,** or **trigone,** is a wide area of the body that connects with the posterior and inferior horns (Fig 10–4).

The **posterior (occipital) horn** extends into the occipital lobe. Its roof is formed by fibers of the corpus callosum. On its medial wall is the **calcar axis,** an elevation of the ventricular wall produced by the calcarine fissure.

The **inferior (temporal) horn** traverses the temporal lobe, whose white substance forms its roof. Along the medial border are the stria terminalis and the tail of the caudate nucleus. The amygdaloid nuclear complex bulges into the upper terminal part of the inferior horn, whose floor and medial wall are formed by the fimbria, hippocampus, and collateral eminence.

The 2 **interventricular foramens** are oval apertures between the column of the fornix and the anterior end of the thalamus. The 2 lateral ventricles communicate with the third ventricle through these foramens, which are sometimes referred to as the foramens of Monro (see Fig 10–1).

Third Ventricle

The third ventricle is a narrow vertical cleft between the 2 halves of the diencephalon (see Figs 10–1 through 10–4). The roof of the third ventricle is formed by a thin tela choroidea, a layer of ependyma, and pia mater from which a small choroid plexus extends into the lumen of the ventricle (see Fig 8–1). This plexus is supplied by the medial posterior choroidal artery from the posterior cerebral artery. The lateral walls are formed mainly by the medial surfaces of the 2 thalami. The lower lateral wall and the floor of the ventricle are formed by the hypothalamus; the anterior commissure and the lamina terminalis form the rostral limit.

The **optic recess** is an extension of the third ventricle between the lamina terminalis and the optic chiasm. The hypophysis is attached to the apex of its downward extension, the funnel-shaped **infundibular recess.** A small **pineal recess** projects into the stalk of the pineal body. A variable, often large extension of the third ventricle above the epithalamus is known as the **suprapineal recess.** The **interthalamic adhesion,** a band of gray matter, crosses the cavity of the ventricle and joins the external walls. This band, which is present in about 60% of all brains, has no functional significance.

Cerebral Aqueduct

The cerebral aqueduct (see Figs 10–1 and 10–4) is a narrow, curved channel running from the posterior third ventricle into the fourth; it contains no choroid plexus.

Fourth Ventricle

The fourth ventricle is a pyramid-shaped cavity bounded ventrally by the pons and medulla oblongata (see Figs 6–16, 10–1, and 10–3); its floor is also known as the **rhomboid fossa.** The **lateral recess** extends as a narrow, curved extension of the ventricle on the dorsal surface of the inferior cerebellar peduncle. The fourth ventricle extends under the **obex** into the central canal of the medulla.

The incomplete roof of the fourth ventricle is formed by the anterior and posterior medullary vela. The **anterior medullary velum** extends between the dorsomedial borders of the superior cerebellar peduncles, and its dorsal surface is covered by the adherent lingula of the cerebellum. The **posterior medullary velum** extends caudally from the cerebellum. The point at which the fourth ventricle passes up into the cerebellum is called the **apex,** or **fastigium.**

The **lateral aperture (foramen of Luschka)** is the opening of the lateral recess into the subarachnoid space near the flocculus of the cerebellum. A tuft of choroid plexus is commonly present in the aperture and partly obstructs the flow of cerebrospinal fluid from the fourth ventricle to subarachnoid space. The **medial aperture (foramen of Magendie)** is an opening in the caudal portion of the roof of the ventricle. Most of the outflow of cerebrospinal fluid from the fourth ventricle passes through this aperture, which varies in size.

The **tela choroidea** of the fourth ventricle is a layer of pia and ependyma that contains small vessels and lies in the posterior medullary velum; it forms the choroid plexus of the fourth ventricle and is supplied by branches of the posterior inferior cerebellar arteries.

MENINGES & SPACES

Three membranes, or meninges, envelop the brain: The dura, the arachnoid, and the pia. The dura, the outer membrane, is separated from the thin arachnoid by a potential compartment, the **subdural space,** that normally contains only a few drops of cerebrospinal fluid. An extensive **subarachnoid space** containing cerebrospinal fluid and the major arteries separates the arachnoid from the *pia,* which completely invests the brain. The arachnoid and the pia known as *leptomeninges,* are connected by thin strands of tissue, the arachnoid trabeculae. The pia together with a narrow extension of the subarachnoid space, accompanies the vessels deep into the brain tissue; this space is called the **perivascular space,** or Virchow-Robin space.

Dura

The cranial dura, or **pachymeninx** (Figs 10–4 and 10–5), is a tough, fibrous structure with an inner **(meningeal)** layer and an outer **(periosteal)** layer. The dural layers over the brain are generally fused, except where they separate to provide space for the venous sinuses (most of the dura's venous sinuses lie between the dural layers) and where the inner layer forms septa between brain portions. The outer layer is firmly attached to the inner surface of the cranial bones and sends vascular and fibrous extensions into the bone itself; the inner layer is continuous with the spinal dura.

One of the dural septa, the curved **falx cerebri,** extends down into the longitudinal fissure between the cerebral hemispheres (Figs 10–5 and 10–6). The anterior falx cerebri is narrower than the posterior end. It attaches to the inner surface of the skull in midplane, from the crista galli to the internal oc-

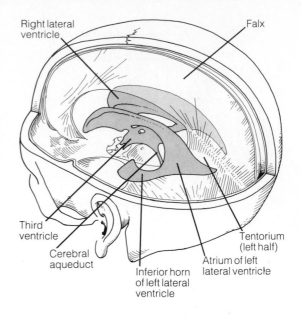

Figure 10-4. Drawing of the ventricles showing their relationship to the dura, tentorium, and skull base.

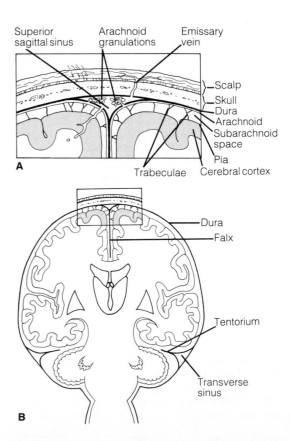

Figure 10-5. *A:* Schematic illustration of a coronal section through the brain and coverings. *B:* Enlargement of the area at the top of *A.*

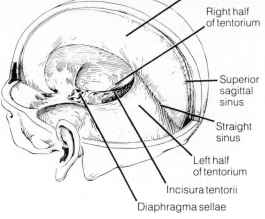

Figure 10–6. Schematic illustration of the dural folds.

cipital protuberance, where it becomes continuous with the tentorium cerebelli.

The **tentorium cerebelli** separates the occipital lobes from the cerebellum. It is a roughly transverse membrane that attaches at the rear and side to the skull at the transverse sinuses; at the front, it attaches to the petrous portion of the temporal bone and to the clinoid processes of the sphenoid bone. Toward the midline, it slopes up and fuses with the falx cerebri. The free, curved, anterior border leaves a large opening, the **incisura tentorii** (tentorial notch), for passage of the upper brain stem, aqueduct, and vessels.

The **falx cerebelli** projects between the cerebellar hemispheres from the inner surface of the occipital bone to form a small triangular dural septum.

The **diaphragma sellae** forms an incomplete lid over the hypophysis in the sella turcica by connecting the clinoid attachments of the 2 sides of the tentorium cerebelli. The pituitary stalk passes through the opening in the diaphragma.

Arachnoid

The arachnoid, a delicate avascular membrane, covers the subarachnoid space, which is filled with cerebrospinal fluid. The inner surface of the arachnoid is connected to the pia by fine (but inconstantly present) **arachnoid trabeculae** (Fig 10–5). The cranial arachnoid closely covers the inner surface of the dura mater but is separated from it by the subdural space, which contains a thin film of fluid. The arachnoid does not dip into the sulci or fissures except to follow the falx and the tentorium.

Arachnoid Granulations (Fig 10–5B) consist of many microscopic villi. They have the appearance of berrylike clumps protruding into the superior

sagittal sinus or its associated venous lacunae and into other sinuses and large veins. With advancing age, the granulations increase in size and number, sometimes pushing against or through the periosteal dura and causing bone resorption and depressions in the skull cap. The granulations are sites of absorption of cerebrospinal fluid.

The **subarachnoid space** between the arachnoid and the pia is relatively narrow over the surface of the cerebral hemisphere, but it becomes much wider in areas at the base of the brain. These widened spaces, the subarachnoid **cisterns,** are often named after neighboring brain structures (Fig 10–7). They communicate freely with adjacent cisterns and the general subarachnoid space.

The **cisterna magna** results from the bridging of the arachnoid over the space between the medulla and the cerebellar hemispheres; it is continuous with the spinal subarachnoid space. The **pontine cistern** on the ventral aspect of the pons contains the basilar artery and some veins. Below the cerebrum lies a wide space between the 2 temporal lobes. This space is divided into the **chiasmatic cisterna** above the optic chiasm, the **suprasellar cistern** above the diaphragma sellae, and the **interpeduncular cistern** between the cerebral peduncles. The space between frontal, parietal, and temporal lobes is called the **cistern of the lateral fissure (cistern of Sylvius).**

Pia

The pia (Fig 10–5) is a thin connective-tissue membrane that covers the brain surface and extends into sulci and fissures and around blood vessels throughout the brain. It also extends into the transverse cerebral fissure under the corpus callosum. There it forms the tela choroidea of the third and lateral ventricles and combines with the

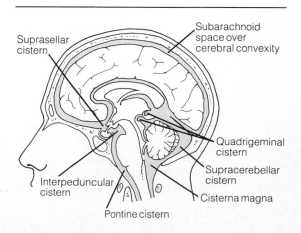

Figure 10–7. Schematic illustration of the brain, showing spaces that contain cerebrospinal fluid.

ependyma and choroid vessels to form the choroid plexus of these ventricles. The pia and ependyma pass over the roof of the fourth ventricle and form its tela choroidea for the choroid plexus there.

Clinical Correlations

The dura may become partly calcified or even ossified with age. In some cases, often in association with longstanding hydrocephalus, the falx is fenestrated.

Several types of herniation of the brain can occur. The tentorium separates the supratentorial and the infratentorial compartments, and the 2 spaces communicate by way of the incisura that contains the midbrain. Both the falx and the tentorium form incomplete separations, and a mass or lesion may displace a portion of the brain around these septa, resulting in either **subfalcial** or **transtentorial herniation.** The latter type may be downward (uncal, or caudal transtentorial, herniation) or upward (rostral transtentorial herniation). The herniation of the cerebellar tonsils into the foramen magnum by a lesion is often called **coning.** Transtentorial herniations, especially the caudal type, are potentially life-threatening because they can distort or compress the brain stem and damage its vital regulatory centers for respiration, consciousness, blood pressure, and other functions (see Chapter 19).

Various types of lesions can occur in one or more intracranial compartments: the brain itself (tumor, bleeding, abscess); the extracellular space (edema); the vascular compartment (venous obstruction, arteriovenous malformation, bleeding); and the spaces containing cerebrospinal fluid (obstructions).

CEREBROSPINAL FLUID

Function

The cerebrospinal fluid provides mechanical support of the brain and acts like a protective water jacket. It controls brain excitability by regulating the ionic composition, carries away metabolites (the brain has no lymphatic vessels), and provides some protection from pressure changes (venous volume versus cerebrospinal fluid volume).

Composition & Volume

Normal cerebrospinal fluid is clear, colorless, and odorless. Its more important average normal values are shown in Table 10–1.

The cerebrospinal fluid is present, for the most part, in a system that comprises 2 communicating parts. The internal portion of the system consists of 2 lateral ventricles, the interventricular foramens, the third ventricle, the cerebral aqueduct, and the fourth ventricle. The external part consists of the subarachnoid spaces and cisterns. Communication between the internal and external portions occurs through the 2 lateral apertures of the fourth ventricle (foramens of Luschka) and the median aperture of the fourth ventricle (foramen of Magendie). In adults, the total volume of cerebrospinal fluid in all the space combined is normally about 150 mL; the internal (ventricular) portion of the system contains about half this amount. Between 400 and 500 mL of cerebrospinal fluid is produced and reabsorbed daily.

Pressure

The normal mean cerebrospinal fluid pressure is 70–180 mm of water; periodic changes occur with heartbeat and respiration. The pressure rises if there is an increase in intracranial volume (eg, with tumors), blood volume (with hemorrhages), or cerebrospinal fluid volume (with hydrocephalus), since the adult skull is a rigid box of bone that cannot accommodate the increased volume without a rise in pressure.

Circulation

Much of the cerebrospinal fluid originates from the choroid plexuses within the lateral ventricles of the brain. The fluid (see Fig 10–8) passes through the interventricular foramens into the midline third ventricle; more cerebrospinal fluid is produced here by the choroid plexus in the ventricle's roof. The fluid then moves through the cerebral aqueduct within the midbrain and passes into the rhombus-shaped fourth ventricle, where the choroid plexus adds more fluid. The fluid leaves the ven-

Table 10–1. Normal cerebrospinal-fluid findings.

Area	Appearance	Pressure (in mm of water)	Cells (per μL)	Protein	Miscellaneous
Lumbar	Clear and colorless	70–180	0–5	15–45 mg/dL	Glucose 50–75 mg/dL.
Ventricular	Clear and colorless	70–190	0–5 (lymphocytes)	5–15 mg/dL	Nonprotein nitrogen 10–35 mg/dL. Kahn and Wassermann (VDRL) tests negative.

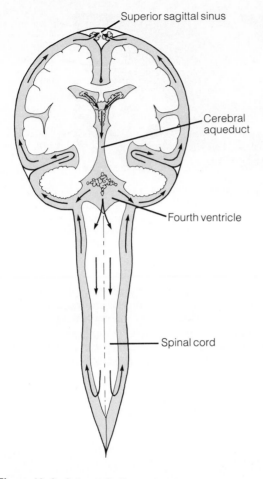

Figure 10-8. Schematic illustration, in a coronal projection, of the circulation (arrows) of cerebrospinal fluid.

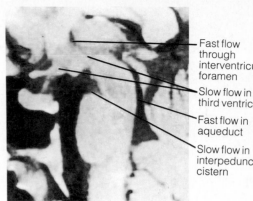

Figure 10-9. Magnetic resonance image of a midsagittal section through a normal head, demonstrating the fast flow of cerebrospinal fluid.

tricular system through the midline and lateral apertures of the fourth ventricle and enters the subarachnoid space. From here it may flow over the cerebral convexities or into the spinal subarachnoid spaces. Some of it is reabsorbed (by diffusion) into the small vessels in the pia or ventricular walls, and the remainder passes via the arachnoid villi into the venous blood (of sinuses or veins) in various areas—mostly over the superior convexity. A minimum pressure of cerebrospinal fluid must be present to maintain reabsorption. There exists, therefore, a continuous circulation of cerebrospinal fluid in and around the brain, in which production and reabsorption are in balance.

A clear concept of the route of the circulation through the ventricles into and through the subarachnoid spaces is of great practical and clinical importance. Magnetic resonance imaging can show that the flow of cerebrospinal fluid is faster

through (and just downstream from) narrow stretches in the pathway (Fig 10-9).

Clinical Correlations

Blocking the circulatory pathway of cerebrospinal fluid usually leads to dilatation of the ventricles upstream (hydrocephalus), since the production of fluid usually continues despite the obstruction (see Figs 10-10 through 10-14 and Table 10-2). There are 2 types of hydrocephalus: noncommunicating and communicating.

In **noncommunicating (obstructive) hydrocephalus,** which occurs more frequently than the other type, the cerebrospinal fluid of the ventricles cannot reach the subarachnoid space because there is obstruction of one or both interventricular foramens, the cerebral aqueduct (the most common site of obstruction, (Figs 10-9 and 10-10), or the outflow foramens of the fourth ventricle (median and lateral apertures). A block at any of these sites leads rapidly to dilatation of one or more ventricles. The production of cerebrospinal fluid continues, and in the acute obstruction phase, there may be a transependymal flow of cerebrospinal fluid. The gyri are flattened against the inside of the skull. If the skull is still pliable, as it is in most children under 2 years of age, the head may enlarge (Fig 10-11).

In **communicating hydrocephalus,** the obstruction is in the subarachnoid space and can be caused by the presence of blood or pus that blocks the return-flow channels or by an enlargement of the supratentorial compartment that closes off the incisura tentorii (Fig 10-14). If the intracranial pressure is raised because of excess cerebrospinal fluid (more production than reabsorption), the central canal of the spinal cord may dilate. In some pa-

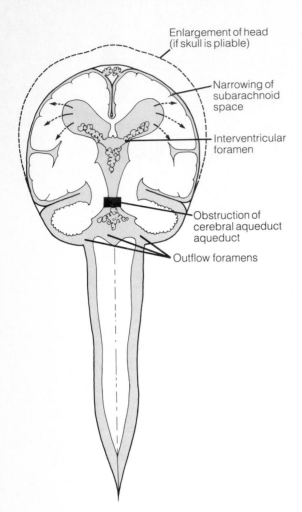

Figure 10-10. Schematic illustration of the effects of obstruction of the cerebral aqueduct causing noncommunicating hydrocephalus. Arrows indicate transependymal flow (compare with Fig 10–8). Other possible sites of obstruction are the interventricular foramen and the outflow foramens of the fourth ventricle.

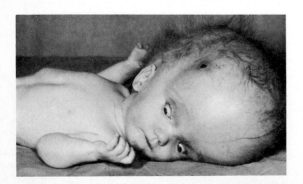

Figure 10-11. Hydrocephalus in a 14-month-old infant.

Figure 10-12. MR image of a midsagittal section through the head of a 3-year-old child with aqueductal stenosis (compare with Fig 1–4). The lateral ventricles are greatly dilated, and the third ventricle is moderately enlarged.

tients, the spaces filled by cerebrospinal fluid are uniformly enlarged without an increase in intracranial pressure. This **normal-pressure hydrocephalus,** may be caused by atrophy of the brain in the elderly (see Chapter 22) or have an uncertain origin (a lesion or trauma causing blood to be present in the subarachnoid space has been suggested).

Various procedures have been developed to by-

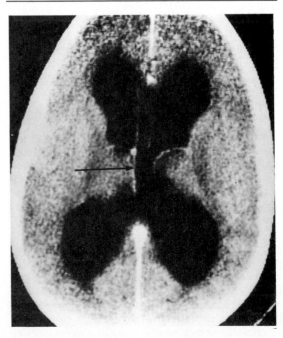

Figure 10-13. CT image of a horizontal section through the head of a 7-year-old child with noncommunicating hydrocephalus due to obstruction of the outflow foramens by a medullablastoma.

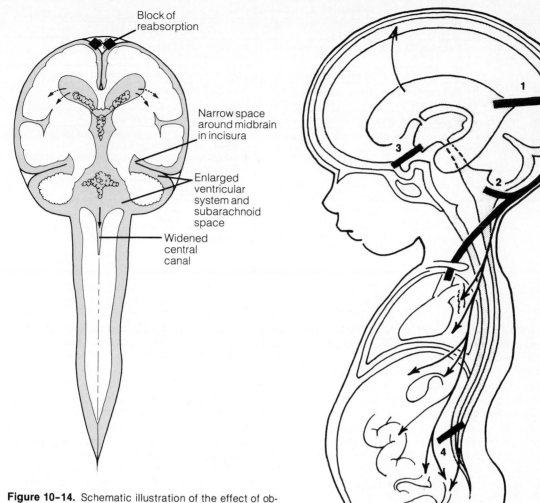

Figure 10–14. Schematic illustration of the effect of obstruction of reabsorption of cerebrospinal fluid causing communicating hydrocephalus. Arrows indicate transependymal flow (compare with Figs 10–8 and 10–10). Another possible site of obstruction is at the narrow space around the midbrain in the incisura.

Figure 10–15. Shunting procedures used to treat noncommunicating hydrocephalus. *1:* Ventriculocaval shunt. *2:* Ventriculocisternal shunt. *3:* Anterior ventriculostomy. *4:* Spinoperitoneal shunt. Lighter lines and arrows indicate other shunts.

pass the obstruction in noncommunicating hydrocephalus or to improve absorption in general. Examples of these shunts are shown in Fig 10–15.

BARRIERS IN THE NERVOUS SYSTEM

Several functionally important types of barriers exist in the nervous system, and all play a role in maintaining a constant environment within and around the brain, so that normal function continues and foreign or harmful substances are kept out. Some are readily visible, such as the 3 investing membranes (meninges), the dura, arachnoid and pia (see Chapter 5); others are distinct only

when examined with an ultramicroscope or electron microscope.

Blood-Brain Barrier

The blood-cerebrospinal-fluid barrier, the vascular endothelial barrier, and the arachnoid barrier together form the blood-brain barrier. This barrier is absent in several specialized regions of the brain: the basal hypothalamus, the pineal gland, the area postrema of the fourth ventricle, and several small

Table 10–2. Hydrocephalus.

Type	Cause	Effect
Non communicating (obstructive)	Obstruction of interventricular foramen	Enlargement of lateral ventricle
	Obstruction of cerebral aqueduct	Enlargement of lateral and third ventricles
	Obstruction of outflow foramens of fourth ventricle	Enlargement of all ventricles
	Sudden obstruction of any of the above	Transependymal flow of CSF
	Chronic obstruction of any of the above	Enlargement of head (if skull is still pliable); flattening of cerebral gyri Enlargement of all ventricles; widening of posterior fossa cisterns Enlargement of all ventricles; widening of all basal cisterns
Communicating	Obstruction of perimesencephalic cistern (occlusion of incisura tentorii)	Enlargement of all ventricles; widening of posterior fossa cisterns
	Obstruction of subarachnoid CSF flow over the cerebral convexities	Enlargement of all ventricles; widening of all basal cisterns

areas of the third ventricle. Highly permeable fenestrated capillaries are present in these regions.

A. Blood-Cerebrospinal-Fluid Barrier: About 60% of the cerebrospinal fluid is formed by active transport (through the membranes) from the blood vessels in the choroid plexus. Epithelial cells of the plexus, joined by tight junctions, form a continuous layer that selectively permits the passage of some substances but not others (see Chapter 11).

B. Vascular-Endothelial Barrier: Collectively, the blood vessels within the brain have a very large surface area that promotes the exchange of oxygen, CO_2, amino acids, and sugars between blood and brain. Because other substances are kept out, the chemical composition of the extracellular fluid of the nervous system differs markedly from that of cell plasma. The blocking function is achieved by tight junctions between endothelial cells. There is evidence that neither the processes of astrocytes nor the basal laminas of endothelial cells prevent diffusion, even for molecules as large as proteins.

C. Arachnoid Barrier: Blood vessels of the dura are far more permeable than those of the brain, but because the outermost layer of cells of the arachnoid forms a barrier, substances diffusing out of dural vessels do not enter the cerebrospinal fluid of the subarachnoidal space. The cells are joined by tight junctions, and their permeability characteristics are similar to those of the blood vessels of the brain itself.

Ependyma

The ependyma lining the cerebral ventricles is continuous with the epithelium of the choroid plexus (Fig 10–16). Except for the ependyma of the lower third ventricle, most ependymal cells do not have tight junctions and cannot prevent the movement of macromolecules between ventricles and brain tissue.

Blood-Nerve Barrier

Large nerves consist of bundles of axons embedded in an **epineurium.** Each bundle is surrounded by a layer of cells called the **perineurium;** connective tissue within each bundle is the **endoneurium.** Blood vessels of the epineurium, which are similar to those of the dura, are permeable to macromolecules but the endoneurial vessels, similar to those of the arachnoid, are not.

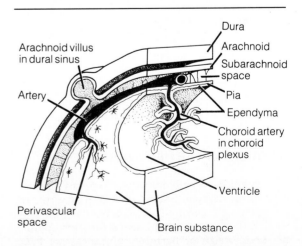

Figure 10–16. Schematic illustration of the relationships and the barriers between the brain, the meninges, and the vessels.

SKULL

The skull (cranium), which is rigid in adults but pliable in newborn infants, surrounds the brain and meninges completely and forms a strong mechanical protection. In adults, skull contents that increase beyond the capacity of the intact cranium can cause tonsillar herniation. Increased cranial pressure in infants may cause the fontanelles to bulge or the head to begin to enlarge abnormally (Fig 10–11).

The skull consists of 2 major portions: the **neurocranium,** which contains the brain and consists of the skull base and cap (**calvaria**); and the skeleton of the face, the **viscerocranium,** (Fig 10–17). The openings in the neurocranium and orbit will be discussed in this chapter.

Basal View of the Skull

The anterior portion of the base of the skull, the hard palate, projects below the level of the remainder of the inferior skull surface. The **choanae,** or posterior nasal apertures, are behind and above the hard palate. The pterygoid plates lie lateral to the choanae (Figs 10–18 and 10–19).

At the base of the lateral pterygoid plate is the **foramen ovale,** which transmits the third branch of the trigeminal nerve, the accessory meningeal artery, and (occasionally) the superficial petrosal nerve. Posterior to the foramen ovale is the **foramen spinosum,** which transmits the middle meningeal vessels. At the base of the styloid process is the

stylomastoid foramen, through which the facial nerve exits.

The **foramen lacerum** is a large irregular aperture at the base of the medial pterygoid plate. Its inferior portion is closed by a fibrocartilaginous plate above the auditory tube. Within its superior aspect is the **carotid canal.** The internal carotid artery, which emerges from this aperture, crosses only the superior part of the foramen lacerum.

Lateral to the foramen lacerum is a groove, the **sulcus tubae auditivae,** that contains the cartilaginous part of the **auditory (eustachian) tube.** It is continuous posteriorly with the canal in the temporal bone that forms the bony part of the auditory tube. Lateral to the groove is the lower orifice of the carotid canal, which transmits the internal carotid artery and the carotid plexus of the sympathetic nerves.

Behind the carotid canal is the large **jugular foramen,** which is formed by the petrous portion of the temporal and occipital bones and can be divided into 3 compartments. The anterior compartment contains the inferior petrosal sinus; the intermediate compartment contains the glossopharyngeal, vagus, and spinal accessory nerves; and the posterior compartment contains the sigmoid sinus and meningeal branches from the occipital and ascending pharyngeal arteries.

Posterior to the basilar portion of the occipital bone is the **foramen magnum,** which transmits the medulla and its membranes, the spinal accessory nerves, the vertebral arteries, the anterior and posterior spinal arteries, and ligaments connecting the occipital bone with the axis. The foramen magnum is bounded laterally by the **occipital condyles.**

Behind each condyle is the condyloid fossa, perforated on one or both sides by the **posterior condyloid canal** (which may transmit an emissary vein from the transverse sinus). Farther forward is the **anterior condylar canal,** or **hypoglossal canal,** which transmits the hypoglossal nerve and a meningeal artery.

Interior of the Skull

A. Calvaria: The inner surface of the calvaria (skullcap) is concave, with depressions for the convolutions of the cerebrum and numerous furrows for the branches of the meningeal vessels. Along the midline is a longitudinal groove, narrow anteriorly and posteriorly wide that contains the superior sagittal sinus. The margins of the groove provide attachment for the falx cerebri. There are several depressions on either side of the groove for the arachnoid granulations of the lateral lacunae. At the rear are the openings of the parietal emissary foramens (when these are present). The sutures of the calvaria (sagittal, coronal, lambdoid, and others) are meshed lines of union between adjacent skull bones.

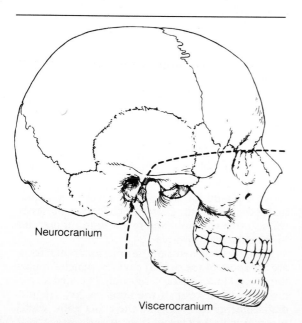

Neurocranium

Viscerocranium

Figure 10–17. Lateral view of the skull.

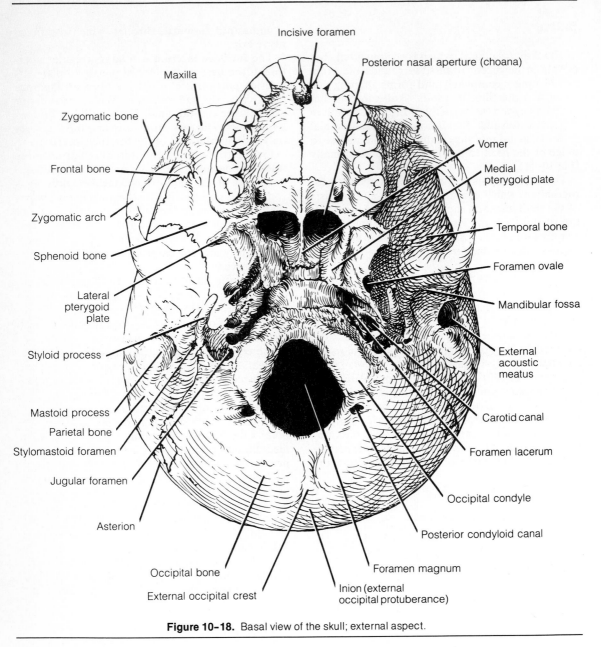

Figure 10–18. Basal view of the skull; external aspect.

B. Floor of the Cranial Cavity: The internal or superior surface of the skull base forms the floor of the cranial cavity (Figs 10–19 and 10–20; Table 10–3). It is divided into 3 fossae: anterior, middle, and posterior. The floor of the anterior fossa lies higher than the floor of the middle fossa, which in turn lies higher than the floor of the posterior fossa.

1. Anterior Cranial Fossa–The floor of this is formed by the orbital plates of the frontal bone, the cribriform plates of the ethmoid, and the lesser wings and anterior part of the sphenoid. It is limited at the rear by the posterior borders of the lesser wings of the sphenoid and by the anterior margins of the chiasmatic groove.

The lateral segments of the anterior cranial fossa are the roofs of the orbital cavities, which support the frontal lobes of the cerebrum. The medial segments form the roof of the nasal cavity. The medial segments lie alongside the **crista galli,** which together with the frontal crest affords attachment to the falx cerebri. A **foramen caecum** is usually

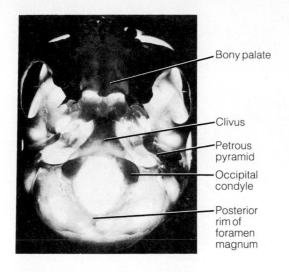

Figure 10-19. Basal view of transilluminated skull, showing areas of thick and thin bone.

Table 10-3. Structures passing through openings in the cranial floor.

Foramens	Structures
Cribriform plate of ethmoid	Olfactory nerves
Optic foramen	Optic nerve, ophthalmic artery, meninges
Superior orbital fissure	Oculomotor, trochlear, and abducens nerves; ophthalmic division of trigeminal nerve; superior ophthalmic vein
Foramen rotundum	Maxillary division of trigeminal nerve, small artery and vein
Foramen ovale	Mandibular division of trigeminal nerve, vein
Foramen lacerum	Internal carotid artery, sympathetic plexus
Foramen spinosum	Middle meningeal artery and vein
Internal acoustic meatus	Facial and vestibulocochlear nerves, internal auditory artery
Jugular foramen	Glossopharyngeal, vagus, and spinal accessory nerves; sigmoid sinus
Hypoglossal canal	Hypoglossal nerve
Foramen magnum	Medulla and meninges, spinal accessory nerve, vertebral arteries, anterior and posterior spinal arteries

present in front of the crista galli; it transmits an emissary vein that connects to the superior sagittal sinus.

The **cribriform plate** of the ethmoid bone lies on either side of the crista galli and supports the olfactory bulb. This plate is perforated by foramens for the olfactory nerves. Internal openings of the anterior and posterior ethmoidal foramens are in the

lateral wall of the olfactory groove. The cranial openings of the **optic canals** lie just behind the flat portion of the sphenoid bone (**planum sphenoidale**).

2. Middle Cranial Fossa—This is deeper than the anterior cranial fossa and is narrow centrally and wide peripherally. It is bounded at the front by the posterior margins of the lesser wings of the sphenoid and the anterior clinoid processes. It is bounded posteriorly, by the superior angles of the petrous portion of the temporal bones and by the dorsum sellae. It is bounded laterally by the temporal squamae and the greater wings of the sphenoid (Figs 10–20 and 10–21).

The narrow medial portion of the fossa presents the **chiasmatic groove** and the **tuberculum sellae** anteriorly; the chiasmatic groove ends on either side at the **optic canal,** which transmits the optic nerve and ophthalmic artery. Behind the optic canal, the **anterior clinoid process** is directed posteriorly and medially and provides attachment for the tentorium cerebelli. In back of the tuberculum sellae is a deep depression, the **sella turcica;** this contains the hypophyseal fossa in which the hypophysis (pituitary) lies. The sella turcica is

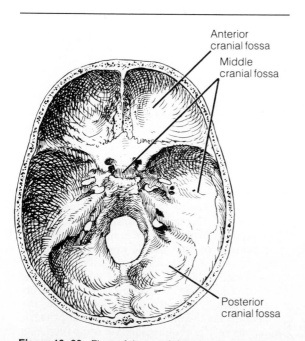

Figure 10-20. Floor of the cranial cavity; internal aspect.

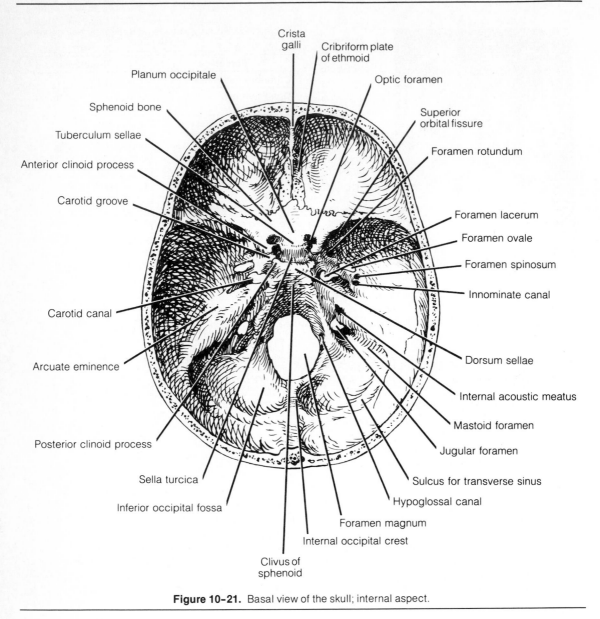

Figure 10–21. Basal view of the skull; internal aspect.

bounded posteriorly by a quadrilateral plate of bone, the **dorsum sellae,** whose sides project anteriorly as the **posterior clinoid processes.** These attach to slips of the tentorium cerebelli. Below each posterior clinoid process is a notch for the abducens nerve.

On either side of the sella turcica is the broad and shallow **carotid groove,** curving upward from the foramen lacerum to the medial side of the anterior clinoid process. This groove contains the internal carotid artery, surrounded by a plexus of sympathetic nerves.

The lateral segments of the middle fossa are deeper than its middle portion; they support the temporal lobes of the brain and show depressions that mark the convolutions of the brain. These segments are traversed by furrows for the anterior and posterior branches of the **middle meningeal vessels,** which pass through the **foramen spinosum.**

The **superior orbital fissure** is situated in the anterior portion of the middle cranial fossa. It is bounded above by the lesser wing, below by the greater wing, and in the middle by the body of the sphenoid. The superior orbital fissure transmits into the orbital cavity the oculomotor nerve, the trochlear nerve, the ophthalmic division of the trigeminal nerve, the abducens nerve, some filaments from the cavernous plexus of the sympathetic nerves, the ophthalmic veins, and the orbital branch of the middle meningeal artery.

The maxillary division of the trigeminal nerve passes through the **foramen rotundum,** which is located behind the medial wall of the superior orbital fissure. Behind the foramen rotundum is the **foramen of Vesalius,** which transmits an emissary vein or a cluster of small venules; it can be large, small, multiple, or absent in different skulls. The **foramen ovale,** which transmits the mandibular division of the trigeminal nerve, the accessory meningeal artery, and the lesser superficial petrosal nerve, is posterior and lateral to the foramen rotundum.

The **foramen lacerum** is medial to the foramen ovale. Its inferior segment is filled by fibrocartilage. Its superior segment transmits the internal carotid artery, which is surrounded by a plexus of sympathetic nerves. The anterior wall of the foramen lacerum is pierced by the pterygoid canal.

The **arcuate eminence,** which marks the position of the superior semicircular canal, lies on the upper surface of the petrous portion of the temporal bone. Medially, there is a groove leading to the hiatus of the facial canal for transmission of the greater petrosal nerve and the petrosal branch of the middle meningeal artery. There is, below, a smaller groove for passage of the lesser petrosal nerve, and near the apex of the petrous bone is the depression for the semicircular ganglion of V and for the irregular orifice of the carotid canal.

3. Posterior Cranial Fossa–This fossa is larger and deeper than the middle and anterior cranial fossae. It is formed by the occipital bone, the dorsum sellae and clivus of the sphenoid bone, and portions of the temporal and parietal bones (Figs 10–19 and 10–20).

The posterior fossa, or **infratentorial compartment,** contains the cerebellum, pons, medulla, and part of the midbrain. It is separated from the middle cranial fossa in and near the midline by the dorsum sellae of the sphenoid bone and on either side by the superior angle of the petrous portion of the temporal bone (**petrous pyramid**). This angle provides attachment for the tentorium cerebelli and is grooved for the superior petrosal sinus.

The **foramen magnum** lies in the center of the fossa. Just above the tubercle is the **anterior condylar canal,** or **hypoglossal canal,** which transmits the hypoglossal nerve and a meningeal branch for the ascending pharyngeal artery. In front of the foramen magnum, the basilar part of the occipital bone and the posterior part of the body of the sphenoid bone support the pons and the medulla. These bones are joined by a synchondrosis in young people. On either side, the petro-occipital fissure is continuous posteriorly with the jugular foramen. The margins of the petro-occipital fissure are grooved for the **inferior petrosal sinus.**

The **jugular foramen** lies between the lateral part of the occipital bone and the petrous portion of the temporal bone. The anterior portion of the foramen transmits the inferior petrosal sinus, the posterior portion transmits the transverse sinus and some meningeal branches from the occipital and ascending pharyngeal arteries, and the intermediate portion transmits the glossopharyngeal, vagus, and spinal accessory nerves.

Above the jugular foramen lies the **internal acoustic meatus** for the facial and acoustic nerves and the internal auditory artery. The inferior occipital fossae, which support the hemispheres of the cerebellum, are separated by the internal occipital crest, which serves for attachment of the falx cerebelli and contains the **occipital sinus.** The posterior fossae are surrounded by deep grooves for the **transverse sinuses.**

Clinical Correlations

Trauma to the skull can result in fractures. By itself, a fracture of the calvaria or the base is not a very serious problem; however, there are often complications. Fractures with meningeal tears can lead to leaks of cerebrospinal fluid and possibly intracranial infection; fractures with vascular tears can lead to extradural (epidural) hemorrhages, especially if branches of large meningeal arteries are torn; and depressed fractures can cause brain contusions with bleeding and tissue destruction. Contusion may also be present on the side opposite to the impact (contrecoup contusion), at a site where the brain has rubbed against bony edges such as the tip of the temporal lobe, the occipital pole, or the orbital surface of the frontal lobe, or where the corpus callosum and pericallosal artery have rubbed against the edge of the falx.

Infection (**osteomyelitis**), **Paget's disease (osteitis deformans),** or skull tumors can affect the skull. Chronic hypertrophic anterior osteitis, in which the squama of the frontal bone is abnormally thickened, is seen in about 5% of human skulls.

CASE 13

A 63-year-old unemployed man was brought to the hospital because he had a fever and was losing consciousness. His landlady stated that he had lost weight for several months and that had lately complained of fever, poor appetite, and cough. On the day of admission, he had been found in a stuporous state, and had felt hot to the touch.

During the general physical examination, the patient was uncooperative and thrashed about in bed. Findings included a rigid neck, a harsh systolic murmur heard along the left sternal margin, a body temperature of 40° C (104° F), and a pulse rate of 140.

The red blood count showed 3.8 million/μL, and the white blood count was 18,000/μ with 80% polymorphonuclear leukocytes. The blood glucose level was 120 mg/dL. Lumbar puncture results showed pressure, 300 mm of water; white blood count, 20,000/μL (with mostly polymorphonuclear leukocytes); glucose, 18 mg/dL; and protein, unknown (test results were lost). Gram's stain of the cerebrospinal fluid sediment revealed gram-positive rod-shaped diplococci (pneumococci).

What is the most likely diagnosis?

CASE 14

A 21-year-old right-handed motorcyclist was brought into the emergency room. He had been found lying unconscious without a helmet in the street, having apparently slipped going around a curve. From the position at the scene it appeared that his head had probably hit the curb. He had several facial abrasions and a swelling above his right ear. While in the emergency room he regained consciousness. He appeared dazed and complained of headache, but did not speak clearly.

Neurologic examination showed no papilledema. His pupils were equally round and reactive to light (PERRL), extraocular movements were normal, and there was questionable left facial weakness. There were no other neurologic deficits. Other findings included a blood pressure of 120/80 mg Hg, a pulse rate of 75/min, and a respiratory rate of 17/min.

What is the differential diagnosis at this time? What neuroradiologic or other diagnostic procedures are indicated?

The patient was kept under observation in the emergency room. Because of a sudden influx of emergency patients, however, repeat neurologic examination was not performed until several hours later. By that time, the patient had become stuporous, his right pupil was dilated, the blood pressure was 150/90 mg Hg, pulse rate 55/min, and respiratory rate 12/min. Emergency surgery was undertaken.

What is the most likely diagnosis?
Cases are discussed further in Chapter 24.

REFERENCES

Fishman RA: *Cerebrospinal Fluid in Diseases of the Nervous System.* Saunders, 1980.
Heimer L: *The Human Brain and Spinal Cord.* Springer-Verlag, 1983.
Rapoport SI: *Blood-Brain Barrier in Physiology and Medicine.* Raven, 1976.
Romanes GJ: *Cunningham's Textbook of Anatomy,* 12th ed. Oxford Univ Press, 1983.
Waddington MM: *Atlas of the Human Skull.* Academic Books, 1983.

Vascularization

11

About 18% of the total blood volume in the body circulates in the brain, which accounts for about 2% of the body weight. The blood transports oxygen, nutrients, and other substances necessary for proper functioning of the brain tissues and carries away metabolites. The brain uses about 20% of the oxygen absorbed in the lungs; the remainder goes to the rest of the body. A constant flow of oxygen must be maintained: loss of consciousness occurs in less than 1 minute after blood flow to the brain has stopped, and irreparable damage to the brain tissue occurs within 5 minutes.

Cerebral angiography is a commonly used neuroradiologic procedure that results in the visualization of cerebral arteries, precapillaries, veins and sinuses. Normal and abnormal angiograms are discussed in Chapter 22.

ARTERIAL SUPPLY OF THE BRAIN

Characteristics of the Cerebral Arteries

The **circulus arteriosus,** or **circle of Willis** (after the English neuroanatomist, Sir Thomas Willis), shows many variations between individuals. The posterior communicating arteries may be large on one or both sides (embryonic type); the posterior cerebral artery may be thin in its first stretch (embryonic type), and the anterior communicating artery may be absent, double, or thin. These variants of the circle (actually an irregular hexagon) make it difficult to predict whether functionally adequate anastomosis will readily occur in any given individual if a major supply vessel on one side suddenly becomes blocked. If some time has elapsed since the blockage, however, the circle may be able to supply blood to both sides.

The course of the large arteries (at least in their initial stretches) is largely ventral to the brain in a relatively small region. The arteries course in the subarachnoid space, often for a considerable distance, before entering the brain itself; rupture of a vessel thus may cause a subarachnoid hemorrhage.

Each major artery supplies a certain territory, separated by boundary zones (watershed areas) from other territories; sudden occlusion in a vessel affects its territory immediately, sometimes irreversibly. Often, a superficial layer of cortex receives blood from the meningeal arteries and thus survives, but in isolation.

Principal Arteries

The arterial blood for the brain enters the cranial cavity by way of 2 pairs of large vessels (Figs 11-1 and 11-2): the internal carotid arteries, which branch off the common carotids; and the **vertebral arteries,** which come from the subclavian arteries. The vertebral arterial system supplies the brain stem, cerebellum, occipital lobe, and parts of the thalamus, while the carotids normally supply the remainder of the forebrain. The carotids are interconnected via the **anterior cerebral arteries** and the **anterior communicating artery;** the carotids are also connected to the **posterior cerebral arteries** of the vertebral system by way of 2 **posterior communicating arteries,** part of the circle of Willis.

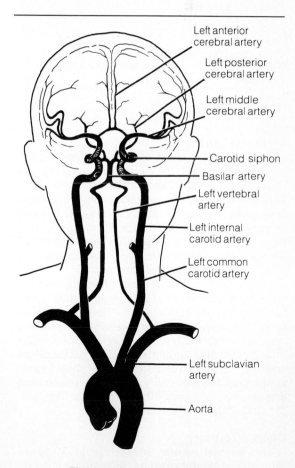

Figure 11-1. Cerebral arteries.

Left anterior cerebral artery

Left posterior cerebral artery

Left middle cerebral artery

Carotid siphon

Basilar artery

Left vertebral artery

Left internal carotid artery

Left common carotid artery

Left subclavian artery

Aorta

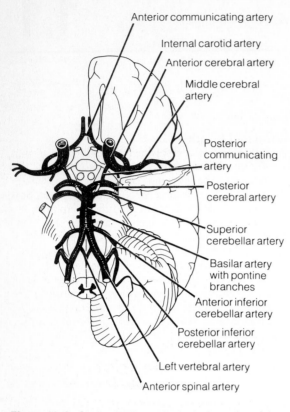

Anterior communicating artery

Internal carotid artery

Anterior cerebral artery

Middle cerebral artery

Posterior communicating artery

Posterior cerebral artery

Superior cerebellar artery

Basilar artery with pontine branches

Anterior inferior cerebellar artery

Posterior inferior cerebellar artery

Left vertebral artery

Anterior spinal artery

Figure 11-2. Circle of Willis and principal arteries of the brain stem.

Vertebral Territory

After passing through the foramen magnum in the base of the skull, the 2 vertebral arteries form a single midline vessel, the **basilar artery** (see Figs 11-2 and 6-11); this vessel terminates in the interpeduncular cistern in a bifurcation as the left and right posterior cerebral arteries. These may be thin, large, or asymmetric, depending on retention of the embryonic pattern (in which the carotid supplies the posterior cerebral arteries).

Several pairs of small circumferential arteries arise from the vertebral arteries and their fused continuation, the basilar artery. These are the **posterior** and **anterior inferior cerebellar arteries,** the **superior cerebellar arteries,** and several smaller branches, such as the **pontine** and **internal auditory arteries.** All these vessels can show considerable asymmetry and variability. The small **penetrating arteries,** which branch off the basilar artery, supply vital centers in the brain stem.

Carotid Territory

The **internal carotid artery** (Fig 11-3) passes through the **carotid canal** of the skull, then curves forward within the cavernous sinus and up and

backward through the dura, forming the **carotid siphon** before reaching the brain. The first branch is usually the **ophthalmic artery.** In addition to their links with the vertebral system, the carotids branch into a large middle and a smaller anterior cerebral artery on each side (Fig 11-4). The 2 anterior cerebral arteries usually meet over a short distance in midplane to form a short but functionally important anterior communicating artery. This vessel forms a link in the anastomoses between the left and right hemisphere, which is especially important when one internal carotid becomes occluded. The **anterior choroidal artery** (Fig 11-5), directly off the internal carotid, carries blood to the choroid plexus of the lateral ventricles as well as to several adjacent brain structures.

Cortical Supply

The middle cerebral artery supplies many deep structures and much of the lateral aspect of the cerebrum; it breaks up into several large branches that course in the depth of the lateral fissure, over the insula, before reaching the convexity of the hemisphere. The anterior cerebral artery and its branches course around the genu of the corpus callosum to supply the anterior frontal lobe and the medial aspect of the hemisphere; they extend quite far to the rear. The posterior cerebral artery curves around the brain stem, supplying mainly the occipital lobe and the choroid plexuses of the third and lateral ventricles and the lower surface of the temporal lobe (Figs 11-6 and 11-7).

Cerebral Blood Flow & Autoregulation

Many physiologic and pathologic factors can affect the blood flow in the arteries and veins of the brain (see Table 11-1). Under normal conditions of autonomic regulation, the pressure in the small cerebral arteries is maintained at 450 mm of water. This ensures adequate perfusion of the cerebral capillary beds despite changes in systemic blood pressure. Increased activity in one cortical area is usually accompanied by a shift in blood volume to that area.

VENOUS DRAINAGE

Types of Channels

The venous drainage of the brain and coverings (Figs 11-8 and 11-9) includes the veins of the brain itself, the dural **venous sinuses,** the dura's **meningeal veins,** and the **diploic veins** between the tables of the skull. Communication exists between most of these channels. Unlike systemic veins, cerebral veins have no valves and seldom accompany the corresponding cerebral arteries.

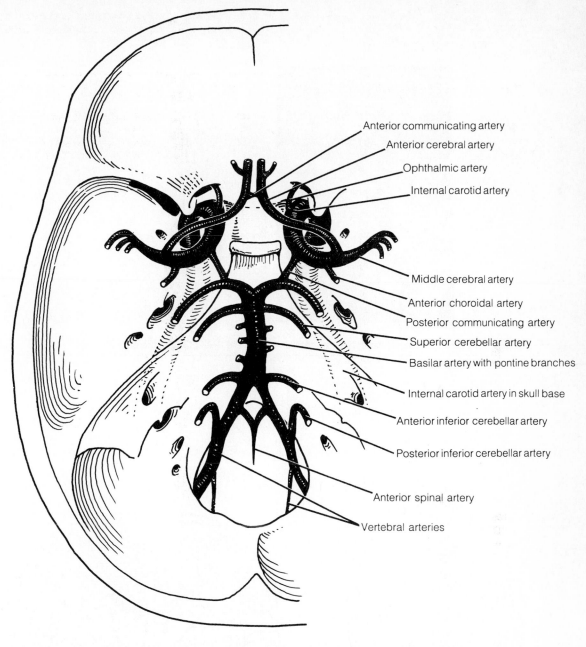

Figure 11-3. Principal arteries on the floor of the cranial cavity (brain removed).

Internal Drainage

The interior of the cerebrum drains into the single midline **great cerebral vein** (of **Galen**), which lies beneath the splenium of the corpus callosum. The internal cerebral veins (with their tributaries, the **septal, thalamostriate,** and **choroidal** veins) empty into this vein, as do the basal veins (of Rosenthal), which wind (one right and one left) around the side of the midbrain, draining the base of the forebrain. The precentral vein from the cerebellum and veins from the upper brain stem also empty into the great vein, which turns upward behind the splenium and joins the inferior sagittal sinus to form the **straight sinus.** The venous drainage of the base of the cerebrum is also into the deep middle cerebral vein (coursing in the lateral fissure) and then to the **cavernous sinus.**

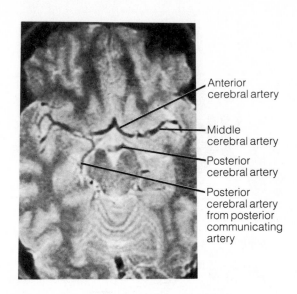

Figure 11–4. MR image of a horizontal section at the level of the circle of Willis.

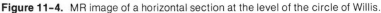

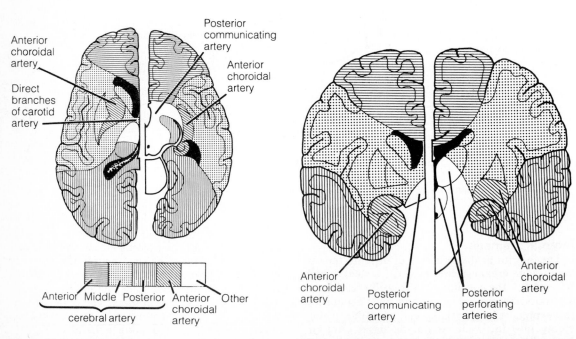

Figure 11–5. Horizontal sections through the cerebrum at 2 levels to show arterial supply.

Figure 11–6. Coronal section through the cerebrum at 2 levels to show major arterial supply.

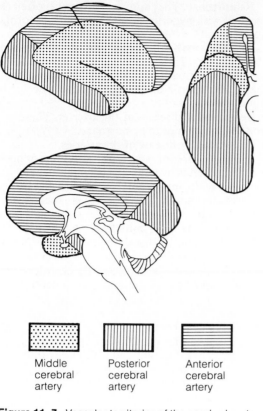

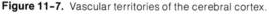

Middle cerebral artery

Posterior cerebral artery

Anterior cerebral artery

Figure 11-7. Vascular territories of the cerebral cortex.

Table 11-1. Factors affecting brain blood flow.

Factor	Increases Flow	Decreases Flow
Physiologic		
Carotid sinus pressure	Higher	Lower
CO$_2$ in blood	Raised	Lowered
O$_2$ in blood	Lowered	Raised
Sympathetic stimulation	Decreased	Increased
Cerebro-vascular tone (auto-nomic ner-vous system)	Dilatation	Constriction
CSF pressure	Decreased	Increased
Mean arterial minus ve-nous blood pressure	Raised	Lowered
Pathologic		
Pathologic changes	Hemangionma	Arteriosclerosis
Anomalies	Arteriovenous malformation	
Drugs	Vasodilation	Vasoconstriction
Other		
	Anemia	Polycythemia
	Hyperthyroidism	Hypothyroidism

Cortical Veins

Venous drainage of the brain surface is generally into the nearest large vein or sinus, from there to the confluence of the sinuses (see Fig 11–8), and ultimately to the **internal jugular vein.**

The veins of the cerebral convex surfaces are divided into superior and inferior groups. The 6–12 **superior cerebral veins** run upward on the hemisphere's surface to the superior sagittal sinus, generally passing under any lateral lacunae. Most of the **inferior cerebral veins** end in the superficial middle cerebral vein. The inferior cerebral veins that do not end in this fashion terminate in the transverse sinus. **Anastomotic veins** can be found; these connect the deep middle cerebral vein with the superior sagittal sinus or transverse sinus.

Venous Sinuses

Venous channels lined by mesothelium lie between the inner and outer layers of the dura; they are called intradural (or dural) sinuses. Their tributaries come mostly from the neighboring brain substance. All sinuses ultimately drain into the internal jugular veins or **pterygoid plexus.** The

sinuses may also communicate with extracranial veins via the **emissary veins.** These latter veins are important because the blood can flow through them in either direction, and because infections of the scalp may extend by this route into the intracranial structures.

Of the venous sinuses, the following are considered most important:

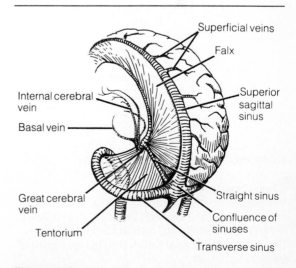

Figure 11-8. Veins and sinuses of the brain, left posterior-lateral view.

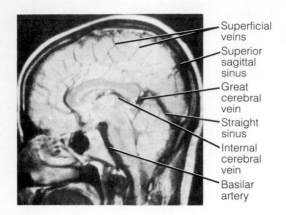

Figure 11-9. MR image (long time sequence; see Chapter 22) of a midsagittal section through the head showing venous channels.

Superficial veins
Superior sagittal sinus
Great cerebral vein
Straight sinus
Internal cerebral vein
Basilar artery

Superior sagittal sinus: Between the falx and the inside of the skullcap.

Inferior sagittal sinus: In the free edge of the falx.

Straight sinus: In the seam between the falx and the tentorium.

Transverse sinuses: Between the tentorium and its attachment on the skullcap.

Sigmoid sinuses: S-curved continuations of the transverse sinuses into the jugular veins. A transverse and a sigmoid sinus together form a lateral sinus.

Sphenoparietal sinuses: Drain the deep middle cerebral veins into the cavernous sinuses.

Cavernous sinuses: On either side of the sella turcica.

Inferior petrosal sinuses: From the cavernous sinus to the jugular foramen.

Superior petrosal sinus: From the cavernous sinus to the beginning of the sigmoid sinus.

The pressure of the cerebrospinal fluid (CSF) varies directly with acute changes in venous pressure. The Queckenstedt test is used with lumbar-puncture manometry to determine whether CSF block is present (see Chapter 5).

CEREBROVASCULAR DISORDERS

Classification

Diseases involving vessels of the brain and its coverings can be classified (Table 11–2) as follows:

Occlusive disorders. These are arterial or venous thrombosis that lead to infarction (tissue death) of parts of the brain.

Transient cerebral ischemia. This can occur without infarction.

Hemorrhage. The rupture of a vessel is often associated with hypertension or vascular malformations.

Vascular malformations and developmental abnormalities. These include aneurysms or arteriovenous malformations, which can lead to hemorrhage. Hypoplasia or absence of vessels occurs in some brains.

Degenerative diseases of the arteries. These can lead to occlusion or to hemorrhage.

Inflammatory disease of the arteries.

The acute onset of most types of infarcts or hemorrhages—cerebrovascular accidents—usually associated with intracranial vascular disease or abnormality can lead to sudden severe focal disturbance of brain function (hemiplegia, unconsciousness, etc). The term **apoplexy,** or **stroke,** is a general one, and further determination of the site and type of the lesion is needed for correct diagnosis and treatment. Cerebrovascular disorders constitute the third most common cause of death in the USA.

Occlusive Disorders

Insufficient blood supply to portions of the brain leads to infarction and swelling, with necrosis of brain tissue (Figs 11–10 through 11–13, Table 11–2). If an infarcted area is later perfused with blood, it becomes a red, or hemorrhagic, infarct; if not, it remains a pale, or white, infarct. Most infarcts are caused by **atherosclerosis** of the vessels, leading to narrowing or to occlusion or **thrombosis;** a **cerebral embolism,** ie, occlusion caused by an **embolus** (a plug of tissue or a foreign substance) from outside the brain; or other conditions such as prolonged hypotension, drug action, spasm, or inflammations of the vessels. Venous infarction may occur when a venous channel becomes occluded.

The extent of an infarct depends on the presence or absence of adequate anastomotic channels. Capillaries from adjacent vascular territories and

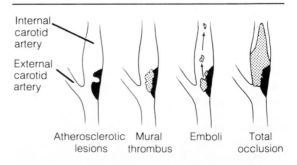

Internal carotid artery
External carotid artery

Atherosclerotic lesions Mural thrombus Emboli Total occlusion

Figure 11-10. Schematic illustration of stages of occlusion of the internal carotid artery. (Modified and reproduced, with permission, from Escourolle R, Poirier J: *Manual of Basic Neuropathology.* Saunders, 1971.)

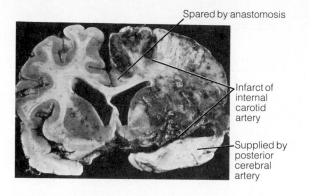
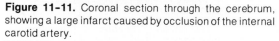

Spared by anastomosis

Infarct of internal carotid artery

Supplied by posterior cerebral artery

Figure 11-11. Coronal section through the cerebrum, showing a large infarct caused by occlusion of the internal carotid artery.

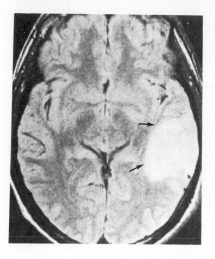

Figure 11-13. MR image of a coronal section of the head, showing an infarct (arrows) caused by occlusion of a branch of the middle cerebral artery.

corticomeningeal capillaries at the surface may reduce the size of the infarct. Although sudden occlusion can lead to irreparable damage, slowly developing local ischemia may be compensated for by extensive anastomoses through one or more routes: the circle of Willis; the ophthalmic artery, whose branches communicate with external carotid vessels; or corticomeningeal anastomoses from meningeal vessels.

Atherosclerosis of the Brain

The principal pathologic change in the arteries of the brain occurs in the vasculature of the neck and brain, although similar changes may be present in other systemic vessels also. The disease is progressive; it is considered by many to be a normal manifestation of the aging process in humans. Disturbances in metabolism—especially of fats—are believed to be a prominent associated change.

Atheromatous changes in the arterial system are found relatively frequently at postmortem examination of the bodies of people who have reached middle age (Fig 11-14). Vessels of all sizes may be

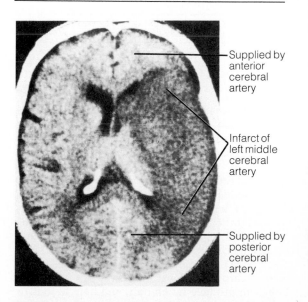

Supplied by anterior cerebral artery

Infarct of left middle cerebral artery

Supplied by posterior cerebral artery

Figure 11-12. CT image of a horizontal section of the head, showing an infarct caused by middle cerebral artery occlusion (compare with Fig 11-5).

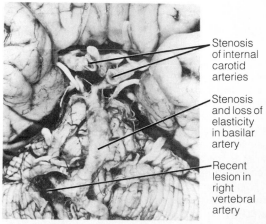

Stenosis of internal carotid arteries

Stenosis and loss of elasticity in basilar artery

Recent lesion in right vertebral artery

Figure 11-14. Atherosclerosis in arteries at the base of the brain.

Table 11-2. Diagnosis of cerebrovascular disorders.

	Intracerebral Hemorrhage	Cerebral Thrombosis Infarct	Cerebral Embolism	Subarachnoid Hemorrhage	Arterio-venous Malformation plus Bleeding	Subdural Hemorrhage	Epidural Hemorrhage
Onset	Generally during activity. Severe headache.	Prodromal episodes of dizziness, aphasia, etc. Transient ischemic attacks with reversible ischemic neurologic deficits.	Usually within seconds or minutes.	Sudden severe headache; possible loss of consciousness.	Sudden stroke in young patient.	Gradual, after minimal trauma.	Abrupt, with severe trauma.
Course	Rapid hemiplegia and other signs and symptoms.	Gradual progression over minutes to hours.	Rapid improvement may occur; patient usually conscious.	Variable; may recur.	Most critical period usually early; patient conscious.	Variable; may progress to coma.	Rapid deterioration; progression from lucid interval to coma.
Special findings	Cardiac hypertrophy; hypertensive retinopathy.	Arteriosclerotic cardiovascular disease frequently present.	Cardiac arrhythmias or infarction (source of emboli usually in heart).	Aneurysms, eg, subhyaloid (preretinal); nuchal rigidity.	Subhyaloid hemorrhages and retinal angioma.	Trauma, bruises.	Severe trauma.
Blood pressure	Severe hypertension.	Hypertension often.	Normal.	Hypertension often.	Normal.	Normal at first.	Normal at first.
CT scan findings	Increased density; possibly blood in ventricles.	In acute phase, less dense avascular area.	In acute phase, less dense avascular area; later changes.	Increased density in basal cisterns.	Abnormal areas; dense cisterns.	Dense (later, lighter) zone (high over convexity).	Dense segment under skull fracture (low over convexity).
MR image	High intensity in characteristic locations.						
CSF	May be bloody.	Clear.	Clear.	Grossly bloody.	Grossly bloody.	May be bloody.	Clear.

affected. A combination of degenerative and proliferative changes can be seen microscopically. The muscularis is the main site of proliferation; the intima may be absent. Disseminated areas of softening of the brain (infarcts) are frequently found.

Frequently the areas most often involved are near branchings or confluences of vessels (Fig 11–15). The most common and severe atherosclerotic lesions are in the carotid bifurcation. Others occur at the origin of the vertebral arteries and in the upper and lower parts of the basilar artery as well as in the internal carotid artery at its trifurcation, the first third of the middle cerebral artery, and the first part of the posterior cerebral artery. Narrowing of vessels severe enough to cause vascular insufficiency can be present in young adulthood, but it is more often present in older persons.

Complete occlusion by atheromatous plaques leads to infarction and the associated infarction and swelling of adjacent areas. There is no specific cure for this disease.

Cerebral Embolism

The sudden occlusion of a brain vessel by a blood clot, a piece of fat, a tumor, a clump of bacteria, another substance—or air—interrupts the blood supply to a portion of the brain abruptly and results in necrosis or infarction (see Fig 11–12 and Table 11–3). A common cause of cerebral embolism is chronic endocarditis. Fracture of a long bone can produce fat emboli, and lung lesions or cuts in large superficial veins can cause an air embolism.

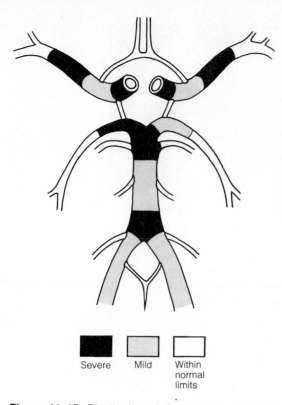

| Severe | Mild | Within normal limits |

Figure 11-15. Distribution of degenerative lesions in large cerebral arteries of the circle of Willis. The severity of the lesions is illustrated by the intensity of the shaded areas, with the darkest areas showing the most severe lesions.

Transient Cerebral Ischemia

Focal cerebral ischemic attacks, especially in middle-aged and older persons, may be caused by transient occlusion of an already narrow vessel. The cause is thought to be a vasospasm, a small embolus that is later carried away, or thrombosis of a diseased vessel (and subsequent anastomosis). Such **transient ischemic attacks (TIAs)** result in reversible ischemic neurologic deficits such as sudden dizziness or weakness, loss of cranial nerve function, or even brief loss of consciousness. These attacks are considered warning signs of future—or imminent—occlusion.

Hypertensive Hemorrhage

Chronic high blood pressure may result in the formation of small areas of vessel distention—**microaneurysms**—mostly in small arteries that arise from much larger vessels. A further rise in blood pressure then ruptures these aneurysms, resulting in an **intracerebral hemorrhage** (see Figure 11-16 and Table 11-2). In order of frequency, the most common sites are the lentiform nucleus, especially the putamen (Fig 11-17), supplied by the lenticulostriate arteries; the thalamus (Fig 11-18), supplied by posterior perforating arteries off the posterior cerebral-basilar artery bifurcation; the pons, supplied by small perforating arteries from the basilar artery; and the cerebellum, supplied by branches of the cerebellar arteries. Such hemorrhages may remain small and become cystic defects, or they may break through into adjacent structures or spaces.

Subarachnoid Hemorrhage

Often seen in normotensive persons, subarachnoid hemorrhages (Figs 11-19 through 11-21; see

Table 11-3. Frequency distribution (in %) of arterial lesions causing cerebrovascular insufficiency.*

Lesion	Left	Right
Stenosis		
Brachiocephalic	—	4
Internal carotid (near bifurcation)	34	34
Anterior cerebral	3	3
Proximal vertebral	22	18
Distal vertebral	4	5
Occlusion		
Brachiocephalic	—	1
Internal carotid (near bifurcation)	8	8
Anterior cerebral	2	1
Posterior vertebral	5	4
Distal vertebal	3	3

*Figures based on Hass WK et al: Joint study of extracranial arterial occlusion. *JAMA* 1968;**203**:916.

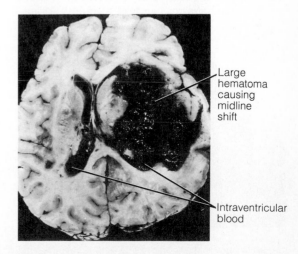

Large hematoma causing midline shift

Intraventricular blood

Figure 11-16. Horizontal section through the head, showing a large intracerebral hematoma.

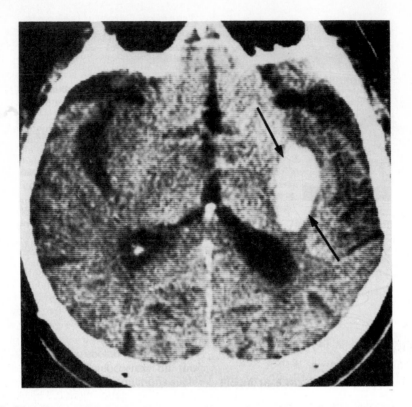

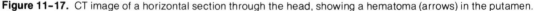

Figure 11-17. CT image of a horizontal section through the head, showing a hematoma (arrows) in the putamen.

also Table 11–2) derive from ruptured aneurysms or vascular malformations. Aneurysms (abnormal distention of local vessels) may be congenital (**berry aneurysm**) or the result of infection (**mycotic aneurysm**). Loss of elasticity because of atherosclerosis (**tubular aneurysm**) may be a contributing factor. One complication of subarachnoid hemorrhage, arterial spasm, can lead to infarct forma-

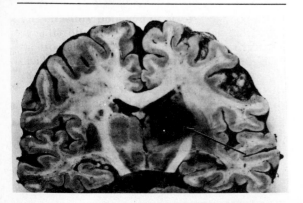

Figure 11-18. Thalamic hemorrhage in the right posterior thalamus and internal capsule in a 64-year-old woman.

tion. Venous aneurysms (eg, of the great cerebral vein) may be present in childhood.

Congenital berry aneurysms are seen most frequently in the circle of Willis or in the middle cerebral trifurcation; aneurysms are seen infrequently in vessels of the posterior fossa. A ruptured aneurysm generally bleeds into the subarachnoid space or, less frequently, into the brain substance itself.

Vascular malformations, especially arteriovenous malformations (AVMs), often occur in younger persons and are found on the surface of the brain, deep in the brain substance, or in the meninges (dural arteriovenous malformations). Bleeding from such malformations can be intracerebral, subarachnoid, or subdural. In some cases, the size of the malformation can be reduced by introducing coagulative emboli (via a catheter) into one or more of the feeder arteries prior to neurosurgical treatment.

Subdural Hemorrhage

Tearing of the bridging veins between brain surface and dural sinus is the most frequent cause of subdural hemorrhage (Figs 11–22 through 11–24; see also Table 11–2). Often it occurs as the result of a relatively minor trauma, and some blood may be present in the subarachnoid space. Children (be-

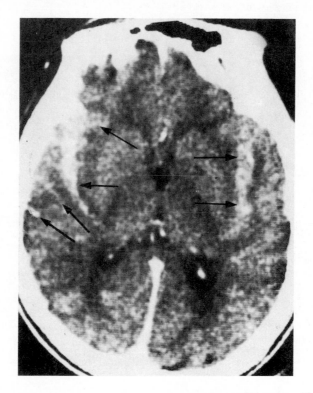

Figure 11-19. CT image of a horizontal section through the head, showing high densities, representing a subarachnoid hemorrhage (arrows), in the sulci.

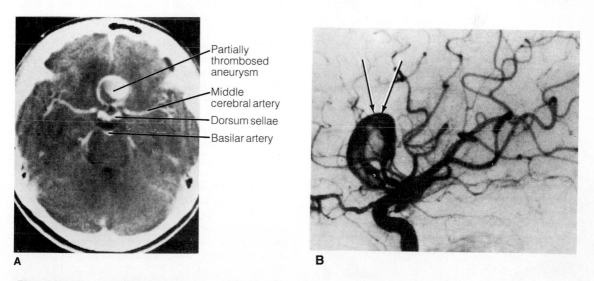

Partially
thrombosed
aneurysm

Middle
cerebral artery

Dorsum sellae

Basilar artery

A

B

Figure 11-20. *A:* CT image of a horizontal section through the head, showing a large aneurysm of the anterior communicating artery. (Reproduced, with permission, from deGroot J: *Correlative Neuroanatomy of Computed Tomography and Magnetic Resonance Imaging,* Lea & Febiger, 1984.) *B:* Corresponding angiogram showing the partially thrombosed aneurysm (arrows).

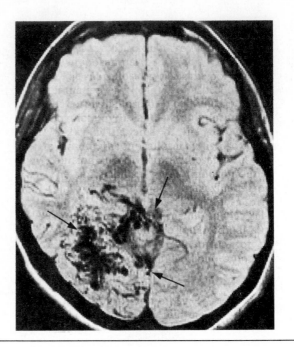

Figure 11-21. MR image of a horizontal section through the head, demonstrating an arteriovenous malformation (arrows).

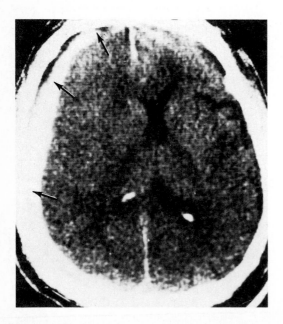

Figure 11-22. CT image of a horizontal section through the head, showing a right subdural hematoma (arrows) causing a shift away from the lesion.

cause they have thinner veins) and adults with brain atrophy (because they have longer bridging veins) are at greatest risk. The bleeding may recur; the subdural blood may be reabsorbed or it may become encapsulated or even calcified.

Epidural Hemorrhage

Bleeding from a torn meningeal vessel (usually an artery) may lead to an extradural (outside the dura) accumulation of blood. Severe trauma and fracture of the skull often cause this type of epidural, or extradural, hemorrhage (Figs 11–25 and 11–26; Table 11–2). Uncontrolled arterial bleeding may lead to compression of the brain and subsequent herniation.

Arteriovenous Shunts

Trauma can cause the rupture of adjacent vessels, allowing arterial blood to flow into nearby veins. For example, in a **carotid-cavernous fistula,** the internal carotid drains into the cavernous sinus and jugular vein, causing ischemia in the cerebral arteries.

Interventional methods, such as inserting a balloon into the shunt via a catheter or surgery, are usually required to correct the problem. Spontaneous correction has occurred occasionally after long

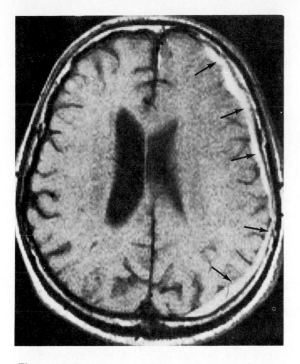

Figure 11–23. MR image of a horizontal section through the head, showing a left subdural hematoma (arrows) causing a midline shift.

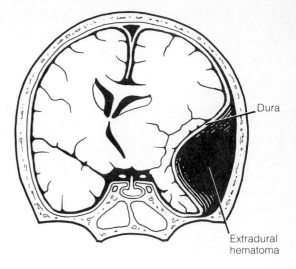

Figure 11–25. Schematic illustration of a epidural hemorrhage.

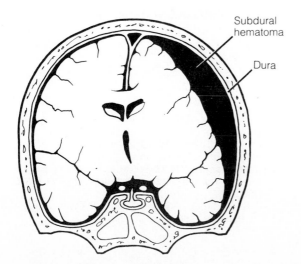

Figure 11–24. Schematic illustration of a subdural hemorrhage.

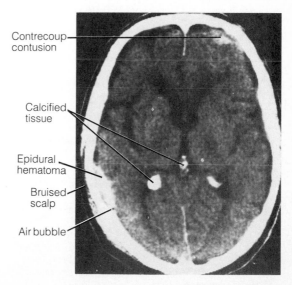

Figure 11–26. CT image of a horizontal section through the head, showing an extradural hematoma and intracerebral contrecoup lesion. (Reproduced, with permission, from deGroot J: *Correlative Neuroanatomy of Computed Tomography and Magnetic Resonance Imaging.* Lea & Febiger, 1984.)

air flights, presumably because of pressure changes.

CASE 15

A 44-year-old woman was admitted after having a seizure. She was lethargic, with a right facial droop, right hemiparesis, and right hyperreflexia. She complained of headache and a painful neck. A few days later, she seemed slightly more alert and made purposeful movements with her left hand— but not her right hand. She was still unresponsive to spoken commands and had a rigid neck. Other findings included bilateral papilledema, a right pupil that was smaller than the left, incomplete extraocular movements on the right side (nerve VI function was normal), decreased right corneal reflex, and right nasolabial droop. The patient's right arm was hypertonic and paretic, but the other extremities were normal. All reflexes appeared within normal range but were slightly higher on the left. The left plantar extensor response was equivocal, but the right was normal.

The blood pressure was 120/85; pulse rate 60; and temperature 38°C (100.4°F). The white blood count was 11,200/μl, and the erythrocyte sedimentation rate was 30 mm/h.

Where is the lesion? What is the cause of the lesion? What is the differential diagnosis?

A CT scan showed a high-density area in the cisterns, especially on the right side. What is the diagnosis now? Would you request a lumbar puncture with analysis of the cerebrospinal fluid?

CASE 16

A 55-year-old salesman exhibiting signs of confusion was brought to the hospital. The history gathered from his landlady disclosed that he had been separated from his family because he drank too much. Although he was apparently in good health, his landlady had entered the apartment on the day of admission because he did not respond to her calls. She found him lying on the floor, incontinent of urine and appearing bewildered; he had also bitten his lip. The landlady remembered that 2 months earlier he had been involved in a fight in a bar; 3 weeks previously he had fractured his wrist falling down stairs.

On examination, the patient was unconcerned, disheveled, and dirty. Bruises on his head and legs were consistent with recent trauma from a fall. The liver was palpable 4 cm below the right costal margin. The patient appeared to fall asleep when left alone. Neurologic examination showed normal optic fundi, normal extraocular movements, and no abnormalities that would result from dysfunction of other cranial nerves. When the left hand was extended, it showed a slow downward drift. The reflexes were normal and symmetric, and there was a left-sided plantar extensor response.

Vital signs, complete blood count, and urinalysis were within normal limits. A lumbar puncture showed an opening pressure of 180 mm of water, xanthochromia, a protein level of 80 mg/dL, and a glucose level of 70 mg/dL. Cell counts in all tubes showed red blood cells, 800/μL; lymphocytes, 20/μL; and polymorphonuclear neutrophils, 4/μL. A CT scan of the head was obtained.

Over the next 36 hours, the patient became deeply obtunded and seemed to develop a left-sided hemiparesis.

What is the differential diagnosis? What is the most likely diagnosis?

Questions and answers pertaining to Section III (Chapters 6–11) can be found in Appendix D.

Cases are discussed further in Chapter 24.

REFERENCES

Barnett HJ et al: *Pathophysiology, Diagnosis, and Management.* Churchill Livingston, 1985.

Fisher CM: Lacunar strokes and infarcts: A review. *Neurology* 1982;**32**:871–876.

Garcia JH: Circulatory disorders and their effects on the brain. In *Textbook of Pathology,* 2nd ed. Davis RL, Robertson DM (editors). Williams & Wilkins, 1990.

Meyer JS (editor): *Modern Concepts of Cerebrovascular Disease.* Sepctrum, 1975.

Ross Russell RW (editor): *Vascular Disease of the Central Nervous System,* 2nd ed. Churchill Livingston, Edinburg, 1983.

Salamon G: *Atlas of the Arteries of the Human Brain.* Sandoz, 1973.

Stephens RB, Stilwell DL: *Arteries and Veins of the Human Brain.* Thomas, 1969.

Thomas DJ, Bannister R: Preservation of autoregulation of cerebral flow in autonomic failure. *J Neurol Sci* 1980;**44**:205.

Wood JH (editor): *Neurobiology of Cerebrospinal Fluid.* Plenum, 1980.

Section IV.
Functional Systems

Control of Movement

12

CONTROL OF MOVEMENT

Evolution of Movement

Movement (motion) is a fundamental property of animal life. In simple, unicellular animals, motion and locomotion (movement from one place to another) depend upon the contractility of protoplasm and the action of accessory organs: cilia, flagella, and so forth. Rudimentary multicellular animals possess primitive neuromuscular mechanisms; in more advanced forms of animal life, motion is based upon the transmission of impulses from a receptor through an afferent neuron and ganglion cell to muscle. This same arrangement is found in the reflex arc of higher animals, including humans, in whom the spinal cord has further developed into a central regulating mechanism. The brain is concerned with the initiation of movement and the integration of complex motions.

Control of Movement in Humans

The motor system controls a complex neuromuscular organism. Commands must be sent to many muscles (sometimes dozens), and several ipsilateral and contralateral joints must also be stabilized. The motor system includes cortical and subcortical areas of gray matter; the corticobulbar, corticospinal, corticopontine, rubrospinal, reticulospinal, vestibulospinal, and tectospinal descending tracts; gray matter of the spinal cord; efferent nerves; and input from the cerebellum and basal ganglia (Fig 12-1). Continuous feedback from sensory systems and cerebellar afferents further influences the motor system. The muscles that produce movement do not function continuously; they require an adequate blood supply and replenishment of glucose as they tire.

The motor system does not function in a mechanical, robotlike fashion, but dynamically, in a highly complex interaction of the afferent, efferent, metabolic, and autonomic systems. (Some aspects of motor control are, in fact, still poorly understood.)

A. Hierarchy: Movement is organized in increasingly complex and hierarchical levels.

Reflexes are controlled at the spinal or higher levels (Table 12-1; see also Chapter 4).

Stereotypical repetitive movements such as walking or swimming are governed by neural networks that include the spinal cord, brain stem, and cerebellum. Normal walking movement can be elicited in experimental animals even after transection of the upper brain stem.

Specific, goal-directed movements are initiated at the level of the cerebral cortex. With repetition, even these movements (writing, playing a musical instrument) can be relearned, so that lower brain centers can take over the control functions.

B. Components: Control over movement is achieved by the functional interconnections between the major motor components of the nervous system: corticospinal (pyramidal) and corticobulbar tracts, basal ganglia, subcortical descending systems (red nucleus, vestibular nucleus, reticular activating system), and cerebellum.

MAJOR MOTOR SYSTEMS

Corticospinal & Corticobulbar Tracts

A. Origin and Composition: The fibers of the corticospinal and corticobulbar tracts arise from the **sensorimotor cortex** (see Figs 12-1 and 6-10) around the central sulcus; about 55% originate in the frontal lobe (areas 4 and 6), and about 35% arise from areas 3, 1, and 2 in the postcentral gyrus of the parietal lobe (see Fig 9-12). About 10% of the fibers originate in other **frontal** or **parietal areas.** The axons arising from the large pyramidal cells in layer V (**Betz cells**) of area 4 contribute only about 5% of the fibers of the corticospinal tract and its pyramidal portion.

The portion of the pyramidal tract that arises from the frontal lobe is concerned with motor function; the portion from the parietal lobe is more concerned with modulation of the ascending sys-

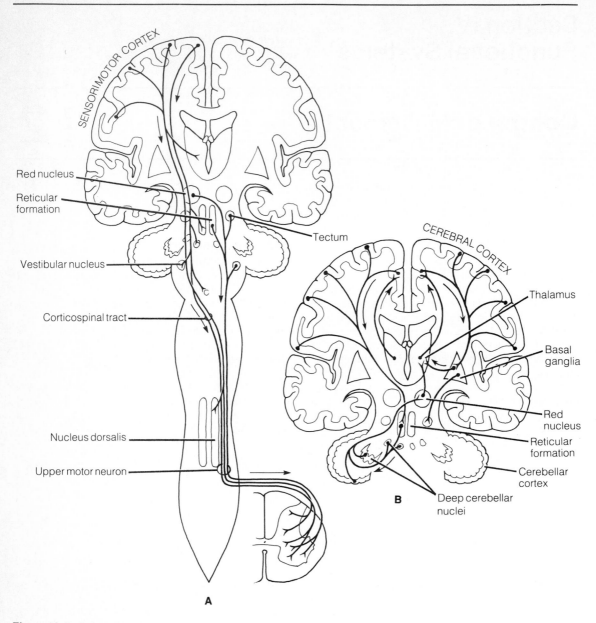

Figure 12-1. Schematic illustration of pathways controlling motor functions. *A:* Arrows denote descending pathways. *B:* Arrows denote cerebellar and basal ganglia circuits.

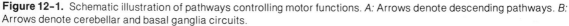

tems. The tracts have endings or collaterals that synapse in the thalamus (ventral nuclei), the brain stem (pontine nuclei, reticular formation and nuclei of cranial nerves), and the spinal cord (anterior horn motoneurons and interneurons; see Fig 12-2). A direct pathway to spinal cord motoneurons exists only for the musculature of the distal extremity.

B. Pathways: The **corticobulbar (corticonuclear) fibers** originate in the region of the sensorimotor cortex where the face is represented (see Figs 9-13 and 9-14). They pass through the posterior limb of the internal capsule and the middle portion of the crus cerebri to their targets, the somatic and brachial efferent nuclei in the brain stem. The **corticospinal tract** originates in the remainder of the sensorimotor cortex and other cortical areas; it follows a similar trajectory through the brain stem and then passes through the pyramids of the medulla (hence the name pyramidal tract), decussates, and descends in the lateral column of the spinal cord (Figs 12-1, 12-2, and 4-13).

Table 12-1. Summary of reflexes.

Reflexes	Afferent Nerve	Center	Efferent Nerve
Superficial reflexes			
Corneal	Cranial V	Pons	Cranial VII
Nasal (sneeze)	Cranial V	Brain stem and upper cord	Cranials V, VII, IX, X, and spinal nerves of expiration
Pharyngeal and uvular	Cranial IX	Medulla	Cranial X
Upper abdominal	T7, 8, 9, 10	T7, 8, 9, 10	T7, 8, 9, 10
Lower abdominal	T10, 11, 12	T10, 11, 12	T10, 11, 12
Cremasteric	Femoral	L1	Genitofemoral
Plantar	Tibial	S1, 2	Tibial
Anal	Pudendal	S4, 5	Pudendal
Deep reflexes			
Jaw	Cranial V	Pons	Cranial V
Biceps	Musculocutaneous	C5, 6	Musculocutaneous
Triceps	Radial	C6, 7	Radial
Periosteoradial	Radial	C6, 7, 8	Radial
Wrist (flexion)	Median	C6, 7, 8	Median
Wrist (extension)	Radial	C7, 8	Radial
Patellar	Femoral	L2, 3, 4	Femoral
Achilles	Tibial	S1, 2	Tibial
Visceral reflexes			
Light	Cranial II	Midbrain	Cranial III
Accommodation	Cranial II	Occipital cortex	Cranial III
Ciliospinal	A sensory nerve	T1, 2	Cervical sympathetics
Oculocardiac	Cranial V	Medulla	Cranial X
Carotid sinus	Cranial IX	Medulla	Cranial X
Bulbocavernosus	Pudendal	S2, 3, 4	Pelvic autonomic
Bladder and rectal	Pudendal	S2, 3, 4	Pudendal and autonomics

About 10% of the pyramidal tract does not cross in the pyramidal decussation but descends in the anterior column of the spinal cord; these fibers decussate at lower cord levels, close to their destination. The pyramidal tract has a somatotopic organization throughout its course. (The origin, termination, and function of this tract have been described more fully in Chapter 4.)

The pyramidal corticospinal and corticobulbar tracts are not solely a system for initiating movement but also for modulating (through their origins and terminations) the function of ascending systems in the thalamus (ventroposterior nucleus), brain stem (dorsal column nuclei), and spinal cord (dorsal horn laminas).

Basal Ganglia

A. Pathways: Many cortical and subcortical components of the motor control system in the cerebrum and brain stem are interconnected, either directly and reciprocally or by way of fiber loops. (The anatomy of these gray masses of the fore-brain has been described in Chapter 9; see Figs 9–16 and 12–1.) The **corpus striatum** (caudate and lentiform nuclei; see Fig 12–3) receives afferents from a large portion of the cerebral cortex, including the sensorimotor cortex (areas 4, 1, 2, and 3), and the more anterior premotor cortex (area 6). It projects to the **globus pallidus** and the **centromedian nucleus** of the thalamus. The globus pallidus in turn projects to the **ventral nuclei** of the thalamus, (which also receive input from the cerebellum, subthalamic nucleus, and substantia nigra). The ventral anterior and ventrolateral nuclei complete the feedback circuit by sending axons back to the cerebral cortex (striatum-pallidus-thalamus). There is thus no direct influence from the caudate nucleus and lentiform nucleus (putamen and globus pallidus; see Fig 12–4) on the spinal cord; however, the subthalamic region, including the prerubral field near the red nucleus, is an important relay and modifying station.

The **substantia nigra** sends fine dopaminergic fibers back to the corpus striatum in another feed-

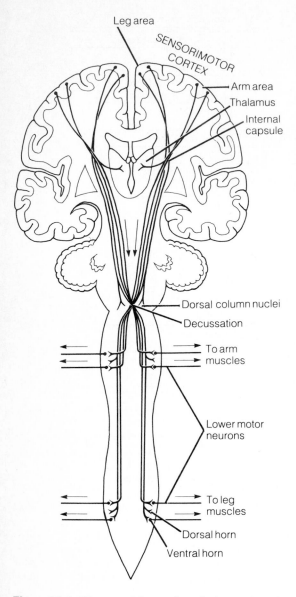

Figure 12–2. Diagram of the corticospinal tract, including descending fibers that provide sensory modulation to thalamus, dorsal column nuclei, and dorsal horn.

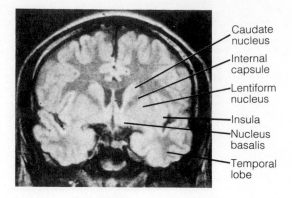

Figure 12–3. MR image of a coronal section through the head at the level of the lentiform nucleus.

rect influence on aspects of motor behavior, the system collaborates as a collective whole with the cerebral cortex in initiating and directing voluntary movement. (This function is independent of the corticospinal tracts; it was formerly known as the *extrapyramidal system.*) The basal ganglia also play a role in generating meaningful motor responses to sensory stimuli or changes in the environment.

Subcortical Descending Systems

Additional pathways—important for certain types of movement—include the rubrospinal, vestibulospinal, tectospinal, and reticulospinal systems (see Fig 12–1 and Chapters 4 and 7).

back circuit (striatonigral-striatum loop). Other fibers form a nigrothalamic system. The **subthalamic nucleus** has interconnections with the globus pallidus (Fig 12–5). Portions of the thalamus project by way of the central tegmental tract to the inferior olivary nucleus; this nucleus in turn sends fibers to the contralateral cerebellar cortex. From the cerebellum, the loop to the thalamus is closed via the dentate and contralateral red nuclei.

B. Function: Although most individual components of the basal ganglia system exercise no di-

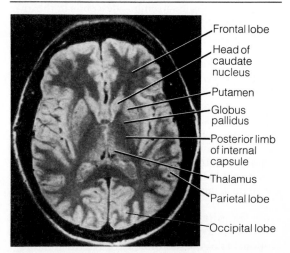

Figure 12–4. MR image of an axial section through the head at the level of the lentiform nucleus.

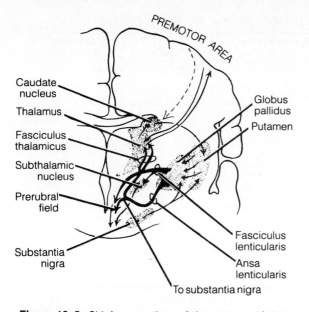

Figure 12-5. Chief connections of the corpus striatum and the subthalamus. (Reproduced, with permission, from Gatz AJ: *Manter's Essentials of Clinical Neuroanatomy and Neurophysiology*, 4th ed. Davis, 1970.)

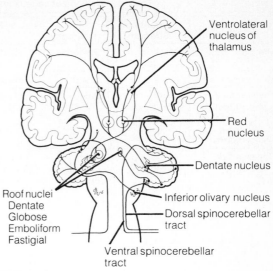

Figure 12-6. Schematic illustration of cerebellar pathways.

A. Pathways: Subcortical descending systems originate in the red nucleus and the tectum of the midbrain, in the reticular formation, and in the vestibular nuclei of the brain stem. The red nucleus receives input from the cerebellar cortex and sends axons to the interneurons of the spinal cord via the crossed **rubrospinal tract** in the lateral column. The sensorimotor cortex projects to several nuclei of the reticular formation in the brain stem, which then sends fibers to the spinal cord in the form of the **reticulospinal tract** in the lateral column. The **vestibulospinal tract** projects to the anterior horn cells (mostly interneurons; extensor muscle motoneurons are supplied directly). The vestibular nuclei do not receive input from the cerebral cortex but from the vestibular nerve and archicerebellum.

B. Function: Experiments in animals suggest that the corticospinal and rubrospinal systems cooperate to control hand and finger movement. They also suggest that the tectospinal, reticulospinal, and vestibulospinal systems play but a limited role in movements of the extremities (their main influence is on the musculature of the trunk) and that the effects of lesions in the corticospinal tract, except for the inability to use the distal extremities, may disappear with time.

Cerebellum

A. Pathways: The cerebellum (Fig 12-6; see also Chapter 6) is interconnected with several regions of the central nervous system: ascending tracts from the spinal cord and brain stem, corticopontocerebellar fibers from the opposite cerebral cortex and cerebellar efferent systems to the contralateral red nucleus, the reticular formation, and the ventral nuclei of the contralateral thalamus (which connects to the cerebral cortex).

B. Function: The cerebellum has 2 major functions: coordination of voluntary motor activity (fine, skilled movements and gross, propulsive movements such as walking, swimming); and control of equilibrium and muscle tone. Experimental work suggests that the cerebellum is essential in motor learning (the acquisition or learning of stereotyped movements) and memory mechanisms (the retention of such learned movements.)

MOTOR DISTURBANCES

Motor disturbances, including weakness (paresis), paralysis, abnormal movements, and abnormal reflexes, can result from lesions of the motor pathways in the nervous system or from lesions of the muscles themselves (Table 12-2).

Muscles

A muscle may be unable to react normally to stimuli conveyed to it by the lower motor neuron, with resulting local weakness, paralysis, or tetanic contraction. The cause of these disturbances may lie in the muscle itself or at the myoneural junction. Myasthenia gravis, myotonia congenita, hypotonia (Fig 12-7), and progressive muscular dystro-

Table 12–2. Signs of various lesions of the human motor system.

Location of Lesion	Voluntary Strength	Atrophy	Muscle Stretch Reflexes	Tone	Abnormal Movements
Muscle (myopathy)	Weak (paretic)	Present	Hypoactive.	Hypotonic.	None.
Motor end-plate	Weak	Slight	Hypoactive.	Hypotonic.	None.
Lower motor neuron (includes peripheral nerve neuropathy	Weak (paretic or paralyzed)	Severe	Hypoactive or absent.	Hypotonic (flaccid).	Fasciculations.*
Upper motor neuron	Weak or paralyzed	Mild (atrophy of disuse)	Hyperactive (spastic). After a massive upper motor neuron lesion (as in stroke), reflexes may be absent at first, with hypotonia and spinal shock.	Hypertonic (clasp-knife).	Withdrawal spasms, abnormal reflexes (eg, Babinski extensor plantar response).
Cerebellar systems	Normal	None	Hypotonic (pendulous).	Hypotonic.	Ataxia, dysmetria, dysdiadochokinesia, gait.
Basal ganglia	Normal	None	Normal.	Rigid (lead-pipe).	Dyskinesias (eg, chorea, athetosis, dystonia, rest tremors, ballismus).
Cortical (parietal)	Usually normal	Usually none	Normal or spastic.	Usually normal.	Apraxia.

*Fasciculations can be spontaneous, grossly visible contractions (twitches) of entire motor units.

phy are typical muscle disorders characterized by muscle dysfunction in the presence of apparently normal neural tissue.

Lower Motor Neurons
A. Description: These nerve cells in the anterior gray column of the spinal cord or brain stem have axons that pass by way of the cranial or peripheral nerves to the motor end-plates of the muscles. The lower motor neuron is called the "final common pathway" for 2 reasons. It is under the influence of the corticospinal, rubrospinal, olivospinal, vestibulospinal, reticulospinal, and tectospinal tracts as well as the segmental or intersegmental reflex neurons, and it is the ultimate pathway through which neural impulses reach the muscle.

B. Lesions: Lesions of the lower motor neurons can be located in the cells of the anterior gray column of the spinal cord or brain stem or in their axons, which constitute the ventral roots of the spinal or cranial nerves. Signs of lower-motor-neuron lesions include weakness, flaccid paralysis of the involved muscles, muscle atrophy with fasciculations and degeneration of muscle fibers over time, and histologic-reaction degeneration (10–14 days after injury; see Chapter 21). Reflexes of the involved muscle are diminished or absent, and no abnormal reflexes are obtainable (Table 12–2).

Upper Motor Neurons
A. Description: The upper motor neuron is a complex of descending systems conveying impulses from the motor areas of the cerebrum and subcortical brain stem to the anterior horn cells of the spinal cord. It is essential for the initiation of voluntary muscular activity. The term itself is used mainly for the portion of the pathway that courses through the brain stem and spinal cord. One major

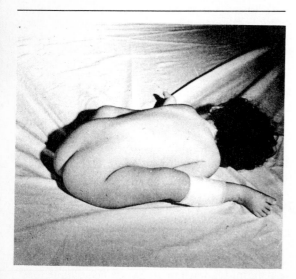

Figure 12–7. Child with hypotonia, hyporeflexia, and muscle weakness.

component, the corticospinal tract, passes through the internal capsule, brain stem, and spinal cord to the lower motor neurons of the cord. Another component, the corticobulbar tract, projects to the brain stem nuclei of the cranial nerves that innervate striated muscles.

B. Lesions: Lesions in the descending motor systems can be located in the cerebral cortex, internal capsule, cerebral peduncles, brain stem, or spinal cord (Table 12–2). Signs of upper-motor-neuron lesions in the spinal cord include spastic paralysis or paresis (weakness) of the involved muscles, hyperactive deep reflexes, no or little muscle atrophy (atrophy of disuse), diminished or absent superficial abdominal reflexes, and abnormal reflexes (eg, Babinski response).

These signs result not only from lesions in the corticospinal or corticobulbar tract itself but also from those of the rubrospinal and reticulospinal tracts; all these tracts course in the lateral white column of the spinal cord. Lesions limited to the corticospinal tract alone cause flaccid paralysis, especially of the extremities.

Discrete lesions in the motor cortex itself have little effect on motor function, with the exception of the distal extensor muscles. Damage to the cerebral cortex incurred in utero, during birth, or in early postnatal life may result in cerebral palsy. This is a heterogeneous group of disorders that often include a form of spastic paralysis; however, the disease may be characterized by other signs such as rigidity, tremor, ataxia, or athetosis. Combinations of these groups of symptoms are common, and the disorder may be accompanied by such other significant defects as speech disorders, apraxia, hemiangioma, and mental retardation.

C. Types of Paralysis: Hemiplegia is a spastic or flaccid paralysis of one side of the body and extremities; it is delimited by the median line of the body. **Monoplegia** is paralysis of one extremity only, while **diplegia** is paralysis of any 2 corresponding extremities, usually both lower extremities (but can be both upper). **Paraplegia** is a symmetric paralysis of both lower extremities. **Quadriplegia,** or **tetraplegia,** is paralysis of all 4 extremities. **Hemiplegia alternans** (crossed paralysis) is paralysis of one or more ipsilateral cranial nerves and contralateral paralysis of the arm and leg.

Basal Ganglia

Defects in function of the basal ganglia (sometimes termed extrapyramidal lesions) are characterized by changes in muscle tone, poverty of voluntary movement (**akinesia**), or involuntary, abnormal movement (**dyskinesia**). (Features of disorders of the basal ganglia are summarized in Table 12–2.)

A. Athetosis: This disorder, which is characterized by slow, writhing movements of the extremities and neck musculature, is not associated with a specific lesion.

B. Chorea: This disorder is characterized by quick, repeated, involuntary movements of the distal-extremity muscles, face, and tongue; it is often associated with lesions in the corpus striatum.

C. Huntington's Chorea: This type of chorea is a late manifestation of a disease with an autosomal dominant pattern of inheritance that also leads to cortical atrophy and dementia. The corpus striatum, especially the caudate nucleus, becomes atrophic. Tremor may result from lesions in the basal ganglia, the cerebellum, or the substantia nigra.

D. Ballismus: Large, flailing movements of one or more extremities characterize ballismus, which is caused by a lesion of the subthalamic nucleus.

E. Parkinson's Disease (Paralysis Agitans): Characteristic signs include rigidity; tremor at rest (pill-rolling tremor); akinesia; slow, monotonous speech; diminutive writing (micrographia); and loss of facial expression (mask face), often without impairment of mental capacity. This progressively worsening disease is associated with loss of pigmented cells in the substantia nigra and its dopaminergic efferents (Figs 12–8 and 12–9). Levodopa alleviates the symptoms and signs but has many adverse side effects. The disease may be arrested by the use of certain drugs when diagnosed early (eg, by positron emission tomography [PET scan]; see Chapter 22.) A rapidly developing Parkinson-like disease has been recently linked to

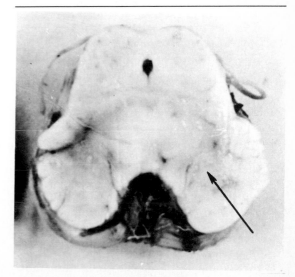

Figure 12–8. Midbrain of a 45-year-old woman with Parkinson's disease, showing depigmentation of the substantia nigra (compare with Fig 18–12).

NORMAL

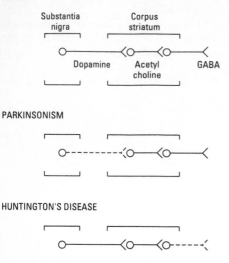

Figure 12–9. Schematic illustration of the processes underlying Parkinsonism. (Reproduced, with permission, from Katzung BG: *Basic and Clinical Pharmacology,* 4th ed. Appleton & Lange, 1989.

the use of certain "designer drugs," eg, MPTP (1-methyl-4-phenyl-1, 2, 5, 6-tetrahydropyridine), a synthetic narcotic related to meperidine.

Cerebellum

Disorders caused by cerebellar lesions (Table 12–2) are characterized by reduced muscle tone and a loss of coordination of smooth movements. Lesions in each of the 3 subdivisions of the cerebellum exhibit characteristic signs.

A. Vestibulocerebellum (Archicerebellum): Loss of equilibrium, often with **nystagmus,** is typical.

B. Spinocerebellum (Paleocerebellum): Truncal ataxia and "drunken" gait are characteristic.

C. Neocerebellum: Ataxia of extremities and **asynergy** (loss of coordination) are prominent. Decomposition of movement occurs, with voluntary muscular movements becoming a series of jerky, discrete motions rather than one smooth motion. **Dysmetria** (past-pointing phenomenon) is also seen, in which the person is unable to estimate the distance involved in muscular acts, so that an attempt to touch an object will overshoot its target. **Dysdiadochokinesia** (the inability to perform rapidly alternating movements), **intention tremor,** and **rebound phenomenon** (loss of interaction between agonist and antagonist smooth muscles) are also typical.

CASE 17

A 63-year-old right-handed secretary/typist consulted her family physician when her right hand and fingers "did not want to cooperate." She also explained that her employers had become dissatisfied with her because her work habits and movements had become slow and her handwriting had become scribbly and illegible over the preceding several months. She was in danger of losing her job even though her intellectual abilities were unimpaired.

Neurologic examination showed moderate slowness of speech and mild loss of facial expression on both sides. The patient had difficulty initiating a movement and then stopping it; once seated, she did not move about much. There was no muscular atrophy and no weakness. Passive movements of both arms, especially those of the right arm, appeared stiff and jerky, and there was a fine tremor in the fingers of the right hand (frequency 3–4 times per second).

The rest of the examination and the laboratory data were within normal limits.

What is the most likely diagnosis? Where is the lesion?

CASE 18

A 49-year-old woman with known severe hypertension had a sudden loss of strength in the left leg and arm; she fell down, and when brought to the emergency room seemed only partially conscious.

Neurologic examination on admission showed an obtunded woman who had difficulty speaking. There was no papilledema and no sensation on the left side of the face or body. The tongue deviated to the left when protruded. Left-central facial weakness was present. The patient complained that she could not see on the left side of both visual fields. Complete paralysis of the left upper and lower extremities was present, and there was no resistance to passive motion. Results of tests of cerebellar function were negative. Deep tendon reflexes were absent in the left upper extremity and increased in the lower extremity. There was a left extensor plantar response, but the response was equivocal on the right. Vital signs and the complete blood count were within normal limits; blood pressure was 190/100.

What is the preliminary diagnosis? Would a lumbar puncture be indicated? Would a neuroradiologic diagnostic procedure be useful?

Cases are discussed further in Chapter 24.

REFERENCES

Alexander J et al: Parallel organization of functionally segregated circuits linking basal ganglia and cortex. *Annu Rev Neurosci* 1986;**9**:357.

Brooks VB (editor): Motor control. In: *Handbook of Physiology,* 2nd ed. Vol 2, section 1. American Physiological Society, 1981.

Carpenter MB, Jayaraman A (editors): *The Basal Ganglia II: Structure and Function.* 2nd International Basal Ganglia Society Symposium, 1986.

Dawnay NAH, Glees FP: Mapping the primate corticospinal pathway. *J Anat* 1981;**133**:124.

Kuypers HGJM, Martin GF (editors): Anatomy of descending pathways to the spinal cord. *Prog Brain Res* 1982;**57**:1–411. [Entire issue.]

Marsden CD, Fahn S (editors): *Movement Disorders 2.* Butterworth, 1987.

Somatosensory Systems

Input from the sensory systems plays a role in the control of motor function, by way of either the connections within the sensorimotor cortex or the cerebellar pathways. Conversely, impulses from the sensorimotor cortex—via the descending pathways—affect the function of sensory neurons in the spinal cord, brain stem, and thalamus.

SENSATION

Sensation can be divided into 4 types: superficial, deep, visceral, and special. **Superficial sensation** is concerned with touch, pain, temperature, and 2-point discrimination. **Deep sensation** includes muscle and joint position sense (proprioception), deep muscle pain, and vibration sense. **Visceral sensations** are relayed by autonomic afferent fibers and include hunger, nausea, and visceral pain (see Chapter 19). The **special senses**—smell, vision, hearing, taste, and equilibrium—are conveyed by certain cranial nerves (see Chapters 7, 14, 15, and 16).

Receptors

Receptors are specialized cells for detecting particular changes in the environment. **Exteroceptors** include receptors affected mainly by the external environment: Meissner's corpuscles, Merkel's corpuscles, and hair cells for touch; Krause's endbulbs for cold; Ruffini's corpuscles for warmth; and free nerve endings for pain (Fig 13–1). Receptors are not absolutely specific for a given sensation; eg, strong stimuli can cause various sensations, even pain, even though the inciting stimuli are not necessarily painful. **Proprioceptors** receive impulses mainly from pacinian corpuscles, joint receptors, muscle spindles, and Golgi tendon organs. Painful stimuli are detected at the free endings of nerve fibers.

Each efferent fiber from a receptor relays stimuli that originate in a receptive field and gives rise to a component of an afferent sensory system. Note that each individual receptor fires either completely or not at all when stimulated. The greater the intensity of a stimulus, the greater the number of end-organs stimulated, the higher the rate of

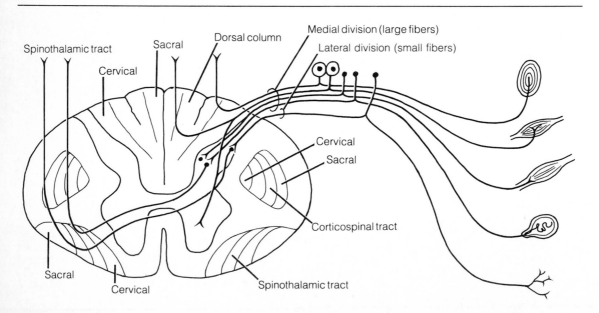

Figure 13–1. Schematic illustration of a spinal cord segment with its dorsal root, ganglion cells, and sensory organs (compare with Fig 4–6).

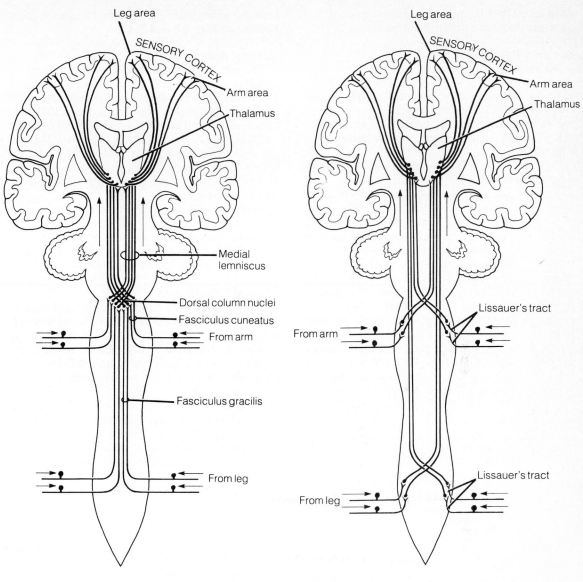

Figure 13-2. Dorsal column system for discriminative touch and position sense (lemniscus system).

Figure 13-3. Spinothalamic tracts for pain and temperature (ventrolateral system).

discharge, and the longer the duration of effect. **Adaptation** denotes the diminution in rate of discharge of some receptors upon repeated or continuous stimulation of constant intensity; the sensation of sitting in a chair or walking on even ground is suppressed.

Connections

A chain of three long neurons and a number of interneurons conducts stimuli from the receptor or free ending (Figs 13-1 through 13-3) to the somatosensory cortex:

A. First-Order Neuron: The cell body of a first-order neuron lies in a dorsal root ganglion or a somatic afferent ganglion of cranial nerves.

B. Second-Order Neuron: The cell body of a second-order neuron lies within the neuraxis (spinal cord and brain stem). Its axon usually decussates and terminates in the thalamus.

C. Third-Order Neuron: The cell body of a third-order neuron, which lies in the thalamus, projects to the sensory cortex—or the thalamus itself in the case of chronic pain. The networks of the brain process information relayed by this type of neuron; they interpret its location, quality, and intensity and make appropriate responses.

Sensory Pathways

Multiple neurons from the same type of receptor often form a bundle (tract), creating a sensory pathway. Sensory pathways ascending in the spinal cord are described in Chapter 4; their continuation within the brain stem is discussed in Chapter 6. The main sensory areas in the cortex are described in Chapter 9.

One major system—the **lemniscal (dorsal column) system** (see Fig 13-2)—carries touch, joint sensation, 2-point discrimination, and vibratory sense from receptors to the cortex. The other important system—the **ventrolateral system** (Fig 13-3)—relays impulses concerning nociceptive stimuli (pain, crude touch) or changes in skin temperature. Significant anatomic and functional differences characterize these 2 pathways: the size of the receptive field, nerve-fiber diameter, course in the spinal cord, and function (Table 13-1). Each system is characterized by **somatotopic distribution,** with convergence in the thalamus (ventroposterior complex) and cerebral cortex (the sensory projection areas; see Figs 9-13 and 9-15). The sensory trigeminal fibers contribute to both the lemniscal and the ventrolateral systems and pro-

vide the input from the face and mucosal membranes (see Figs 6-8 and 7-12).

Cortical Areas

The **primary somatosensory cortex** (areas 3, 1, and 2) is organized in functional somatotopic columns that represent points in the receptive field. Within each column are inputs from thalamic, commissural, and associational fibers, all of which end in layers IV, III, and II (see Fig 9-10). The output is from cells in layers V and VI; however, the details of the processing occurring in each column and its functional significance (how it is felt) are largely unknown.

Additional cortical areas—secondary projection areas—also receive input from receptive fields in the columns; the somatotopic map of these areas is more diffuse, however. A separation of sensory modalities occurs within the somatosensory cortex.

Clinical Correlations

Interruption in the course of first- and second-order neurons produces characteristic **sensory deficits;** these are sometimes difficult to define in unconscious or malingering patients or in young children. Small deficits are sometimes ignored by the patient unless a sensitive area such as the fingertips is involved.

Thalamic lesions are often characterized by outbursts of severe, poorly localized pain (thalamic pain) associated with weakness, ataxia, hyperkinesia, paresthesia, and loss of the ability to discriminate or localize simple crude sensations. Slight stimuli may evoke severe and disagreeable sensations (thalamic syndrome).

PAIN

Pathways

The free nerve endings in peripheral and cranial nerves are probably the specific receptors, or **nociceptors,** for pain (Figs 13-1, 13-3, and 6-8). The pain fibers in peripheral nerves are of small diameter and are readily affected by local anesthetic. The thinly myelinated and unmyelinated fibers make up the A-delta fibers, which convey discrete, sharp, short-lasting pain, and the C fibers, which transmit chronic, burning, and often unbearable pain.

Injured tissue may release prostaglandins, which lower the threshold of peripheral nociceptors and thereby increase the sensibility to pain (**hyperalgesia**). Aspirin and other nonsteroidal anti-inflammatory drugs inhibit the action of prostaglandins and relieve pain (**hypalgesia,** or **analgesia**).

Pain Systems

The central ascending pathway for sensation consists of 2 systems: the **spinothalamic tract** and

Table 13-1. Differences between lemniscal and ventrolateral systems.

	Lemniscal (Dorsal Column) Pathway	Ventrolateral Pathway
Course in spinal cord	Dorsal and dorsolateral funiculi	Ventral and ventrolateral funiculi
Size of receptive fields	Small	Small and large
Specificity of signal conveyed	Each sensation carried separately; precise localization of sensation	Multimodal (several sensations carried in one fiber system)
Diameter of nerve fiber	Large-diameter primary afferents	Small-diameter primary afferents
Sensation transmitted	Fine touch, joint sensation, vibration	Pain, temperature, crude touch, visceral pain
Synaptic chain	Two or 3 synapses to cortex	Multisynaptic
Speed of transmission	Fast	Slow
Tests for function	Vibration, 2-point discrimination, stereognosis	Pinprick, heat and cold testing

the phylogenetically older **spinoreticulothalamic system.** The first pathway conducts the sensation of sharp, stabbing pain; the second conveys deep, poorly localized, burning pain. Both pathways are interrupted when the ventrolateral quadrant of the spinal cord is damaged by trauma or in surgery, such as a cordotomy (Fig 13–4), deliberately performed to relieve pain; contralateral loss of all pain sensation results below the lesion. Small lesions higher in the neuraxis involve one of the pathways because they course upward separately; the lesion reduces the sensation of the type of pain associated with that pathway. Isolated lesions in the spinothalamic tract in the brain stem or thalamus may, paradoxically, produce thalamic pain in some cases.

Referred Pain

The cells in Lamina V of the posterior column that receive noxious sensations from afferents in the **skin** also receive input from nociceptors in the **viscera** (Fig 13–5). When visceral afferents receive a strong stimulus, the cortex may misinterpret the source. A common example is referred pain in the shoulder caused by gallstone colic: the spinal segments that relay pain from the gallbladder also receive afferents from the shoulder region (con-

vergence theory). Similarly, pain in the heart caused by **acute anoxia (myocardial infarct)** is conducted by fibers that reach the same spinal cord segments where pain afferents from the ulnar nerve (lower arm area) synapse. Another theory, the pacilitation theory, in which the visceral pain facilitates input from a somatic structure, has not been proved conclusively.

Relief of Pain

A. Spinal Cord Stimulation: Recent analysis of the laminar organization of the spinal cord gray matter has shown that most cells of laminas I and II and some in lamina V respond to noxious stimuli by way of small-diameter afferent fibers (see Fig 4–11). Laminas III, IV and VI show a narrow range of response to nonnoxious stimuli via large-diameter afferents, and lamina V has a broad range of responses. The large-diameter fibers prevent the lamina V afferents from transmitting signals. Stimulating (eg, by rubbing) these fibers helps to suppress the sensation of pain, especially sharp pain. (Parents of small children seem to know this instinctively: they rub the injured spot, thus activating the large-diameter fibers.) One therapeutic procedure formerly used to inhibit pain was to

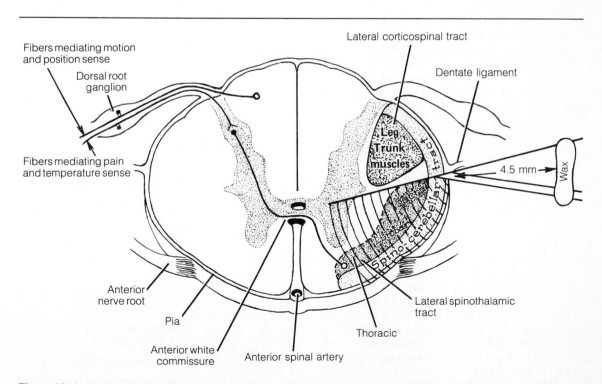

Figure 13–4. Ideal cordotomy at upper dorsal spinal cord segments. Surgical interruption of the lateral spinothalamic tract may provide relief from intractable pain of the opposite half of the body below the level of cordotomy. (Redrawn and reproduced, with permission, from Kahn EA and Rand RW: On the anatomy of anterolateral cordotomy. *J Neurosurg* 1952;**9:**611.)

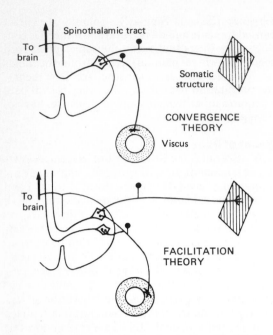

Figure 13-5. Diagram of convergence and facilitation theories of referred pain. (Reproduced, with permission, from Ganong WF: *Review of Medical Physiology*, 14th ed. Appleton & Lange, 1989.)

stimulate the dorsal columns electrically by means of permanently implanted electrodes; this alleviated sharp pain but chronic, emotionally burdensome, deep, burning pain was not relieved.

B. Endorphins: Another system of pain suppression can be activated by stimulating the endorphin receptor region in the periaqueductal gray matter of the midbrain (Fig 13–6). This region contains **opiate receptors,** membrane-bound proteins that specifically bind opiate agonists (eg, morphine) or antagonists (eg, naloxone). There are several endogenous opiumlike compounds within the body: **enkephalin** and β-**endorphins** (a fragment of the pituitary hormone β-**lipotropin**), among others. These peptides bind to opiate receptors, as does morphine. In most cases, pain (especially chronic pain) is relieved. Endogenous endomorphin production is empirically aided by a diet rich in **tryptophan (serotonin).**

Deep, chronic pain is relieved when periaqueductal gray cells activate serotonergic neurons in the midline pons (nucleus raphe magnus). These neurons send descending fibers to the spinal cord, ending on laminas I and V of the posterior horn, and act to inhibit pain. A method currently used to treat unbearable pain is to implant electric stimulators in the periaqueductal gray matter and connect them to a subcutaneous inductor coil. The patient can activate the stimulation with an external bat-

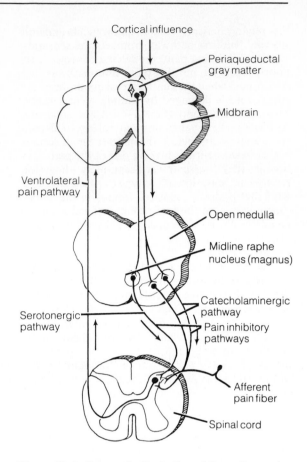

Figure 13-6. Schematic illustration of the pathways involved in pain control. (Courtesy of Al Basbaum.)

tery-operated induction coil as needed to provide many hours of pain relief.

C. Surgery: Various surgical procedures (Fig 13–4 and Table 13–2) attempt to alleviate intolerable pain. Although most of these are somewhat effective, a large number of patients with deep, chronic pain may not be helped.

D. Placebos: People have known throughout

Table 13-2. Procedures for pain relief.

Surgery
   Single nerve section
   Sympathectomy (for visceral pain)
   Rhizotomy (root section at 2 or more levels)
   Cordotomy (see Fig 13–4)
   Mesencephalic tractotomy (for trigeminal pain)
   Thalamotomy

Stimulation
   Dorsal column
   Periaqueductal gray matter
   Medial lemniscus near thalamus

history that treatment itself often influences the course of a disease, even if the treatment is not specific or suggestive. This placebo ("I will please") effect is defined as consistent improvement following the administration of a substance without pharmacologic effect. Conversely, a **nociebo** ("I will harm") effect occurs when a consistent worsening occurs after administration of an inactive substance.

The placebo effect is probably mediated by not one but several mechanisms, most of which are not yet clearly understood. Hypnosis, the environment, the suggestions and attitude of the person giving the placebo, and the patient's confidence in its effectiveness seem to act together to produce the effect. Some studies have reported a success rate of 70–90% with the use of placebos. Careful diagnostic evaluation must always precede administration of a placebo; in any case, "primum, non nocere" (first, do not harm) must remain the guiding principle of therapy.

CASE 19

A 41-year-old woman was referred after complaining of numbness and tingling in her right hand for more than a year. These sensations started gradually, at first only in the fingers, but ultimately extending to the entire right hand and forearm. She was unable to do fine work such as sewing, and she sometimes dropped objects because of weakness that had developed in that hand during the last year. Three weeks before her admission to the hospital, she had burned 2 fingers of her right hand on her electric range; she had not felt the heat.

Neurologic examination showed considerable wasting and weakness of the small muscles in the right hand. The deep tendon reflexes in the right upper extremity were absent or difficult to elicit. The knee and ankle jerks, however, were abnormally brisk, especially on the right side; the right plantar response was extensor. Abdominal reflexes were absent on both sides. Pain and temperature senses were lost in the right hand, forearm, and shoulder and an area of the left shoulder. Touch, joint, and vibration senses were completely normal.

A plain-film radiograph of the spine was read as normal.

Where is the lesion? What is the differential diagnosis? Which neuroadiologic procedure(s) would be helpful? What is the most likely diagnosis?

CASE 20

A 41-year-old man was admitted to the hospital with complaints of progressive weakness and unsteadiness of his legs. His disability had begun more than a year earlier with creeping and tingling feelings in his feet. Gradually, these sensations had become more disagreeable, and he developed burning pains on the soles of his feet; the rest of his feet became numb. His legs had become so weak that they felt tired if he walked more than 100 meters, and he had lately begun to stumble frequently when walking.

For about 6 months he had had tingling feelings in his fingers and hands; his fingers felt clumsy, and he often dropped things. He had lost more than 6 kg (about 14 pounds) during the previous 6 months. The patient had smoked about 30 cigarettes daily for many years, and he drank 15 glasses of beer and half a bottle of whiskey or more a day. After losing his job a year before, he had worked at several unskilled jobs and was now employed as a bartender.

Neurologic examination showed a poorly muscled man with conspicuous atrophy and hypotonic muscles in the calves and forearms. There was gross weakness of movement at both ankles and wrists and slightly weakened movement of the knees and elbows. The patient's gait was unsteady and of the high-stepping type. There was loss of touch and pain sensation on the feet and distal thirds of the legs and on the hands and distal halves of the forearms, giving a "sock-and-glove" distribution of sensory loss. The soles of the feet and the calf muscles were hyperalgesic when squeezed. Ankle and biceps reflexes were absent, and knee jerks and triceps reflex were diminished.

What is the differential diagnosis? What is the most likely diagnosis?

Cases are discussed further in Chapter 24.

REFERENCES

Basbaum AI, Fields HL: Endogenous pain control systems. *Annu Rev Neurosci* 1984;7:309.

Besson J-M, Chaouch A: Peripheral and spinal mechanisms of nociception. *Physiol Rev* 1987;**67**:67.

Bowker RM, et al: Descending serotonergic, peptidergic and cholinergic pathways from the raphe nuclei: A multiple transmitter complex. *Brain Res* 1983;**288**:33.

THE EYE

The functions (and clinical correlations) of the cranial nerves (III, IV, VI) involved in moving the eyes have been discussed in Chapter 7, along with the gaze centers and pupillary reflexes. The vestibulo-ocular reflex is briefly explained in Chapter 16. This chapter discusses the form, function, and lesions of the optic system, from the retina to the cerebrum.

Anatomy & Physiology

The optical components of the eye (Fig 14–1) are the cornea, the pupillary opening of the iris, the lens, and the retina. Light passes through the first four components, the anterior chamber, and the vitreous to reach the retina; the point of fixation (direction of gaze) normally lines up with the fovea. The retina (Fig 14–2) and the optic nerve (grown as a portion of the brain itself) transform light to electrical impulses.

The transformation from absorbed light rays to action potential occurs along a chain of 3 elements. The **rods** and **cones** (Fig 14–3) are first-order neurons that connect with the **bipolar cells** of the retina; these in turn synapse with ganglion cells near the surface of the retina, the **ganglion cells** are third-order neurons whose myelinated axons form the optic nerve fibers.

When light is absorbed by the photosensitive elements of the rods and cones, the structure of the latter changes, triggering a series of events that initiate a local graded potential (Fig 14–4). When this reaches the ganglion cells, it forms an all-or-none potential that is transmitted over the fibers in the optic nerve.

The electrical activity of the eye can be studied by electroretinography, placing one recorder on the cornea and the other on the skin of the head. Fig 14–5 shows the effect of a light stimulus under experimental conditions. The **a-wave** represents the photoreceptors' response to light. The **b-wave,** the most sensitive element of the electroretinogram (ERG), is probably related to the depolarization of the bipolar cells. The **c-wave** corresponds to the hyperpolarization of the photoreceptors. The ERG can be used to determine the wavelength of the light stimulus, the response of the rods apart from that of the cones, and the state of adaptation.

The retinal area for central, fixated vision during good light is the macula; the remainder of the ret-

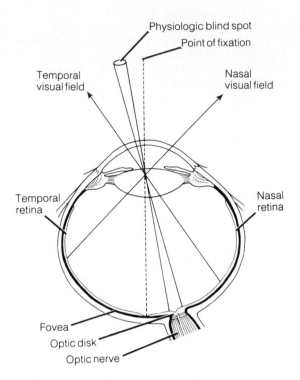

Figure 14–1. Horizontal section of the left eye; representation of the visual field at the level of the retina. The focus of the point of fixation is the fovea, the physiologic blind spot on the optic disk, the temporal (lateral) half of the visual field on the nasal side of the retina, and the nasal (medial) half of the visual field on the temporal side of the retina. (Reproduced, with permission, from Simon RP, Aminoff MJ, Greenberg DA: *Clinical Neurology,* Appleton & Lange, 1989.)

ina is concerned with paracentral and peripheral vision. The inner layers of the retina in the macular area are pushed apart, forming the **fovea centralis,** a small central pit composed of closely packed cones, where vision is sharpest and color discrimination most acute.

The rods and cones of the retina react specifically to physical light. The cones are stimulated by relatively high intensity light; they are responsible for sharp vision and color discrimination. The more numerous rods react to low-intensity light and function in twilight and at night.

The deepest part of the eye—the **fundus oculi**—

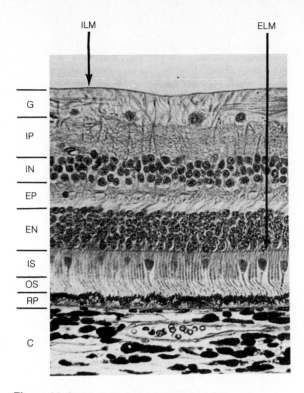

Figure 14–2. Section of the retina of a monkey. Light enters from the top and traverses the following layers: ILM, internal limiting membrane; G, ganglion cell layer; IP, internal plexiform layer; IN, internal nuclear layer (bipolar neurons); EP, external plexiform layer; EN, external nuclear layer (nuclei of rods and cones); ELM, external limiting membrane; IS, inner segments of rods (narrow lines) and cones (triangular dark structures); OS, outer segments of rods and cones; RP, retinal pigment epithelium; C, choroid. × 655.

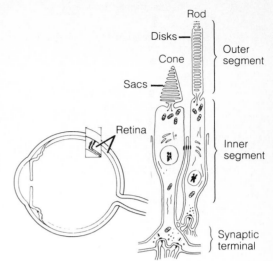

Figure 14–3. Schematic diagram of a rod and cone in the retina.

can be examined with the help of an ophthalmoscope (Fig 14–6).

A. Adaptation: If a person spends a considerable period of time in brightly lighted surroundings and then moves to a dimly lighted environment, the retinas slowly become more sensitive to light as the individual becomes accustomed to the dark. This decline in visual threshold, known as **dark adaptation,** is nearly maximal in about 20 minutes, although there is some further decline over longer periods. On the other hand, when one passes suddenly from a dim to a brightly lighted environment, the light seems intensely and even uncomfortably bright until the eyes adapt to the increased illumination and the visual threshold rises. This adaptation occurs over a period of about 5 minutes and is called light adaptation, although, strictly speaking, it is merely the disappearance of dark adaptation. The pupillary light reflex, which constricts the pupils (see Chapter 7),

is normally a protective accompaniment to sudden increases in light intensity.

B. Color Vision: The portion of the spectrum that stimulates the retina to produce sight ranges from 400 to 800 nm. Stimulation of the normal eye by either this entire range of wavelengths or by mixtures from certain different parts of the range produces the sensation of white light. Monochromatic radiation from one part of the spectrum is perceived as a specific color or hue. The Young-Helmholtz theory postulates that the retina contains 3 types of cones, each with a different photopigment maximally sensitive to one of the primary colors (red, blue, and green), and that the sensation of any given color is determined by the relative frequency of impulses from each type of cone.

Each of the photopigments has been identified and characterized by recombinant DNA techniques. The amino-acid sequences of all 3 are about 41% homologous with rhodopsin. The green-sensitive and red-sensitive pigments are very similar—about 40% homologous with each other—and are coded by the same chromosome. The blue-sensitive pigment is only about 43% homologous with the other 2 and is coded by a different chromosome. The absorption rates of these photopigments overlap somewhat.

Binocular fusion of color is possible, allowing a subjective sensation of yellow when one eye is exposed to red light and the other to green.

In normal color (trichromatic) vision, the human eye can perceive the 3 primary colors and mix these in suitable portions to match white or

Incident light

↓

Structural change in the
retinene₁ of photopigment

↓

Metarhodopsin II

↓

Activation of transducin

↓

Activation of phosphodiesterase

↓

Decreased intracellular cGMP

↓

Closure of Na⁺ channels

↓

Hyperpolarization

↓

Decreased release of
synaptic transmitter

↓

Response in bipolar cells
and other neural elements

Figure 14-4. Probable sequence of events involved in phototransduction in rods and cones. (Reproduced, with permission, from Ganong WF: *Review of Medical Physiology,* 14th ed. Appleton & Lange, 1989.)

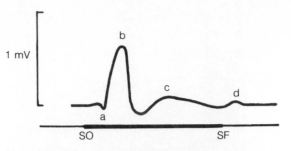

Figure 14-5. Human electroretinogram (ERG). SO, light stimulus on; SF, light stimulus off. (Redrawn and reproduced, with permission, from Ziv: Electroretinography. *N Engl J Med* 1961;**264:**5.)

any color of the spectrum. Color blindness can result from a weakness of one cone system or from dichromatic vision, in which only 2 cone systems are present. In the latter case, only one pair of primary colors is perceived, with the 2 colors being complementary to each other. Most dichromats are red-green blind and confuse red, yellow, and green. Color blindness tests use special cards or colored pieces of yarn.

C. Accommodation: The lens is held in place by fibers between the lens capsule and the ciliary body (Figs 14–1 and 14–7). In the unaccommodated state, these elastic fibers are taut and keep the lens somewhat flattened. In the accommodated state, contraction of the circular ciliary muscle slackens the tension on the elastic fibers, and the lens, which has an intrinsic capacity to become rounder, assumes a more biconvex shape. The cili-

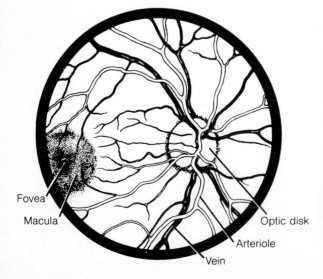

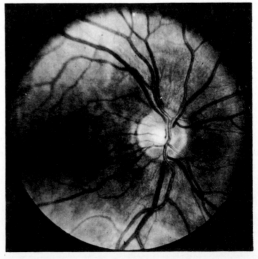

Figure 14-6. The normal fundus as seen through an ophthalmoscope. (Photo by Diane Beeston; reproduced, with permission, from Vaughan D, Asbury T, Tabbara KF: *General Ophthalmology,* 12th ed. Appleton & Lange, 1989.)

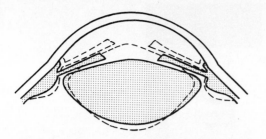

Figure 14-7. Accommodation. The solid lines represent the shape of the lens, iris, and ciliary body at rest, and the dotted lines represent the shape during accommodation. (Reproduced, with permission, from Ganong WF: *Review of Medical Physiology,* 14th ed. Appleton & Lange, 1989.)

ary muscle is a smooth muscle that is innervated by the parasympathetic system (cranial nerve III; see Chapter 7); it can be paralyzed with atropine or a similar drug.

D. Refraction: When viewing a distant object the normal (emmetropic) eye is unaccommodated and the object is in focus. A normal eye readily focuses an image of a distant object on its retina, 24 mm behind the cornea; the focal length of the optics and the distance from cornea to retina are well matched, a state known as **emmetropia** (Fig 14-8). To bring closer objects into focus, the eye must in-

crease its refractive power by accommodation. The ability of the lens to do so decreases with age as the lens loses its elasticity and hardens. The effect on vision usually becomes noticeable at around the age of 40 years; by the 50s, accommodation is generally lost **(presbyopia).** Each eye is permanently focused at a constant distance, and reading becomes difficult. Holding the reading material far enough away (if possible) helps, but then the image may be too small to distinguish the letters. A positive lens helps alleviate the difficulty.

Tests of Eye Function

In assessing **visual acuity,** distant vision is tested with Snellen or similar cards (Fig 14-9) for persons with fairly normal vision. Finger counting and finger movement tests are used for those with subnormal vision, and light perception and projection for those with markedly subnormal vision. Near vision is tested with standard reading cards.

Perimetry is used to determine the visual fields (Fig 14-10). The field for each eye (monocular field) is plotted with a device or by the confrontation method to determine the presence of a scotoma or other field defect (see below). For equal-sized targets, the visual field for white is most extensive; the size of the visual fields for blue, red, yellow, and green decreases in that order. Normally the visual fields overlap in an area of binocular vision (Fig 14-11).

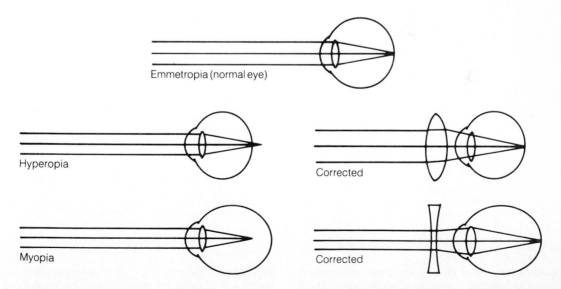

Figure 14-8. Emmetropia (normal eye) and hyperopia and myopia (common defects of the eye). In hyperopia, the eyeball is too short, and light rays come to a focus behind the retina. A biconvex lens corrects this by adding to the refractive power of the lens of the eye. In myopia, the eyeball is too long, and light rays focus in front of the retina. Placing a biconcave lens in front of the eye causes the light rays to diverge slightly before striking the eye, so that they are brought to a focus on the retina. (Reproduced, with permission, from Ganong WF: *Review of Medical Physiology,* 14th ed. Appleton & Lange, 1989.)

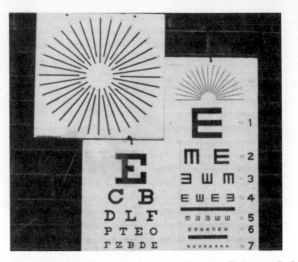

Figure 14–9. Snellen card test. (Reproduced, with permission, from Vaughan D, Asbury T: *General Ophthalmology,* 12th ed. Appleton & Lange, 1989.)

Clinical Correlations

A. Errors of Refraction: In **myopia** (nearsightedness, see Fig 14–8), the refracting system is too powerful for the length of the eyeball, causing the image of a distant object to focus in front of, instead of at, the retina. The object will be in focus only when it is brought nearer to the eye. Myopia can be corrected by placing an appropriate negative (minus) lens in front of the eye.

In **hyperopia** (farsightedness), the refracting power is too weak for the length of the eyeball, causing the

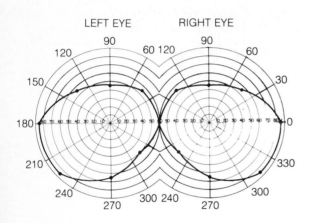

Minimum Legal Visual Field

Minimal Normal Field:

Temporally	85°
Down and temporally	85°
Down	65°
Down and nasally	50°
Nasally	60°
Up and nasally	55°
Up	45°
Up and temporally	55°
Full field	= 500°

Figure 14–10. Visual field charts. Small white objects subtending 1 degree are moved slowly to chart fields on the perimeter. The smaller the object, the more sensitive the test (with a gross error of refraction, 1 degree is reliable). Red has the smallest normal field and gives the most sensitive field test. (Reproduced, with permission, from Vaughan D, Asbury T, Tabbara KF: *General Ophthalmology,* 12th ed. Appleton & Lange, 1989.)

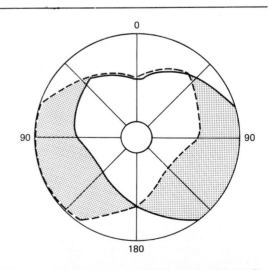

Figure 14–11. Monocular and binocular visual fields. The dotted line encloses the visual field of the left eye; the solid line, that of the right eye. The common area (heart-shaped clear zone in the center) is viewed with binocular vision. The shaded areas are viewed with monocular vision. (Reproduced, with permission, from Ganong WF: *Review of Medical Physiology,* 14th ed. Appleton & Lange, 1989.)

image to appear on the retina before it focuses. An appropriate positive (plus) lens placed in front of the eye provides additional refracting power.

Astigmatism, another optical problem, occurs when the curvature of either the lens or cornea is greater in one axis or meridian. For example, if the refracting power of the cornea is greater in its vertical axis than in its horizontal axis, the vertical rays will be refracted more than the horizontal rays, and a point source of light looks like an ellipse. A lens with an astigmatism that exactly complements that of the eye is used to correct the condition.

Scotomas are abnormal blind spots in the visual fields (the normal, physiologic, blind spot corresponds to the position of the optic disk, which lacks receptor cells). There are numerous types: Positive scotomas are apparent to the patient as dark spots, while negative scotomas (blank spots) may exist without the patient's knowledge. Motile scotomas result from opacities floating in the vitreous. In absolute scotoma, perception of light is completely lost over the defective area; in relative scotoma, it is not. Central scotomas (loss of macular vision) are caused by axial neuritis; the point of fixation is involved, and central visual acuity is correspondingly impaired. Cecocentral scotomas involve the point of fixation and extend to the normal blind spot; paracentral scotomas are adjacent to the point of fixation. Ring (annular) scotomas encircle the point of fixation. Scintillating scotomas are subjective experiences of bright colorless or colored lights in the line of vision. Other scotomas are caused by patchy lesions, as in hemorrhage and glaucoma.

B. Lesions of the Visual Apparatus: Inflammation of the optic nerve (**optic neuritis,** or **papillitis**) (Fig 14–12), is associated with various forms of retinitis, such as simple, syphilitic, diabetic, hemorrhagic, and hereditary. One form of retinitis, **retrobulbar neuritis,** occurs far enough behind the optic disk so that no changes are seen on examination of the fundus; the most common cause is multiple sclerosis.

Papilledema (choked disk; Fig 14–13) is usually a symptom of increased intracranial pressure caused by a mass (eg, brain tumor). The increased pressure is transmitted to the optic disk through the extension of the subarachnoid space around the optic nerve (see Fig 14–1). Papilledema caused by a sudden increase in intracranial pressure develops within 24–48 hours. Visual acuity is not affected in papilledema unless secondary atrophy occurs; the visual fields then contract. Most lesions of the retina or optic nerve produce a central scotoma, although contractions of the visual field or even blindness may occur.

Optic atrophy is associated with decreased visual acuity and a change in color of the optic disk to

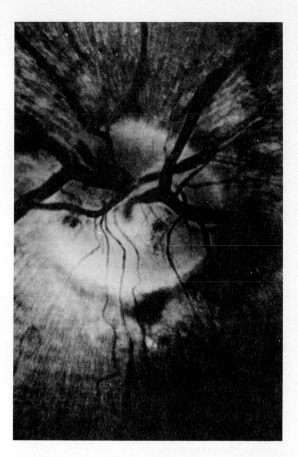

Figure 14–12. Optic neuritis (papillitis) with disk changes, including capillary hemorrhages and minimal edema (Compare with Fig 14–16). (Courtesy of WF Hoyt. Reproduced, with permission, from Vaughan D, Asbury T, Tabbara KF: *General Ophthalmology,* 12th ed. Appleton & Lange, 1989.)

light pink, white, or gray (Fig 14–14). Primary (simple) optic atrophy is caused by a process that involves the optic nerve; it does not produce papilledema. It may be caused by tabes dorsalis or multiple sclerosis, or it may be inherited. Secondary optic atrophy is a sequel of papilledema and may be due to neuritis, glaucoma, or increased intracranial pressure.

Tay-Sachs disease is an autosomal recessive, metabolic disorder that occurs in Jewish children and is associated with mental deficiency, optic atrophy, a dark cherry-red spot in place of the macula lutea, and blindness.

Holmes-Adie syndrome is characterized by a tonic pupillary reaction and the absence of one or more tendon reflexes. The pupil is said to be myotonic, with an extremely slow—and almost imperceptible—contraction to light; dilatation occurs slowly upon removal of the stimulus.

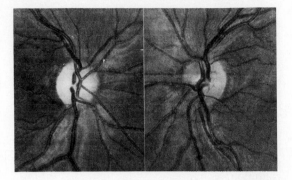

Figure 14-14. Optic atrophy. Note avascular white disk and avascular network in surrounding retina. (Courtesy of WF Hoyt. Reproduced, with permission, from Vaughan D, Asbury T, Tabbara KF: *General Ophthalmology*, 12th ed. Appleton & Lange, 1989.)

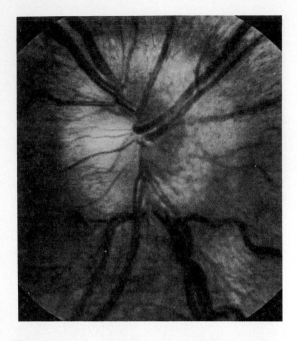

Figure 14-13. Papilledema, causing moderate disk elevation without hemorrhages. (Courtesy of WF Hoyt. Reproduced, with permission, from Vaughan D, Asbury T: *General Ophthalmology*, 11th ed. Appleton & Lange, 1986.)

VISUAL PATHWAYS

Anatomy

The **optic nerve** conveys visual impulses; it consists of about a million nerve fibers and contains axons arising from the inner, ganglion-cell layer of the retina. The information from the retina's receptors—about 126 million rods and cones—is integrated, coded, and summarized within the retina. These fibers (Fig 14–15) cross the **lamina cribrosa** of the sclera and then course through the optic canal of the skull to form the **optic chiasm.** The fibers from the nasal half of the retina decussate; those from the lateral (temporal) half do not. Each **optic tract** carries fibers from half of each retina to a **lateral geniculate body.** From there, the right halves of each retina project by way of the optic radiation to the right occipital lobe; the left halves project to the left calcarine cortex. There is a more extensive representation for the area of central vision (see Fig 14–16). **Meyer's loop** is the sweep of geniculocalcarine fibers (optic radiation) that curve around the lateral ventricle, reaching forward into the temporal lobe.

Clinical Correlations

The accurate determination of visual defects in a patient is of considerable importance in localizing a lesion in the eye, retina, optic nerve, optic pathways, or visual cortex.

Amblyopia (dim vision) is a defect of visual acuity; the cause may be in the eye or the visual pathway.

Amaurosis (complete blindness) may be hereditary or acquired. The use of the term is sometimes restricted to blindness occurring without any apparent ocular lesion, possibly because of a disease of the brain, retina, or optic nerve.

Field defects (shown in Fig 14–6) can affect one or both visual fields. If the lesion is in the optic chiasm or farther distal, both eyes show field defects. A chiasmatic lesion, often a large pituitary tumor, produces **bitemporal hemianopia,** characterized by blindness in the lateral or temporal halves of either eye (Fig 14–16B). Lesions behind the chiasm cause a field defect in the temporal half of one eye, together with a field defect in the nasal (medial) half of the other eye. The result is a **homonymous hemianopia** (Fig 14–16C and D), in which the site of the lesion is on the side opposite to the field defect.

Contraction of the visual field is a common defect that often has psychogenic causes. In severe cases, it may result in tunnel, or gun-barrel, vision. The tendency for the fields to remain small rather than to enlarge appropriately when the patient moves away from the screen is characteristic of psychogenic field defects.

Foster Kennedy's syndrome may be caused by tumors at the base of the frontal lobe. It is characterized by contralateral papilledema and ipsilateral blindness and anosmia with atrophy of the optic and olfactory nerves.

Abnormalities of pupillary size may be caused by lesions in the pathway for the pupillary light re-

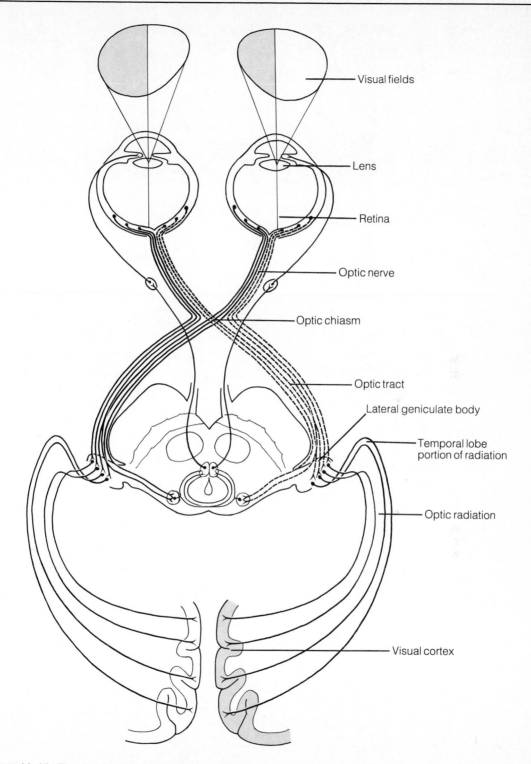

Figure 14–15. The visual pathways. The lines represent nerve fibers that extend from the retina to the occipital cortex and carry afferent visual and pupillary impulses from the left half of the visual field.

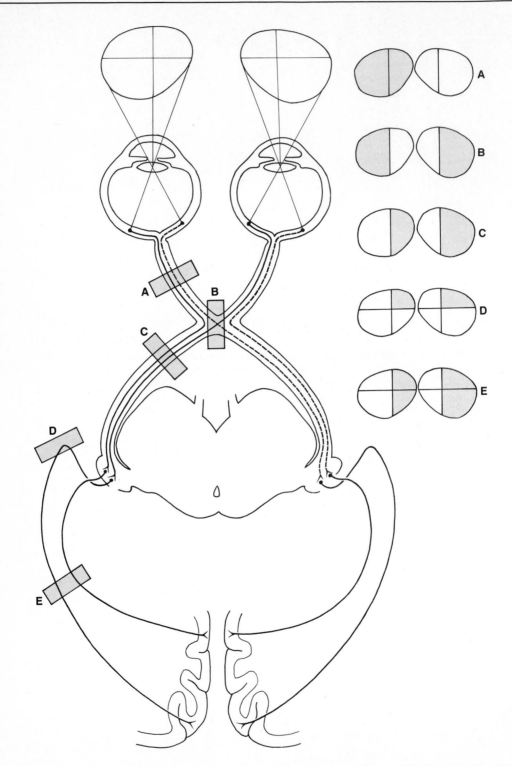

Figure 14–16. Typical lesions of the visual pathways. Their effects on the visual fields are shown on the right side of the illustration. *A:* Blindness in one eye. *B:* Bitemporal hemianopia. *C:* Homonymous hemianopia. *D:* Quadrantanopia. *E:* Homonymous hemianopia.

Table 14-1. Local effects of drugs on the eye.

Parasympathomimetics Used as miotics (to constrict pupil) for control of intraocular pressure in glaucoma	Parasympatholytics Used as mydriatics (to dilate pupil) to aid in eye examination or as cycloplegics (to relax ciliary muscles)	Sympathomimetics Used for mydriasis; do not cause cycloplegia
Pilocarpine Carbachol Methacholine Cholinesterase Inhibitors: Physostigmine (eserine) Isoflurophate	Mydriatic: Eucatropine Cyctoplegic and Mydriatic: Homatropine Scopolamine (hyoscine) Atropine Cyclopentolate	Phenylephrine Hydroxyamphetamine Epinephrine Cocaine

flex (see Fig 7–9) or to the action of a drug that affects the balance between parasympathetic and sympathetic innervation of the eye (Table 14–1).

Argyll-Robertson pupils, usually caused by neurosyphilis, are small, sometimes unequal or irregular pupils. The lesion is thought to be in the posterior commissure.

In **Horner's Syndrome,** one pupil is small (miotic) and there are other signs of dysfunction of the sympathetic supply to the pupil and orbit (see Chapter 19 and Figs 19–5 and 19–6).

Nyctalopia (night blindness) is sometimes associated with vitamin A deficiency, which affects the regeneration of rhodopsin in the retinal elements.

THE VISUAL CORTEX

Anatomy

The primary visual cortex (striate, or calcarine, cortex; area 17) is located on the medial surface of the occipital lobe, above and below the calcarine fissure (Figs 14–15 and 14–17). Areas 18 and 19, which extend concentrically outside the primary cortex, are called the **visual association cortex.**

The primary visual cortex receives its blood from the calcarine branch of the posterior cerebral artery. The remainder of the occipital lobe is supplied by other branches of this artery. The arterial supply can be (rarely) interrupted by emboli or by compression of the artery between the free edge of the tentorium and enlarging or herniating portions of the brain.

Histology. The primary visual cortex appears to contain 6 layers. It contains a line of myelinated fibers within lamina IV (the line of Gennari, or the external line of Baillarger; see Fig 14–18). The stellate cells of lamina IV receive input from the lateral

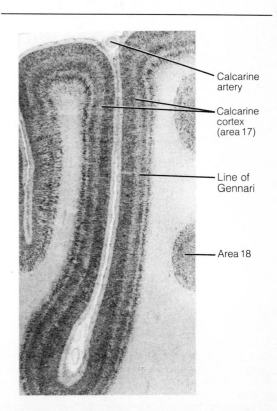

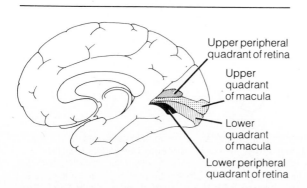

Figure 14-17. Medial view of the right cerebral hemisphere, showing projection of the retina on the calcarine cortex.

Figure 14-18. Light micrograph of the primary visual cortex (calcarine cortex) on each side of the calcarine fissure.

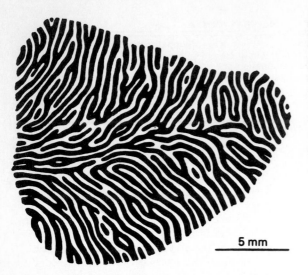

Figure 14–19. Reconstruction of ocular dominance columns in a subdivision of layer IV of a portion of the right visual cortex of a rhesus monkey. Dark stripes represent one eye, light stripes represent the other. (Reproduced, with permission, from LeVay S, Hubel DH, Wiesel TN: The pattern of ocular dominance columns in macaque visual cortex revealed by a reduced silver stain. *J Comp Neurol* 1975;**159**:559.)

geniculate nucleus, and the pyramidal cells of layer V project to the superior colliculus. Layer VI cells send a recurrent projection to the lateral geniculate nucleus.

Physiology

The visual cortex contains vertical ocular dominance columns, each 0.8 mm in diameter. Columns receiving input from one eye alternate with columns receiving input from the other (Fig 14–19). The ocular dominance columns can be mapped by injecting radioactive amino acid in one eye. The amino acid is incorporated into protein and transported by axoplasmic flow to the ganglion cell terminals, across the geniculate synapses, and along the optic radiation fibers to the visual cortex. Layer IV becomes evenly labeled. Above and below this layer, however, labeled columns alternate with unlabeled columns that receive input from the uninjected eye. Ocular dominance columns can also be demonstrated by radioautography following injection of 2-deoxyglucose into one eye while the other eye is closed.

Like the ganglion cells in the retina, the lateral geniculate cells and the cells in layer IV of the visual cortex respond in a typical way to stimuli in their receptive fields, as shown in Fig 14–20. Illuminating the center of these cells with a linear stimulus, such as a bar of light, is an effective way to test them. They have circular receptive fields, with an excitatory center and inhibitory surrounding zone, or vice versa. The bar of light is equally effective at any angle, and it has no preferred orientation. Simple cells are strikingly different; they respond to a bar of light only when the bar has a particular orientation. Complex cells respond best to a moving linear stimulus.

CASE 21

A 50-year-old woman had experienced a sudden loss of consciousness 3 months prior to admission. She said that her husband described the incident as an epileptiform attack and that she had a headache

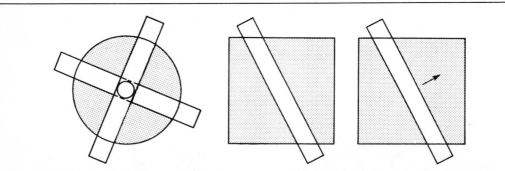

Figure 14–20. Receptive fields of cells in visual pathways. *Left:* Ganglion cells, lateral geniculate cells, and cells in layer IV of cortical area 17 have circular fields with an excitatory center and an inhibitory surround or an inhibitory center and an excitatory surround. There is no preferred orientation of a linear stimulus. *Center:* Simple cells respond best to a linear stimulus with a particular orientation in a specific part of the cell's receptive field. *Right:* Complex cells respond to linear stimuli with a particular orientation, but they are less selective in terms of location in the receptive field. They often respond maximally when the stimulus is moved laterally, as indicated by the arrow. (Modified from Hubel DH: The visual field cortex of normal and deprived monkeys. *Am Sci* 1979;**67**:532. Reproduced, with permission, from Ganong WF: *Review of Medical Physiology,* 14th ed. Appleton & Lange, 1989.)

for a few hours following it. The day after, she had felt much better. More recently, however, she thought that her memory was failing because she had several episodes during which her thoughts "would become all jumbled up" and her right hand would feel heavy. Two weeks earlier, she began to suffer from a constant frontal headache. She felt her glasses needed changing, and the ophthalmologist referred her to the neurological service. While giving her history, the patient appeared to be moderately alert but with impaired memory, and she made some silly jokes about her health.

Neurologic examination showed that olfaction was totally lost on the left side but normal on the right. The right optic papilla was congested and edematous, and the left optic disk was abnormally pale. Visual acuity was normal in the right eye but impaired in the left. The muscles of facial expression were slightly weaker on the right than on the left side. Deep tendon reflexes on the right side of the body were brisker than those on the left. The remainder of the findings was within normal limits.

Where is the lesion? What is the differential diagnosis? Would a neuroradiologic procedure be useful? What is the most likely diagnosis?
Cases are discussed further in Chapter 24.

REFERENCES

Enoch JM (editor): *Optics of Vertebrate Retinal Receptors.* Springer-Verlag, 1982.

Hubel DH, Wiesel TN: Brain mechanisms of vision. *Sci Am* (Sept) 1979;**241**:150.

Kandel ER, Schwartz JS: *Principles of Neural Science,* 2nd ed. Elsevier, 1985.

Miller NR (editor): *Walsh and Hoyt's Clinical Neuro-Ophthalmology,* 4th ed. Vol 1. Williams & Wilkins, 1984.

Rodieck RW: Visual pathways. *Ann Rev Neurosci* 1979; **2**:193.

Van Essen DC: Visual areas of the mammalian cerebral cortex. *Ann Rev Neurosci* 1979;**2**:227.

The Auditory System

ANATOMY & FUNCTION

The **cochlea** is the specialized organ that registers and transduces sound waves. It lies within the cochlear duct, a portion of the membranous labyrinth within the temporal bone of the skull base (Fig 15–1; see also Chapter 10). Sound waves converge through the **pinna** and **outer ear canal** to strike the **tympanic membrane** (Figs 15–1 and 15–2). The vibrations of this membrane are transmitted by way of 3 **ossicles (malleus, incus,** and **stapes)** in the **middle ear** to the oval window, where the sound waves are transmitted to the **cochlear duct.** Two small muscles can affect the strength of the auditory signal: the **tensor tympani,** which attaches to the eardrum, and the **stapedius** muscle, which attaches to the stapes. These muscles may dampen the signal; they also help prevent damage to the ear from very loud noises. The **inner ear** contains the **organ of Corti** within the cochlear duct (Fig 15–3). Sound waves stimulate the organ of Corti through the vibrations of the tectorial membrane against the kinocilia of the hair cells (Figs 15–3 and 15–4). The mechanical distortions of the kinocilium of each haircell are transformed into electric signals that course into the neurons of the cochlear nerve.

AUDITORY PATHWAYS

Peripheral branches of bipolar nerve cells in the spiral ganglion innervate the cochlear organ of Corti; central branches course in the cochlear portion of nerve VIII and terminate in the ventral and dorsal **cochlear nuclei** in the brain stem (Fig 15–5; see also Chapter 6). Second-order fibers ascend from the cochlear nuclei on both sides; the crossing fibers pass through the trapezoid body. The ascending fibers course in the **lateral lemnisci** within the brain stem; these tracts therefore carry impulses derived from both ears (Fig 15–6). Cell groups along the course of each lateral lemniscus (nuclei of the trapezoid body, lateral lemniscus, and inferior colliculus) probably receive collateral fibers, some of which end in the cerebellum or re-

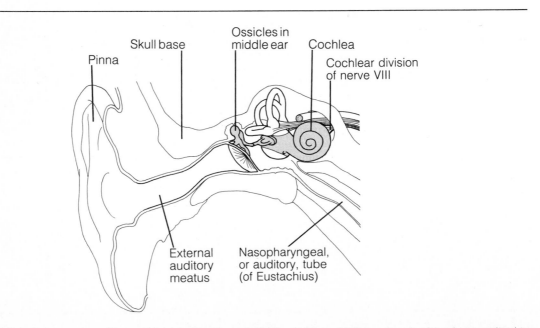

Figure 15–1. The human ear. The cochlea has been turned slightly, and the middle ear muscles have been omitted to make the relationship clear.

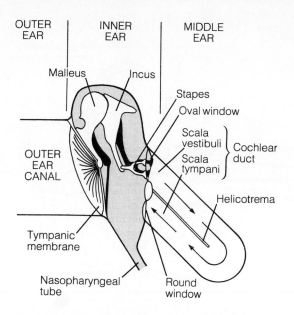

Figure 15-2. Schematic view of the ear. As sound waves hit the tympanic membrane, the position of the ossicles (shown in black) changes.

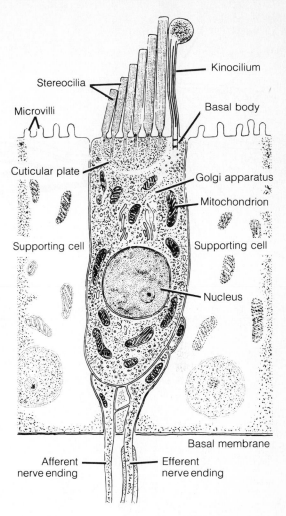

Figure 15-4. Structure of hair cell. (Reproduced, with permission, from Hudspeth AJ: The hair cells of the inner ear. *Sci Am* 1983;**248**:54.

ticular formation. Others cross to the opposite nucleus; they are involved in determining the difference in signal strength from each auditory input, and may thus determine the location of the sound. Reflex connections pass to eye muscle nuclei and other motor nuclei of the cranial and spinal nerves via the **tectobulbar** and **tectospinal tracts.** These connections are activated by strong, sudden sounds; the result is reflex turning of the eyes and head toward the site of the sound. In the lower

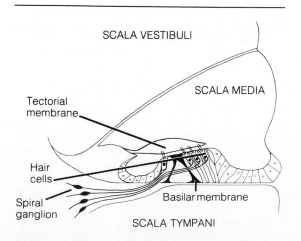

Figure 15-3. Cross section through one turn of the cochlea.

pons, the **superior olivary nuclei** receive input from both ascending pathways. Efferent fibers from these nuclei course along the cochlear nerve back to the organ of Corti. The function of this **olivocochlear bundle** is to modulate the sensitivity of the cochlear organ.

The lateral lemnisci end in the **medial geniculate bodies** by way of the **inferior colliculus** and **inferior quadrigeminal brachium;** additional fibers terminate directly in these thalamic nuclei. The third-order fibers project to the upper and medial portion of the superior temporal gyrus (area 41; Figs 15-6 and 9-11).

Tonotopia, a precise localization of high-frequency to low-frequency sound-wave transmission exists along the entire pathway from cochlea to auditory cortex.

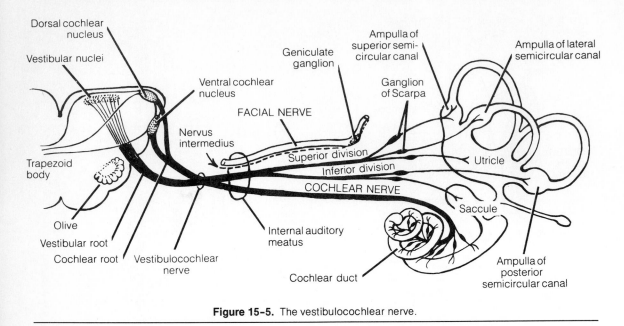

Figure 15–5. The vestibulocochlear nerve.

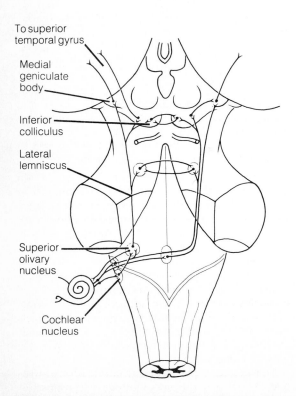

Figure 15–6. Diagram of main auditory pathways superimposed on a dorsal view of the brain stem.

Clinical Correlations

A. Tinnitus: Ringing, buzzing, hissing, roaring, or "paper-crushing" noises in the ear are frequently an early sign of peripheral cochlear disease (eg, hydrops, or edema, of the cochlea).

B. Deafness: Deafness in one ear can be caused by an impairment in the conduction of sound through the external ear canal and ossicles to the endolymph and tectorial membrane; this is called conduction deafness. **Nerve (sensoneural)**, deafness can be caused by interruption of cochlear nerve fibers from the hair cells to the brain stem nuclei (Fig 15–7). Tests used to distinguish between nerve and conduction deafness are shown in Table 15–1. Nerve deafness is often located in the inner ear or in the cochlear nerve in the internal auditory meatus; conduction deafness is the result of middle or external ear disease. Progressive ossification of the ligaments between the ossicles, **otosclerosis,** is a common type of hearing loss in adults. A delicate surgical procedure, **fenestration,** exposes the cochlear duct to the outside air (a membrane is interposed), improving the air conduction of auditory signals.

A peripheral lesion in the eighth nerve with loss of hearing, such as a **cerebellopontine angle tumor,** usually involves both the cochlear and vestibular nerves (Fig 15–8). Central lesions can involve either system independently. Because the auditory pathway above the cochlear nuclei represents parts of the sound input to both ears, a unilateral lesion in the lateral lemniscus, medial geniculate body, or auditory cortex does *not* result in marked loss of hearing on the ipsilateral side. The brain stem audi-

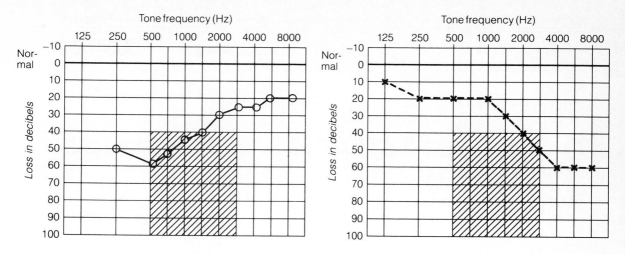

Figure 15–7. *Left:* Middle ear, or conduction, deafness. Representative air conduction curve shows greatest impairment of pure tone thresholds in lower frequencies. *Right:* Perception, or nerve, deafness. Representative bone conduction curve of pure tone thresholds shows greatest deficit at higher frequencies.

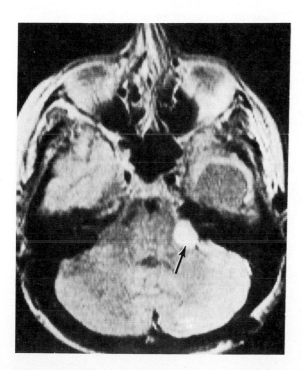

Figure 15–8. Magnetic resonance image of a horizontal section through the head at the level of the lower pons and internal auditory meatus. A left acoustic nerve schwannoma with its high intensity is shown in the left cerebellopontine angle (arrow).

tory evoked response (BAER) test (see Chapter 23) aids in localizing a lesion.

Hearing loss becomes a significant handicap when there is difficulty in communicating by speech. Beginning impairment has been defined as an average hearing-level loss of 16 decibels (dB) at frequencies of 500, 1000, and 2000 Hz: Sounds of these frequencies cannot be heard when their strength is 16 dB or less (a loud whisper). A person is usually considered to be deaf when the hearing level loss for these 3 frequencies is at or above 82 dB (the noise level of heavy traffic). Early hearing loss often appears initially at a high frequency (4000 Hz), in both children with conduction impairment and adults with **presbycusis** (lessening of hearing in old age). An artificial hearing aid may improve sound perception by amplifying the strength of the incoming sound, and an experimental procedure, artificial cochlear implantation, has had promising results.

C. Hearing Scotomas: Deafness to certain pitches and noises is not infrequent in multiple sclerosis; this is probably the result of the demyelinated areas that develop within the cochlear nerve of the auditory pathways. Devotees of loud music often have a generalized hearing loss, sometimes hearing scotomas caused by destruction in the organ of Corti. There is no demonstrable physical explanation for the deafness found in hysteria or schizophrenia.

CASE 22

A 64-year-old woman was admitted for evaluation of progressive hearing loss, facial weakness,

Table 15-1. Common tests with a tuning fork to distinguish between nerve and conduction hearing loss.

Method	Normal	Conduction Hearing Loss (one ear)	Nerve (sensorineural) Hearing Loss (one ear)
Weber Base of vibrating tuning fork placed on vertex of skull.	Sound equal on both sides.	Sound louder in diseased ear because masking effect of environmental noise is absent on diseased side.	Sound louder in normal ear.
Rinne Base of vibrating tuning fork placed on mastoid process until subject no longer hears it, then held in air next to ear.	Hears vibration in air after bone conduction is over.	Does not hear vibrations in air after bone conduction is over.	Hears vibration in air after bone conduction is over.

and increasing headaches, all on the right side. Her hearing loss had been present for at least 5 years, and 2 years prior to admission, she had noted the gradual development of unsteadiness in walking. During recent months, she began to experience weakness and progressive numbness of the right side of the face as well as occasional double vision. There was no nausea or vomiting.

Neurologic examination showed beginning bilateral papilledema, decreased pain and touch sensation in the right half of the face, moderate right peripheral facial weakness, absence of both the right corneal reflex and blinking with the right eye. Tests of air and bone conduction showed hearing was markedly decreased on the right side. Caloric labyrinthine stimulation was normal on the left; there was no response on the right. Examination of the motor system, reflexes, and sensations yielded normal results, with the exception of 2 findings: a broad-based gait and the inability to walk with feet tandem.

What is the differential diagnosis? What is the most likely diagnosis?

Cases are discussed further in Chapter 24.

REFERENCES

Hart RG, Gardner DP, Howieson J: Acoustic tumors: Atypical features and recent diagnostic tests. *Neurology* 33;**211**:1983.

Hudspeth AJ: The cellular basis of hearing: The biophysics of hair cells. *Science* 230;**745**:1985.

Kim Do, Molnar CE: Cochlear mechanics. Pages 45–56 in: *The Nervous System.* Vol 3. Eagles EL (editor). Raven, 1975.

Morest DK: Structural organization of the auditory pathways. Pages 19–30 in: *The Nervous System.* Vol 3. Eagles EL (editor). Raven, 1975.

Patuzzi R, Robertson D: Tuning in the mammalian cochlea. *Physiol Rev* Vol 68, 1988.

Schubert ED: *Hearing: Its Function and Dysfunction.* Springer-Verlag, 1980.

Smith CA: Inner Ear. Pages 1–18 in: *The Nervous System.* Vol 3. Eagles EL (editor). Raven, 1975.

The Vestibular System

16

ANATOMY

The membranous **labyrinth,** filled with endolymph and surrounded by perilymph, lies in the bony labyrinthine space within the temporal bone of the skull base (Fig 16–1). Two special sensory systems receive their input from structures in the membranous labyrinth: the auditory system from the cochlea (see Chapter 15), and the vestibular system from the remainder of the labyrinth. The **static labyrinth** gives information regarding the position of the head in space; the specialized sensory areas lie in the **macula** and the **utricle** (Fig 16–1). The **kinetic labyrinth** sends information regarding head movement from special areas within the **ampullae** (the 3 semicircular canals).

VESTIBULAR PATHWAYS

The peripheral branches of the bipolar cells in the **vestibular ganglion** course from the specialized neuroepithelium in the ampullae, and from the maculae of the utricle and the saccule. The central branches enter the brain stem and end in the **vestibular nuclei** (Figs 16–1 and 16–2; see also Chapter 6).

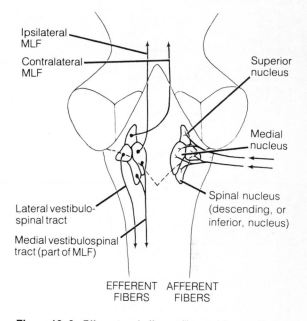

Figure 16–2. Efferent and afferent fibers of the vestibular nuclei. MLF, medial longitudinal fasciculus.

Some vestibular connections go from the superior and lateral vestibular nuclei to the cerebellum. Others course from the lateral nuclei into the ipsilateral spinal cord via the lateral **vestibulospinal tracts** from the superior and medial vestibular nuclei to nuclei of the eye muscles, and to the motor nuclei of the upper spinal nerves via the **medial longitudinal fasciculi** (MLF) of the same and opposite sides (Fig 16–3). The **medial vestibulospinal tract** (the descending portion of the MLF) connects to the anterior horn of the cervical and upper thoracic cord; this tract is involved in the labyrinthine righting reflexes that adjust the position of the head in response to signals of vestibular origin. Some vestibular nuclei send fibers to the reticular formation. The ascending fibers travel by way of the thalamus (ventral posterior nucleus) to the parietal cortex (area 40).

FUNCTIONS

The vestibular nerve conducts 2 types of information to the brain stem: the position of the head in space, and the angular rotation of the head.

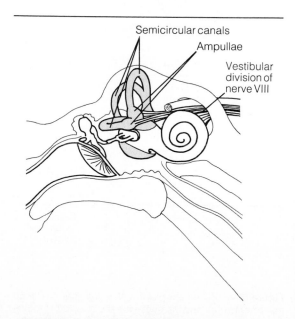

Figure 16–1. The human ear (compare with Fig 15–1).

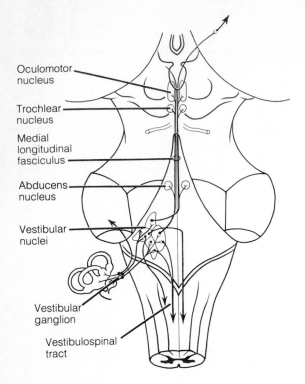

Figure 16–3. Simplified diagram of main vestibular pathways superimposed on a dorsal view of the brain stem (cerebellar connections are not shown).

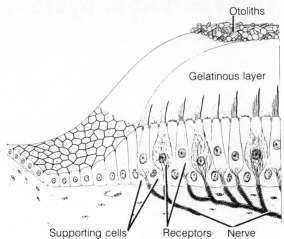

Figure 16–4. Macular structure. (Reproduced, with permission, from Junqueira LC, Carneiro J, Kelley RO: *Basic Histology,* 6th ed. Appleton & Lange, 1989.)

The pressure of the **otoliths** (calcareous particles) on the sensitive areas in the **macula** and **saccule** is transduced to impulses in the inferior division of the vestibular nerve (Figs 16–1 and 16–4).

Each of the 3 semicircular canals (superior, posterior, and lateral) contains a widened portion, the **ampulla** (Fig 16–5). Within each ampulla, a flexible **crista** changes its shape and direction according to the movement of the endolymph within the canal, so that any rotation of the head can affect the crista and its afferent nerve fibers (Fig 16–6). Acting together, the semicircular canals send impulses along the superior division of the vestibular nerve to the central vestibular pathways.

The entire vestibular apparatus thus provides information that contributes to the maintenance of **equilibrium** and, together with information from the visual and proprioceptive systems, provides a complex position sense in the brain stem and cerebellum.

When the head moves, a compensatory adjustment of gaze, the **vestibulo-ocular reflex,** is required to keep the eyes fixed on one object. Clockwise rotation of the eyes is caused by counterclockwise rotation of the head. The pathways for the reflex are via the medial longitudinal fascic-

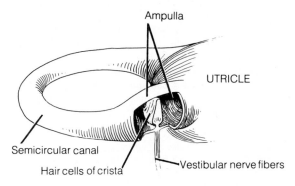

Figure 16–5. Diagram of a crista in an opened ampulla.

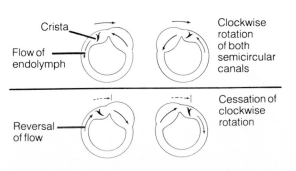

Figure 16–6. Schematic illustration of the effects of head movements (*top*) and the subsequent cessation of movement (*bottom*) on the crista and the direction of endolymph flow.

ulus and involve the vestibular system and the motor nuclei for eye movement (see Fig 7–7).

Clinical Correlations

Nystagmus is an involuntary back-and-forth, up-and-down, or rotating movement of the eyeballs, with a slow pull and a rapid return jerk. (The name comes from the rapid jerking component, which is a compensatory adjustment to the slow reflex movement.) Nystagmus can be induced in normal individuals; if it occurs spontaneously it is a sign of a lesion (Table 16–1). The lesions that cause nystagmus affect the complex neural mechanism that tends to keep the eyes constant in relation to their environment and is thus concerned with equilibrium. **Physiologic nystagmus** can be elicited by turning the eyes far to one side or by stimulating one of the semicircular canals (usually the lateral) with cool (30 °C) or warm 40 °C) water injected into one external ear canal (Fig 16–7). Cool water produces nystagmus toward the opposite side; warm water produces nystagmus to the same side. (A mnemonic for this is COWS: cool, opposite; warm, same.) **Peripheral vestibular nystagmus** results from stimulation of the peripheral vestibular apparatus and is always accompanied by vertigo. Fast spinning of the body, sometimes seen on the playground, is an example: if the child is suddenly stopped, its eyes show nystagmus for a few seconds. Professional skaters and dancers learn not to be bothered by nystagmus and vertigo. **Central nervous system nystagmus** is seldom associated with vertigo; it occurs with lesions in the region of the fourth ventricle. **Optokinetic (railroad, or freeway), nystagmus** occurs when there is continuous movement of the visual field past the eyes, as when traveling by train. **Toxic nystagmus** may follow treatment with certain drugs. Streptomycin and other drugs may even cause degeneration of the vestibular organ and nuclei.

Vertigo, an illusory feeling of giddiness with disorientation in space that usually results in a disturbance of equilibrium, is often a sign of labyrinthine disease originating in the middle or internal

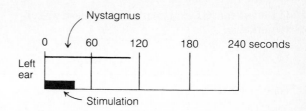

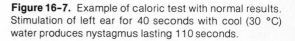

Figure 16–7. Example of caloric test with normal results. Stimulation of left ear for 40 seconds with cool (30 °C) water produces nystagmus lasting 110 seconds.

ear. Adjustment to peripheral vestibular damage is rapid (within a few days). Even though a labyrinth is not intact or functioning, balance is still remarkably good when vision is present: visual information can even compensate for the loss of both labyrinths. Vertigo can also result from tumors or other lesions of the vestibular system (eg, **Meniere's syndrome,** or **paroxysmal labyrinthine vertigo**) or from reflex phenomena (eg, **seasickness**). Seasickness is caused by continuous, irregular movement of the endolymph in susceptible individuals. It is characterized by disturbances in equilibrium and by nausea and vomiting that are not related to diet. Vertigo is sometimes relieved or induced by placing the head in certain positions; it can often be prevented by medication.

Vestibular ataxia, with clumsy, uncoordinated movements, may result from the same lesions that produce vertigo. Nystagmus is often present. Vestibular ataxia must be distinguished from other types: **cerebellar ataxia** (see Chapters 6 and 12) and **sensory ataxia** (caused by lesions in the proprioceptive pathways; see Chapter 4).

Interruption of the pathway between the nuclei of nerves VIII, VI and III (the medial longitudinal fasciculus, pathway of the vestibulo-ocular reflex) results in **internuclear ophthalmoplegia,** an inability to adduct the eye ipsilateral to the lesion.

CASE 23

A 38-year-old male clerk saw his doctor because he experienced sudden episodes of nausea and dizziness. These attacks had started 3 weeks earlier and seemed to be getting worse. The abnormal episodes at first lasted only a few minutes, during which "the room seemed to spin." Lately they had been lasting for many hours. A severe attack caused him to vomit and to hear abnormal sounds (ringing, buzzing, paper-rolling) in the left ear. He thought that he was becoming deaf on that side.

The neurologic examination was within normal limits except for a slight sensorineural hearing loss

Table 16–1. Types of nystagmus.

Induced	Optokinetic ("railway" or "freeway") Ocular ("miners", with eyes in extreme position) Caloric (COWS) Postrotatory (opposite to the direction of rotation)
Pathologic	Peripheral vestibular (away from the lesion): cerebropontine angle tumor, Meniere's syndrome Central vestibular (away from the lesion): brain stem lesion Cerebellar, with ataxia of the eye muscles

in the left ear. CT examination of the head was unremarkable.

What is the probable diagnosis?
Cases are further discussed in Chapter 24.

REFERENCES

Baloh RW, Honrubia V: *Clinical Neurophysiology of the Vestibular System.* Davis, 1979.

Brandt T, Daroff RB: The multisensory physiological and pathological vertigo syndromes. *Ann Neurol* 1980;7:195.

Harada Y: *The Vestibular Organs.* Kugler & Ghedini, 1988.

Luxon LM: Diseases of the eighth cranial nerve. In: *Peripheral Neuropathy,* 2nd ed. Dyck PJ et al (editors). Saunders, 1984.

Reticular Formation

ANATOMY

The reticular formation (Fig 17–1) consists of interconnected regions in the tegmentum of the brain stem, the lateral hypothalamic area; and the medial, intralaminar, and reticular nuclei of the thalamus. Thalamic efferents project to most of the cerebral cortex. The term itself derives from the characteristic appearance of loosely packed cells of varying sizes and shapes that are embedded in a dense meshwork of cell processes, including dendrites and axons.

FUNCTIONS

Arousal

Regulation of arousal and the level of consciousness is a generalized function of the reticular formation. The neurons of the activating portion of the reticular formation are excited by a wide variety of sensory stimuli that are conducted by way of collaterals from the somatosensory, auditory, visual, and visceral sensory systems. The reticular formation is therefore nonspecific in its response and performs a generalized regulatory function. When a novel stimulus is received, attention is focused on it while general alertness increases. This **behavioral arousal** is independent of the modality of stimulation and is accompanied by electroencephalographic changes from low-voltage to high-

voltage activity over much of the cortex. The nonspecific thalamic regions project to the cortex, specifically to the distal dendritic fields of the large pyramidal cells. When the stimulus is repeated, the arousal response becomes habituated (dies down). In fact, slow repetitive stimuli, such as those in counting sheep or inducing hypnosis, will reduce cortical activity and lull a person to sleep. If the reticular formation is depressed by anesthesia or destroyed, sensory stimuli still produce activity in the specific thalamic and cortical sensory areas, but they do not produce generalized cortical arousal.

Consciousness

Many regions of the cerebral cortex produce generalized arousal when stimulated (this is the basis for the saying, "pinch yourself to see if you're dreaming"). Arousal, which is abolished by lesions in the mesencephalic reticular formation, does not require an intact corpus callosum. The cortex and the mesencephalic reticular-activating system are mutually sustaining areas involved in maintaining consciousness. Lesions that destroy a large area of the cortex, a small area of the midbrain, or both produce coma (see Fig 17–2).

The loss of consciousness in **syncope** (fainting) is usually brief in duration and sudden in onset; more prolonged and profound loss of consciousness is described as **coma.** A patient in coma is unresponsive and cannot be aroused. There may be no reaction—or only a primitive defense movement such as corneal reflex or limb withdrawal—to to painful stimuli. A patient in **semicoma** (a milder grade of coma) may attempt to push away an offending stimulus. **Stupor, obtundation,** and **confusion** are still lesser grades and are characterized by variable degrees of disorientation and impaired reactivity. Acute confusional states must be distinguished from dementia (see Chapter 21). In the former case, the patient is disoriented, inattentive, and sleepy but reacts appropriately to certain stimuli.

Coma may be of intracranial or extracranial origin. **Intracranial** causes include head injuries, cerebrovascular accidents, central nervous system infections, tumors, convulsive disorders, degenerative diseases, and increased intracranial pressure. **Extracranial** causes include vascular disorders (shock or hypotension caused by severe hemorrhage or myocardial infarction), metabolic disorders (diabetic acidosis, hypoglycemia, uremia, hepatic coma, addisonian crisis, electrolyte imbal-

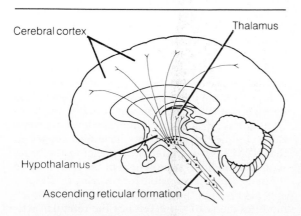

Figure 17-1. Ascending reticular system.

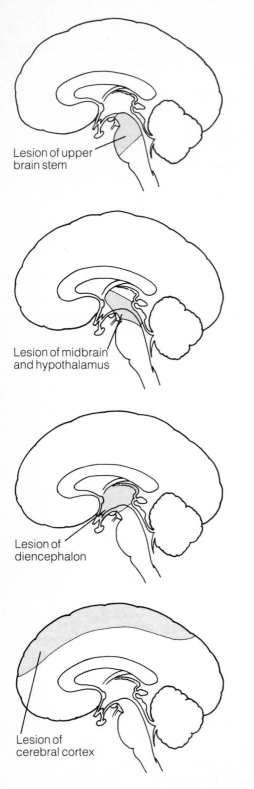

Lesion of upper
brain stem

Lesion of midbrain
and hypothalamus

Lesion of
diencephalon

Lesion of
cerebral cortex

Figure 17-2. Lesions that cause coma or loss of consciousness.

ance), intoxication (with alcohol, barbiturates, narcotics, bromides, analgesics, ataractics, carbon monoxide, heavy metals), and miscellaneous disorders (hyperthermia, hypothermia, electric shock, anaphylaxis, severe systemic infections). The **Glasgow Coma Scale** (Table 17–1) offers a practical method of assessing changes in the level of consciousness, based upon eye opening and verbal and motor responses.

Sleep

A. Periodicity: The daily cycle of arousal, which includes periods of sleep and of waking, is regulated by reticular formation structures in the hypothalamus and brain stem. The sleep process of this 24-hour circadian rhythm is an active physiologic function. Nerve cells in the reticular formation of the pons begin to discharge just prior to the onset of sleep. Lesions of the pons just forward of the trigeminal nerve produce a state of hyperalertness and much less sleep than normal.

B. Stages: The sleep cycle consists of several stages that follow one another in an orderly fashion (Fig 17–3), each taking about 90 minutes. The stages can be defined by characteristic wave patterns on electroencephalograms (see Chapter 23). There are 2 distinct types of sleep: slow-wave sleep and rapid eye movement sleep.

Slow-wave sleep is further divided into stages. Stage 1 of **slow-wave (spindle) sleep** is characterized by easy arousal. Stages 2–4 are progressively deeper, and the electroencephalographic pattern becomes more synchronized. In stage 4, the deepest stage of slow-wave sleep, blood pressure, pulse rate, respiratory rate, and the amount of oxygen consumed by the brain are very low. The control mechanisms for slow-wave sleep are not known.

Rapid eye movement (REM) sleep is characterized by the sudden appearance of an asynchronous pattern on electroencephalograms. The sleepers make intermittent rapid eye movements, are hard to awake, show a striking loss of muscle tone in the limbs, and have vivid visual imagery and complex dreams. There is a specific need for REM sleep, which is triggered by neurons in the dorsal midbrain and pontine tegmentumm.

In experiments involving cats, a waking pattern was found if a transection was made at the junction of the medulla and spinal cord (**encephale isole**); a slow-wave pattern was found if the transection was at a higher midbrain level (**cerveau isole**). Studies involving cats have also suggested that REM sleep is initiated by nuclei in the brain stem. The **midline raphe system** of the pons may be the main center responsible for bringing on sleep; it may act through the secretion of serotonin, which modifies many of the effects of the reticular activating system. Paradoxic REM sleep follows when a second secretion (norepinephrine), produced by

Table 17-1. Glasgow Coma Scale. A practical method of assessing changes in level of consciousness, based upon eye opening and verbal and motor responses. The response can be expressed by the sum of the scores assigned to each response. The lowest score is 3, and the highest score is 15.*

	Examiner's Test	Patient's Response	Assigned Score
Eye opening	Spontaneous	Opens eyes on own.	4
	Speech	Opens eyes when asked to do so in a loud voice.	3
	Pain	Opens eyes when pinched.	2
	Pain	Does not open eyes.	1
Best motor response	Commands	Follows simple commands.	6
	Pain	Pulls examiner's hand away when pinched.	5
	Pain	Pulls a part of body away when pinched.	4
	Pain	Flexes body inappropriately to pain (decorticate posturing).	3
	Pain	Body becomes rigid in an extended position when pinched (decerebrate posturing).	2
	Pain	Has no motor response to pinch.	1
Verbal response (talking)	Speech	Carries on a conversation correctly and tells examiner where and who he or she is and the month and year.	5
	Speech	Seems confused or disoriented.	4
	Speech	Talks so examiner can understand words but makes no sense.	3
	Speech	Makes sounds examiner cannot understand.	2
	Speech	Makes no noise.	1

*Slightly modified and reproduced, with permission, from Rimel RN, Jane JA, Edlich RF: Injury scale for comprehensive management of CNS trauma. *JACEP* 1979; 8:64.

the **locus ceruleus,** supplants the raphe secretion. The effects resemble normal wakefulness.

Destruction of the rostral reticular nucleus of the pons abolishes REM sleep, usually without affecting slow-wave sleep or arousal. REM sleep is suppressed by dopa or monoamine oxidase inhibitors, which increase the norepinephrine concentration in the brain. Lesions of the raphe nuclei in the pons cause prolonged wakefulness. The raphe nuclei contain appreciable amounts of serotonin, and it has been shown that treatment with p-chlorophenylalanine (which inhibits serotonin synthesis) causes wakefulness in cats. When cats are treated with compounds that increase serotonin, there is an increase in the amount of slow-wave sleep.

C. Clinical Correlations:
1. Somnambulism and nocturnal enuresis– Somnambulism (sleepwalking) and nocturnal enuresis (bed-wetting) are particularly apt to occur during arousal from slow-wave sleep. Somnambulists walk with their eyes open and avoid obstacles, but they cannot recall the episode (which may last several minutes) when they are awakened.

2. Hypersomnia and apnea–Hypersomnia (excessive daytime sleepiness) and recurrent apnea during sleep may occur. Affected patients are apt to be obese middle-aged men who snore loudly. Functional obstruction of the oropharyngeal airway during sleep has been implicated in these patients, and symptoms in severe cases may be relieved by tracheostomy.

3. Narcolepsy–Narcolepsy is a chronic clinical syndrome characterized by intermittent episodes of uncontrollable sleep. Sudden transient loss of muscle tone in the extremities or trunk (**cataplexy**) and pathologic muscle weakness during emotional reactions may also occur. There may be **sleep paralysis,** the inability to move in the interval between sleep and arousal, and **hypnogogic hallucinations** may occur at the onset of sleep. Sleep attacks can occur several times daily under appropriate or inappropriate circumstances, with or without forewarning. The attacks last from minutes to hours.

Narcolepsy usually persists throughout life. Although the attacks of somnolence and sleep may be relieved by medical treatment, the cataplexy and attacks of muscular weakness that accompany emotional reactions (eg, laughing and crying) are usually not affected by drug therapy. The nocturnal sleep of narcoleptics is usually unremarkable.

CASE 24

A 64-year-old right-handed man was admitted with subacute weakness and numbness of the left arm and leg. The patient was slightly confused and

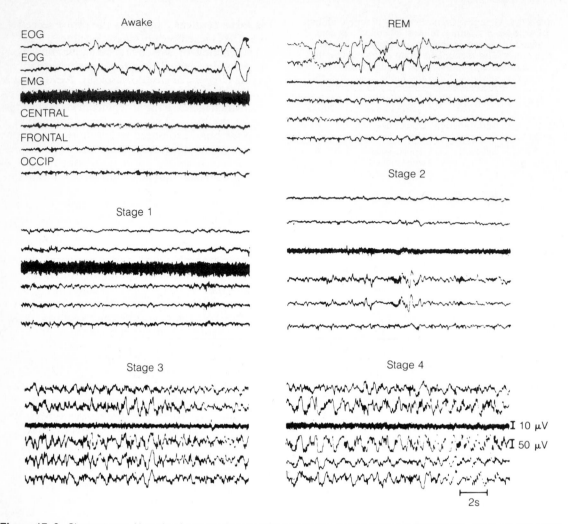

Figure 17-3. Sleep stages. Note that low muscle tone with extensive eye movement in REM sleep. EOG, electro-oculogram registering eye movements; EMG, electromyogram registering skeletal muscle activity. Central, Frontal, Occip, 3 electroencephalographic leads. (Reproduced, with permission, from Kales A et al: Sleep and dreams: Recent research on clinical aspects. *Ann Intern Med* 1968;**68**:1078.)

unable to speak clearly. In the previous several months, he had experienced a dozen or so transient episodes of unsteadiness of gait with weakness in both legs, together with dizziness and ringing in the left ear. Once or twice while walking in the park, he had had to stop because of sharp pains in his left leg. These pains went away after a few minutes.

Neurologic examination showed a well-muscled, cooperative patient with barely intelligible speech (**dysarthria**). Findings included a left pupil that was slightly larger than the right, weakness of the right lateral rectus muscle, nystagmus on left and right gaze, decreased pain sensation in the right side of the face, decreased right corneal reflex, paralysis of the right side of the lower face, decreased gag reflex, an inability to swallow on command, and the tongue in midline location but weak in lateral movement. The patient's strength was uniformly decreased in all extremities but more so on the right. Results of finger-to-nose and heel-to-shin tests were abnormal. Deep tendon reflexes were hyperactive, with clonus of the quadriceps muscle and bilateral plantar extensor responses. Pain sensation was decreased in the left leg; vibratory and position senses were decreased in both legs. There were no visual field defects. Laboratory findings were normal, but blood pressure was 200/90, and pulses in the lower extremities ranged from decreased to absent. The patient refused any radiologic tests.

What is the differential diagnosis? What is the most likely diagnosis?

Cases are discussed further in Chapter 24.

REFERENCES

Globus GG, Maxwell G, Savodnik P (editors): *Consciousness and the Brain.* Plenum Press, 1976.

Plum F, Posner JB: *The Diagnosis of Stupor and Coma,* 3rd ed. Vol 19: *Contemporary Neurology Series.* Davis, 1980.

18

The Limbic System

The **great limbic lobe,** described by Broca in 1874, was so named because this cortical complex formed a limbus (border) between the diencephalon and the more lateral neocortex of the telencephalic hemispheres (Fig 18–1). This limbic lobe was said to consist of a ring of cortex outside the corpus callosum, largely made up of the subcallosal and cingulate gyri, as well as the parahippocampal gyrus (Fig 18–2). Later anatomic studies showed that the **hippocampal formation** (a more primitive cortical complex) was situated even closer to the diencephalon, in part below, in part on top of, the neocortical corpus callosum. The formation consists of the **hippocampus (cornu Ammonis);** the **dentate gyrus;** the **supracallosal gyrus,** which is the gray matter on top of the corpus callosum and is sometimes called the **indusium griseum;** the **fornix;** and a primitive precommisural area known as the **septal area** (Fig 18–3).

Histology. The 3 concentric cortical regions (hippocampal formation, great limbic lobe, and neocortex) have different cytoarchitectonic features. The most primitive cortex, the **archicortex,** has 3 layers and consists of the **allocortex** plus the **paleocortex.** The cortex of the transitional limbic lobe—the **mesocortex,** or **juxtallocortex**—has as many as 5 layers. The remaining cortex, known as the **neocortex,** or **isocortex,** has 5 or 6 layers. In phylogenetically recent species such as humans, the extent of the neocortex is much greater than in lower forms (Fig 18–4). Note that in the lower forms, the concentric arrangement is more obvious.

Comparative neuroanatomic studies up to 1948 suggested that both the hippocampal formation and the limbic lobe were concerned with olfaction; these parts of the brain were called the **rhinencephalon,** or smell brain (Fig 18–4). More recent work

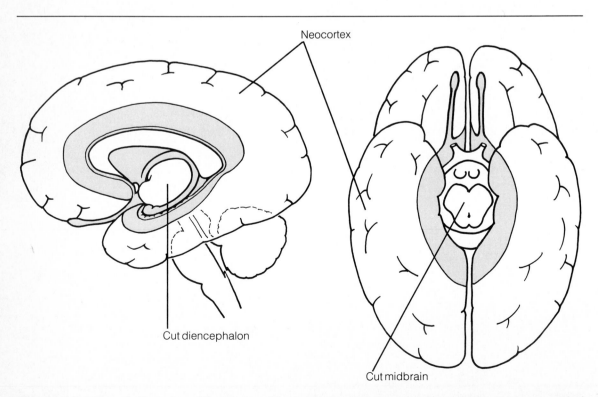

Neocortex

Cut diencephalon

Cut midbrain

Figure 18–1. Schematic illustration of the location of the limbic system between the diencephalon and the neocortical hemispheres.

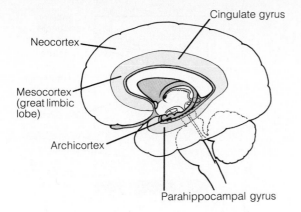

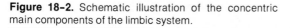

Figure 18-2. Schematic illustration of the concentric main components of the limbic system.

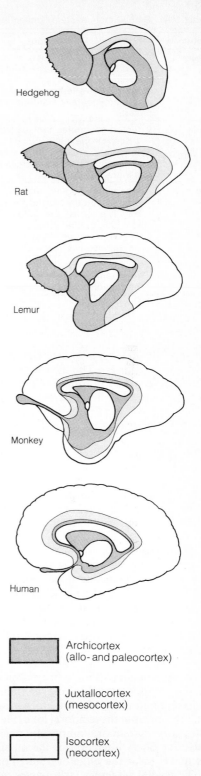

has shown that many of the structures are only indirectly related to the sense of smell but are directly involved in primitive, vital, visceral functions. Such names as the visceral brain, vital brain, emotional brain, and limbic brain were discontinued in favor of the more neutral **limbic system.** In general, this system includes phylogenetically ancient portions of the cerebral cortex, related subcortical structures, and fiber pathways that interconnect with the diencephalon and brain stem (Table 18-1).

Current research indicates that the basic functions of the limbic system contribute to the continuation of the species as well as to the preservation of the individual. These functions include feeding behavior; aggression; the expression of emotion; and the autonomic, behavioral, and endocrinal aspects of sexual response. Smell plays an important

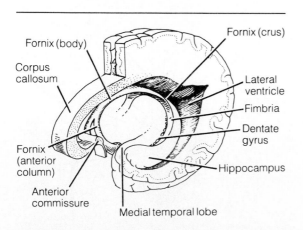

Figure 18-3. Schematic illustration (left oblique view) of the position of the hippocampal formation within the left hemisphere.

Figure 18-4. Diagrams of the medial aspect of the right hemisphere in 5 species. Note the relative increase in size of the human neocortex (isocortex).

Table 18-1. Some limbic system connections.

Structure	Connections
Amygdala	To hypothalamus (direct), septal area and hypothalamus (via stria terminalis) From primitive temporal cortex, opposite amygdala (via anterior commissure)
Habenula	To interpeduncular nucleus (via fasciculus retroflexus) From septal area (via stria medullaris thalami), opposite habenula (via habenular commissure)
Hippocampus	To mamillary bodies, anterior thalamus, septal area, and tuber cinereum (via fornix); subcallosal area (via longitudinal striae) From dental gyrus, septum (via fornix), limbic lobe (via cingulum)
Septal area	To habenula, hypothalamus medial forebrain bundle From olfactory bulb, amygdala, fornix

role in triggering these types of behavior and sometimes recalls memories. The neocortex, on the other hand, is involved in somatic functions such as motor control and interpretation of sensation and in mental capacities for reasoning, remembering, and converting information into action.

ANATOMY

The phylogenetically oldest portions of the cerebral hemisphere include the olfactory system, the hippocampal formation, and their connections.

Olfactory System

Ten to 15 **olfactory nerves** (Fig 18–5) convey the sensation of smell from the upper nasal mucosa through the cribriform plate to the olfactory bulb. The **olfactory bulb** and **olfactory tract (peduncle)** lie in the **olfactory sulcus** on the orbital surface of the frontal lobe. As the tract passes posteriorly, it divides into lateral and medial olfactory striae (Fig 18–6).

The **lateral olfactory stria** is a projection bundle of fibers that passes laterally along the floor of the lateral fissure and enters the **olfactory projection area** near the uncus in the temporal lobe (Fig 18–7). The olfactory system is completely uncrossed. Commissural fibers interconnect the anterior olfactory nuclei (near the olfactory bulbs) on both sides. The **medial olfactory stria** passes medially and up toward the subcallosal gyrus near the inferior of the corpus callosum. Other fibers reach the **anterior perforated substance,** a thin layer of gray matter with many openings that permit the small

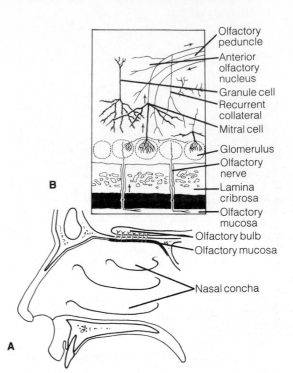

Figure 18-5. *A:* The olfactory nerves (lateral view). *B:* Neural elements in the olfactory bulb.

lenticulostriate arteries to enter the brain; it extends from the olfactory striae to the optic tract. These fibers and the medial stria serve olfactory reflex reactions.

Hippocampal Formation

The **dentate gyrus** is a thin, scalloped strip of cortex that lies on the upper surface of the para-

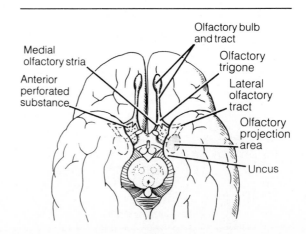

Figure 18-6. Olfactory connections projected on the basal aspect of the brain (intermediate olfactory tract not labeled).

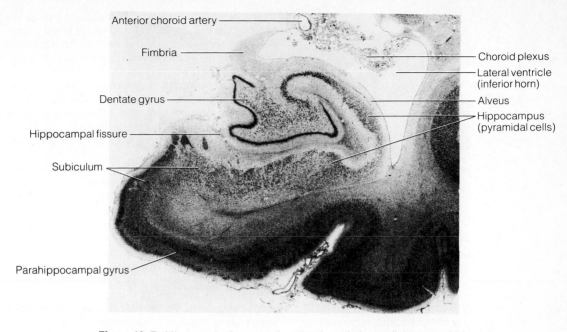

Anterior choroid artery

Fimbria

Dentate gyrus

Hippocampal fissure

Subiculum

Parahippocampal gyrus

Choroid plexus

Lateral ventricle (inferior horn)

Alveus

Hippocampus (pyramidal cells)

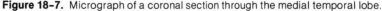

Figure 18-7. Micrograph of a coronal section through the medial temporal lobe.

hippocampal gyrus. It connects with the supracallosal gyrus.

The **hippocampus,** a primitive cortical structure, extends the length of the floor of the inferior horn of the lateral ventricle and becomes continuous with the fornix below the splenium of the corpus callosum (see Fig 18–3). For purposes of study, the hippocampus (also called cornu Ammonis, or Ammon's horn) has been divided into several sectors, partly on the basis of fiber connections and partly because pathologic processes occur mostly in a portion of the hippocampus (H_1 [CA_1 and CA_2], the Sommer sector; see Fig 18–8).

The dentate gyrus and the hippocampus itself show the histologic features of an archicortex with 3 layers: dendrite, pyramidal cell, and axon. The transitional cortex from the archicortex of the hippocampus to the neocortex (in this area called the subiculum) is juxtallocortex, or mesocortex, with 4 or 5 distinct cortical layers (Figs 18–7 and 18–8).

Hippocampal input and **output** (Fig 18–9) have been well studied in recent years. The dentate gyrus receives its input from the overlying subiculum and the adjacent temporal lobe cortex. The granule cells of the dentate gyrus send axons (mossy fibers) to the pyramidal cells of the hippocampus, mostly in the H_3 region. These cells in turn project to the fornix, which is a major efferent pathway. A collateral branch from the H_3 cells projects to the H_1 region.

The **fornix** is an arched white fiber tract extending from the hippocampal formation to the dien-

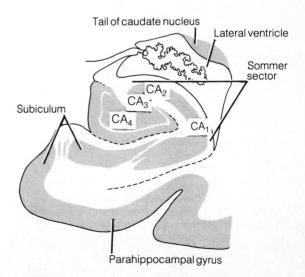

Tail of caudate nucleus

Lateral ventricle

Sommer sector

CA_2

CA_3

Subiculum

CA_4

CA_1

Parahippocampal gyrus

Figure 18-8. Schematic illustration of a coronal section showing the components of the hippocampal formation and subiculum (compare with Fig 18–7). CA_1 through CA_4 are sectors of the hippocampus (cornu ammonis) and are used for localization.

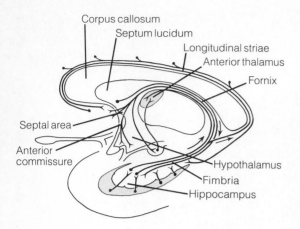

Figure 18-9. Schematic illustration of pathways between the hippocampal formation and the diencephalon.

cephalon and septal area. Its fibers start as the alveus, a white layer on the ventricular surface of the hippocampus that contains fibers from the dentate gyrus and hippocampus (Figs 18–7 and 18–10). From the alveus, fibers lead to the medial aspect of the hippocampus and form the **fimbria,** a flat band of white fibers that ascends below the splenium of the corpus callosum and bends forward to course above the thalamus, forming the crus of the fornix. The hippocampal commissure, or commissure of the fornix, is a variable collection of transverse fibers connecting the 2 crura of the fornix. The 2 crura lie close to the undersurface of the corpus callosum and join anteriorly to form the body of the fornix. From the body, the 2 columns of the

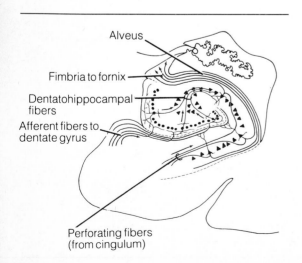

Figure 18-10. Schematic illustration of the major connections to, within, and from the hippocampal formation. (Compare with Fig 18–8.)

fornix bend inferiorly and posteriorly to enter the anterior part of the lateral wall of the third ventricle. They terminate in the mamillary bodies of the hypothalamus and in several other areas of the diencephalon (Fig 18–9).

The hippocampus thus projects to the septal area, the anterior thalamus, and the hypothalamus (mamillary bodies and tuber cinereum); it also projects indirectly to the midbrain. Some fibers in the fornix course from the septal area to the hippocampus.

The **subcallosal gyrus** is the portion of gray matter that covers the inferior aspect of the rostrum of the corpus callosum. It continues posteriorly as the **cingulate gyrus** and **parahippocampal gyrus** (Fig 18–2). In the area of the genu of the corpus callosum, the subcallosal gyrus also contains fibers coursing into the supracallosal gyrus (Fig 18–10). The **supracallosal gyrus (indusium griseum)** is a thin layer of gray matter that extends from the subcallosal gyrus and covers the upper surface of the corpus callosum. The **medial** and **lateral longitudinal striae** are delicate longitudinal strands that extend along the upper surface of the corpus callosum to and from the hippocampal formation.

Anterior Commissure

The anterior commissure is a band of white fibers that crosses the midline to join both cerebral hemispheres (see Fig 18–9). It contains 2 fiber systems, an interbulbar system that joins both anterior olfactory nuclei near the olfactory bulbs, and an intertemporal system that connects the temporal lobe areas of both cerebral hemispheres.

Septal Area

The septal area, or septal complex, is an area of gray matter lying above the lamina terminalis, near and around the anterior commissure (Figs 18–9 and 18–11). A portion of it, the **septum lucidum,** is a double sheet of gray matter below the genu of the corpus callosum. In humans, the septum separates the anterior portions of the lateral ventricles.

Amygdala & Hypothalamus

The amygdala (**amygdaloid nuclear complex**) lies in the medial temporal pole, between the uncus and the parahippocampal gyrus (Figs 18–11 and 18–12). Its fiber connections include the semicircular **stria terminalis** to the septal area and anterior hypothalamus and a direct **amygdalofugal pathway** to the middle portion of the hypothalamus. Some fibers of the stria pass across the anterior commissure to the opposite amygdala. The stria terminalis courses along the inferior horn and body of the lateral ventricle to the septal and preoptic areas and the hypothalamus.

The fornix and **medial forebrain bundle,** cours-

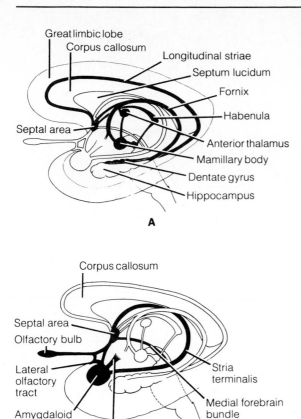

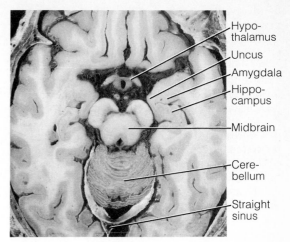

Figure 18–12. Horizontal section through the head at the level of the midbrain and amygdala. (Reproduced, with permission, from DeGroot, J: *Correlative Neuroanatomy of Computed Tomography and Magnetic Resonance Imaging,* Lea & Febiger, 1984.)

Figure 18–11. Diagram of the principal connections of the limbic system. *A:* Hippocampal system and great limbic lobe. *B:* Olfactory and amygdaloid connections.

ing within the hypothalamus, are also considered part of the limbic system.

FUNCTIONS & DISORDERS

A variety of experimental studies in both animals and humans indicate that stimulating or damaging some components of the limbic system causes profound changes. Stimulation alters somatic motor responses, leading to bizarre eating and drinking habits, changes in sexual and grooming behavior, and defensive postures of attack and rage. There are changes in autonomic responses, altering cardiovascular or gastrointestinal function, and in personality, with shifts from passive to aggressive behavior. Damage to some areas of the limbic system may also affect memory or olfactory function.

Autonomic Nervous System

The hierarchical organization of the autonomic nervous system (see Chapter 19) includes the limbic system; most of the limbic system output connects to the hypothalamus, often to the medial forebrain bundle. The specific sympathetic or parasympathetic aspects of autonomic control are not well localized in the limbic system, however.

Stimulation of various limbic system structures produces changes in cardiovascular or gastrointestinal functions, and there are reports of gastric ulcer formation and emotional changes.

Septal Area

The septal area, or complex, is relatively large in such animals as the cat and rat. Because it is a pivotal region with afferent fibers from the olfactory and limbic systems and efferent fibers to the hypothalamus, epithalamus, and midbrain, no single function can be ascribed to the area. Experimental studies have shown the septal area to be a substrate mediating the sensations of self-stimulation or self-reward. Test animals will press a bar repeatedly, even endlessly, to receive a (presumed) pleasurable stimulus in the septal area. Additional areas of pleasure have been found in the hypothalamus and midbrain; the stimulation of yet other areas reportedly evokes the opposite response. Recent studies in humans indicate that antipsychotic drugs may act by modifying dopaminergic inputs from the midbrain to the septal area. Other studies suggest that an ascending pathway to the septal area may be involved in the euphoric feelings described by narcotics addicts.

Olfactory System

Olfactory system fibers, or collaterals, course to many limbic system structures: the septal area, the ipsilateral and contralateral amygdaloid complex, and the medial forebrain bundle in the hypothalamus. Through this pathway the olfactory system influences many hypothalamic functions and limbic system activities.

Olfactory sensation often has emotional associations, leading to the use of such phrases as a "revolting stench" or a "fine bouquet of wine". Some smells, on the other hand, may induce autonomic reactions such as nausea, vomiting, and changes in skin color.

The olfactory nerves may serve as portals of entry for cryptogenic infections of the meninges and brain such as meningitis and encephalitis. Disorders of the sense of smell may be caused by many pathogenic lesions. **Foster Kennedy's syndrome,** which involves the olfactory nerve, is often caused by a meningioma near the olfactory tracts and optic nerves. **Bilateral anosmia** (loss of the sense of smell) commonly occurs with colds and rhinitis. **Unilateral anosmia** may be of diagnostic significance in locating brain lesions, such as tumors at the base of the frontal lobe. **Hyperosmia** (an abnormally acute sense of smell) is present in some patients with hysteria and is sometimes noted in cocaine addicts. Parosmia (a perverted sense of smell) occurs in some patients with schizophrenia, hysteria, or lesions of the uncinate gyrus. **Cacosmia** (unpleasant odors) is usually caused by decomposition of tissues and is noticed by the patient on exhalation. **Olfactory hallucinations** are present in some psychoses and as uncinate fits (see below) that are caused by irritative lesions of the uncus and hippocampus.

Behavior

Several of the hypothalamic regions associated with typical patterns of behavior such as eating, drinking, sexual behavior, and aggression receive input from limbic system structures, especially the amygdaloid and septal complexes. Lesions in these areas can modify, inhibit, or unleash these behaviors. Some of the behavioral patterns are quite different; for example, lesions in the lateral amygdala induce unrestrained eating (bulimia), while those in the medial amygdala induce anorexia, accompanied by hypersexuality (Fig 18–13). Electrical stimulation of the amygdala in humans may produce fear, anxiety, or rage and aggression. Amygdalectomy, which has been performed to suppress these antisocial traits in patients, has sometimes been followed by hypersexuality.

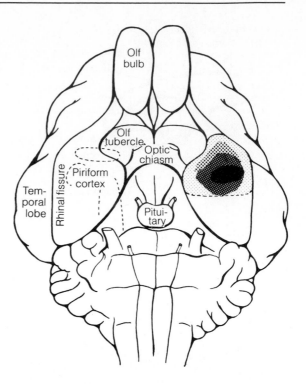

Figure 18–13. Site of lesions producing hypersexuality in male cats. Destroying the black area always produced hypersexuality. The incidence of hypersexuality in animals with lesions in the surrounding lighter zones was not as high. Olf = olfactory. (Reproduced, with permission, from Green J et al: Rhinencephalic lesions and behavior in cats. *J Comp Neurol* 1957;**108**:505.)

Memory

The three types of memory are **immediate recall, short-term memory,** and **long-term memory.** The hippocampus is involved in converting short-term memory (up to 60 minutes) to long-term memory (several days or more). The anatomic substrate for long-term memory probably includes the temporal lobes. Patients with bilateral removal of the hippocampus (as part of a bilateral temporal lobectomy for epilepsy) demonstrate **anterograde amnesia,** in which events prior to surgery are retained but no new long-term memories can be established. This lack of memory storage is also present in patients with bilateral interruption of the fornices (eg, by removal of a colloid cyst at the interventricular foramen).

Other Disorders of the Limbic System

A. Klüver-Bucy Syndrome: This is an example of the disturbance of limbic system activities in patients with large, bilateral temporal lobe lesions. The major characteristics of this syndrome are **hyperorality,** the indiscriminate eating or chewing of objects and all kinds of food; **hypersexuality,**

sometimes described as a lack of sexual inhibition; **psychic blindness,** or visual agnosia, in which objects are no longer recognized; and **personality changes,** to either passivity or aggression.

B. Temporal Lobe Epilepsy: The temporal lobe (especially the hippocampus and amygdala) has a lower threshold for epileptic seizure activity than do the other cortical areas. The seizures, called **psychomotor (temporal lobe) seizures,** differ from the jacksonian seizures that originate in or near the motor cortex (see Chapter 20). Temporal lobe epilepsy may include abnormal sensations, especially bizarre olfactory sensations, sometimes called uncinate fits; repeated involuntary movements such as chewing, swallowing, and lip smacking; disorders of consciousness; memory loss; hallucinations; and disorders of recall and recognition.

The underlying cause of the seizures may sometimes be difficult to determine. A tumor (eg, astrocytoma or oligodendroglioma) may be responsible, or glial scar formation after trauma to the temporal poles may trigger seizures. Small hamartomas or areas of temporal sclerosis have been found in patients with temporal lobe epilepsy. Although drugs are often given to control the seizures, they may be ineffective.

C. Wernicke-Korsakoff Syndrome: There are 2 separate components of the Wernicke-Korsakoff Syndrome. **Wernicke's encephalopathy syndrome** includes ataxia, confusion, and ophthalmoplegia. The associated lesion consists of edema, demyelination, and small hemorrhages; these are found in the mamillary bodies, in the walls of the third and fourth ventricles and aqueduct, and sometimes in the dorsomedial thalamic nucleus. The cause is chronic thiamine deficiency, which is common in alcoholics. **Korsakoff's amnestic syndrome** (also associated with alcoholism) includes the inability to store new information (loss of short-term memory), confabulation (to mask the loss of memory) and, in some cases, peripheral neuropathy. There may be apathy or a quiet confused state, which can progress to coma. The progress of this syndrome may be halted by repeated administration of thiamine.

CASE 25

A 59-year-old unemployed male was brought to the hospital by his wife because he had been confused at times and had suffered 2 shaking "fits." His wife said that he did not seem to be himself. Two days earlier, he had developed a severe head-

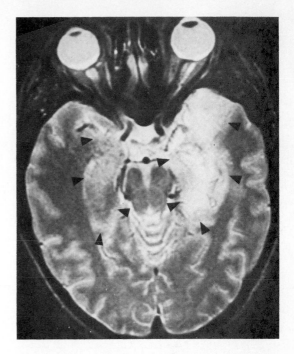

Figure 18–14. MR image of horizontal section through the head at the level of the temporal lobe. The large lesion in the left temporal lobe and a smaller one on the right side are indicated by arrowheads.

ache, generalized malaise, and a temperature of 103 °F (39.4 °C) and refused to eat. On the morning of admission, he had fainted. Examination showed that the patient was mildly confused, had dysphasia, and was generally in poor health. There was no stiffness of the neck. The serum glucose level was 165 mg/dL. Lumbar puncture findings showed pressure, 220 mm of water; white blood count 153/μL, mostly lymphocytes; protein, 51 mg/dL; and glucose, 101 mg/dL. An electroencephalogram showed focal slowing over the temporal region on both sides, with some sharp periodic bursts. Brain biopsy revealed the features of an active granuloma, without pus formation. Results of CT scanning are shown in Fig 18–14.

What is the differential diagnosis?

Over the next 8 days, the patient became increasingly drowsy and dysphasic. A repeat scan showed extensive defects of both temporal lobes. The patient died on the tenth day after admission, despite appropriate drug treatment.

Cases are discussed further in Chapter 24.

REFERENCES

Ben-Ari Y (editor): *The Amygdaloid Complex.* Elsevier, 1981.

Cofer CN (editor): *The Structure of Human Memory.* Freeman, 1976.

deGroot J: The limbic system: An anatomical and functional orientation. Chap 6, pp 89–106, in: *American Handbook of Psychiatry.* Vol 6. Arieti S (editor). Basic Books, 1975.

Doty RL: *Mammalian Olfaction, Reproductive Processes, and Behavior.* Academic Press, 1976.

Eslinger PJ, Damasio AR, Van Hoesen GW: Olfactory dysfunction in man: A review of anatomical and behavioral aspects. *Brain Cogn* 1982;**2**:259.

Isaacson RL: *The Limbic System,* 2nd ed. Plenum, 1982.

Livingston KE, Hornykiewicz O (editors): *Limbic Mechanisms.* Plenum, 1978.

Moulton DG, Beidler LM: Structure and function in the peripheral olfactory system. *Physiol Rev* 1987;**47**:1.

The Autonomic Nervous System

The autonomic (visceral) nervous system (ANS) is concerned with control of the target tissues: the cardiac muscle, the smooth muscle in viscera, and the glands. It also helps maintain a constant internal body environment (homeostasis). The autonomic nervous system consists of efferent pathways, afferent pathways, and groups of neurons in the brain and spinal cord that regulate the system's functions. Autonomic reflex activity in the spinal cord is modulated by brain centers, so that there is a hierarchical organization within the central nervous system itself.

AUTONOMIC OUTFLOW

The efferent components of the autonomic system are the sympathetic and parasympathetic divisions, which arise from preganglionic cell bodies in different locations. A 2-neuron chain characterizes the structure of the autonomic outflow. The cell body of the primary neuron (the **presynaptic,** or **preganglionic,** neuron) within the central nervous system is located in the lateral gray column of the spinal cord or in the brain stem nuclei (see Chapter 7). It sends its axon out to synapse with the secondary neuron (the **postsynaptic,** or **postganglionic,** neuron) located in one of the autonomic ganglia. From there, the postganglionic axon passes to its terminal distribution in a target organ. Since the postganglionic fibers outnumber the preganglionic neurons by a ratio of about 32:1, a single preganglionic neuron may control the autonomic functions of a rather extensive terminal area.

Sympathetic Division

The sympathetic (**thoracolumbar**) division of the autonomic nervous system arises from preganglionic cell bodies located in the lateral cell columns of the 12 thoracic segments and the upper 2 lumbar segments of the spinal cord (Fig 19–1).

A. Preganglionic Efferent Fiber System: Preganglionic fibers are mostly myelinated. Coursing with the ventral roots, they form the **white communicating rami** of the thoracic and lumbar nerves, through which they reach the ganglia of the sympathetic chains or trunks (Fig 19–2). These **trunk ganglia** lie on the lateral sides of the bodies of the thoracic and lumbar vertebrae. Upon entering the ganglia, the fibers may synapse with a number of ganglion cells, pass up or down the

sympathetic trunk to synapse with ganglion cells at a higher or lower level, or pass through the trunk ganglia and out to one of the collateral (intermediary) sympathetic ganglia (eg, the **celiac** and **mesenteric ganglia**).

The **splanchnic nerves** arising from the lower 7 thoracic segments pass through the trunk ganglia to the **celiac** and **superior mesenteric ganglia.** There, synaptic connections occur with ganglion cells whose postganglionic axons then pass to the abdominal viscera via the **celiac plexus.** The splanchnic nerves arising from spinal cord segments in the lowest thoracic and upper lumbar region convey fibers to synaptic stations in the **inferior mesenteric ganglion** and to small ganglia associated with the **hypogastric plexus** through which postsynaptic fibers are distributed to the lower abdominal and pelvic viscera.

B. Postganglionic Efferent Fiber System: The mostly unmyelinated postganglionic fibers form the **gray communicating rami.** The fibers may course with the spinal nerve for some distance or go directly to their target tissues.

The gray communicating rami join each of the spinal nerves and distribute the vasomotor, pilomotor, and sweat gland innervation throughout the somatic areas. Branches of the **superior cervical sympathetic ganglion** enter into the formation of the sympathetic plexuses about the internal and external carotid arteries for distribution of sympathetic fibers to the head (Fig 19–3). The superior **cardiac nerves** from the 3 pairs of cervical sympathetic ganglia pass to the **cardiac plexus** at the base of the heart and distribute accelerator fibers to the myocardium. Vasomotor branches from the upper 5 thoracic ganglia pass to the thoracic aorta and to the posterior **pulmonary plexus,** through which dilator fibers reach the bronchi.

Parasympathetic Division

The parasympathetic (craniosacral) division of the autonomic nervous system (Figs 19–2 and 19–4) arises from preganglionic cell bodies in the gray matter of the brain stem and the middle 3 segments of the sacral cord (S2–S4). Most of the preganglionic fibers run without interruption from their central origin either to the wall of the viscus they supply or to the site where they synapse with terminal ganglion cells associated with the **plexuses of Meissner** and **Auerbach** in the wall of the intestinal tract. The parasympathetic distribution is confined entirely to visceral structures.

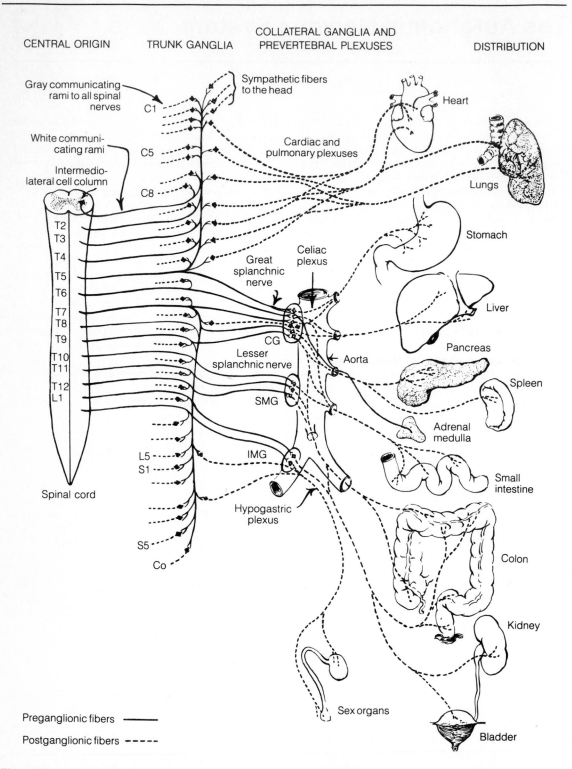

Figure 19–1. Sympathetic division of the autonomic nervous system (left half). CG, celiac ganglion; SMG, superior mesenteric ganglion; IMG, inferior mesenteric ganglion.

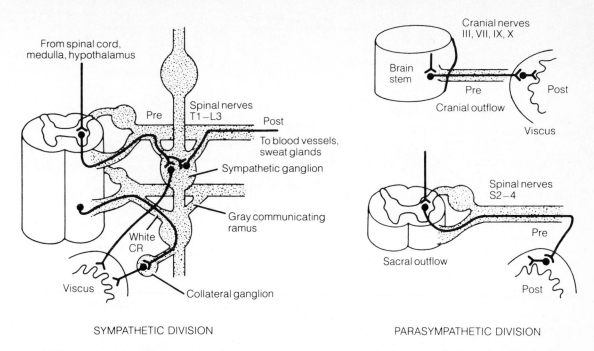

Figure 19-2. Types of outflow in autonomic nervous system. Pre, preganglionic neuron. Post, postganglionic neuron. RC, ramus communicans. (Reproduced, with permission, from Ganong WF: *Review of Medical Physiology,* 14th ed. Appleton & Lange, 1989.)

There cranial nerves convey preganglionic parasympathetic (visceral efferent) fibers: The **vagus nerve** (cranial nerve X) distributes its autonomic fibers to the thoracic and abdominal viscera via the **prevertebral plexuses.** The **pelvic nerve (nervus erigens)** distributes parasympathetic fibers to most of the large intestine and to the pelvic viscera and genitals via the **hypogastric plexus;** the **oculomotor, facial,** and **glossopharyngeal nerves** (cranial nerves III, VII, and IX) distribute parasympathetic or visceral efferent fibers to the head (Fig 19–3; see also Chapters 6 and 7).

Autonomic Plexuses

The autonomic plexuses (Figs 19–1 and 19–4) are large networks of nerves that serve as areas of redistribution for the sympathetic and parasympathetic (and afferent) fibers that enter into their formation.

The **cardiac plexus,** located about the bifurcation of the trachea and roots of the great vessels at the base of the heart, is divided into superficial and deep parts. It is formed from the cardiac sympathetic nerves and cardiac branches of the vagus nerve, which it distributes to the myocardium and walls of the vessels leaving the heart.

The right and left **pulmonary plexuses** are intimately joined with the cardiac plexus and are located about the primary bronchi and pulmonary arteries at the roots of the lungs. They are formed from both the vagus and the upper thoracic sympathetic nerves and are distributed mainly to the vessels and bronchi of the lung.

The **celiac (solar) plexus** is located in the epigastric region of the abdomen over the abdominal aorta near the origin of the celiac and superior mesenteric arteries. It is formed from vagal fibers reaching it via the esophageal plexus, sympathetic fibers arising from celiac ganglia, and sympathetic fibers coursing down from the thoracic aortic plexus. The distribution of the celiac plexus includes most of the abdominal viscera, which it reaches by way of numerous subplexuses along the various visceral branches of the aorta. These subplexuses include the phrenic, hepatic, splenic, superior gastric, suprarenal, renal, spermatic or ovarian, abdominal aortic, and superior and inferior mesenteric plexuses.

The **hypogastric plexus** is located in front of the fifth lumbar vertebra and the promontory of the sacrum. It receives sympathetic fibers from the aortic plexus and lumbar trunk ganglia and parasympathetic fibers from the pelvic nerve. Its 2 lateral portions, the **pelvic plexuses,** lie on either side of the rectum. Distribution to the pelvic viscera and genitals is effected by subplexuses that extend along the visceral branches of the hypogastric artery. These subplexuses of the hypogastric plexus include the

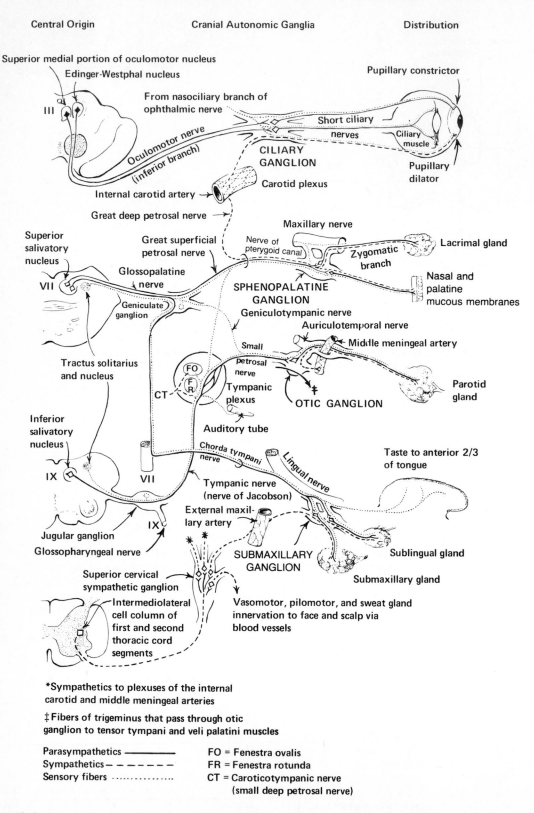

Figure 19-3. Autonomic nerves to the head. FO, oval window; FR, round window; CT, caroticotympanic (small deep petrosal) nerve.

CENTRAL ORIGIN   PREVERTEBRAL PLEXUSES   DISTRIBUTION AND TERMINAL GANGLIA

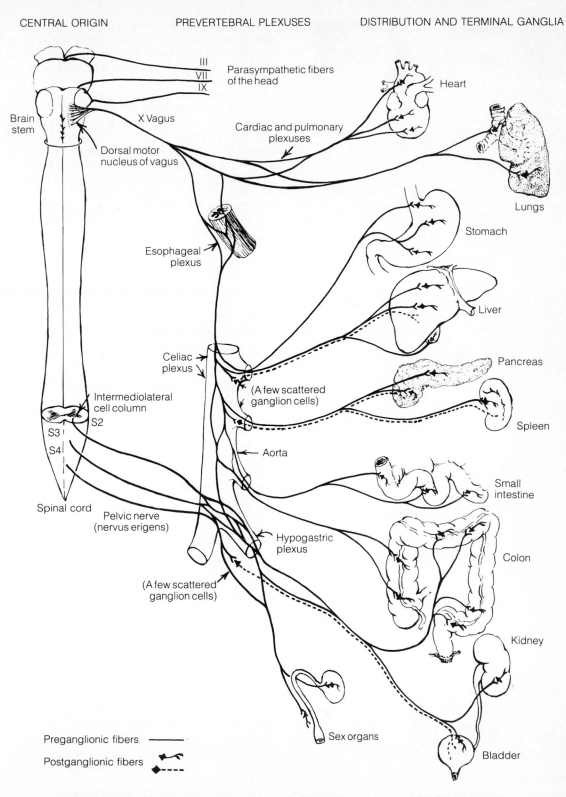

Brain stem

III
VII
IX

Parasympathetic fibers of the head

Heart

X Vagus

Cardiac and pulmonary plexuses

Dorsal motor nucleus of vagus

Lungs

Esophageal plexus

Stomach

Liver

Celiac plexus

Pancreas

(A few scattered ganglion cells)

Intermediolateral cell column

S2

Spleen

S3

S4

Aorta

Small intestine

Spinal cord

Pelvic nerve (nervus erigens)

Hypogastric plexus

Colon

(A few scattered ganglion cells)

Kidney

Sex organs

Bladder

Preganglionic fibers _____

Postganglionic fibers

Figure 19-4. Parasympathetic division of the autonomic nervous system (only left half shown).

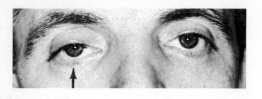

Figure 19-5. Horner's syndrome in the right eye, associated with a tumor in the superior sulcus of the right lung.

middle hemorrhoidal plexus, to the rectum; the vesical plexus, to the bladder, seminal vesicles, and ductus deferens; the prostatic plexus, to the prostate, seminal vesicles, and penis; the vaginal plexus, to the vagina and clitoris; and uterine plexus, to the uterus and uterine tubes.

Clinical Correlations

Horner's syndrome consists of unilateral enophthalmos, ptosis, miosis, and flushing of the face (Fig 19-5). It is caused by ipsilateral involvement of the sympathetic pathways in the carotid plexus, the cervical sympathetic chain, the upper thoracic cord, or the brain stem (Fig 19-6).

Spinal shock is a syndrome possibly caused by a sudden release of sympathetic vasomotor tone resulting from transection of or severe injury to the spinal cord or from an overdose of spinal anesthetic. Spinal shock may lead to neurogenic bladder, as discussed earlier (see Chapter 4 and Figs 19-9 to 19-11).

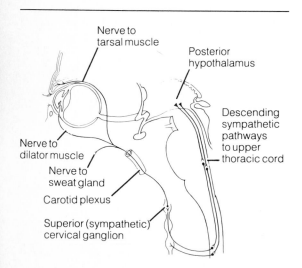

Figure 19-6. Sympathetic pathways to the eye and orbit. Interruption of these pathways inactivates the dilator muscle and thereby produces miosis, inactivates the tarsal muscle and produces the effect of enophthalmos, and reduces sweat secretion in the face (Horner's syndrome).

Raynaud's disease affects the toes, the fingers, the edges of the ears, and the tip of the nose and spreads to involve large areas. Beginning with local changes when the parts are pale and cold, it may progress to local asphyxia characterized by a blue-gray cyanosis and, finally, symmetric dry gangrene. It is a disorder of the peripheral vascular innervation. **Scleroderma,** a thickening of the skin, that can be diffuse or circumscribed may be accompanied by or follow Raynaud's disease or other disturbances of peripheral vessel innervation.

Causalgia, a painful condition of the hands or feet, is caused by irritation of the median or sciatic nerve through injury. It is characterized by severe burning pain, glossy skin, swelling, redness, sweating, and trophic nail changes. Causalgia is frequently relieved by sympathetic blocks or sympathectomy of the involved areas.

Hirschsprung's disease (megacolon) consists of a tremendous dilatation of the colon, accompanied by chronic constipation. It is associated with congenital lack of parasympathetic ganglia and the existence of abnormal nerve fibrils in an apparently normal segment of large bowel wall.

AUTONOMIC INNERVATION OF THE HEAD

The autonomic supply to visceral structures in the head deserves special consideration (see Fig 19-3). The skin of the face and scalp (smooth muscle, glands, and vessels) receives postsynaptic sympathetic innervation only, from the superior cervical ganglion via a plexus that extends along the branches of the external carotid artery. The deeper structures (intrinsic eye muscles, salivary glands, and mucous membranes of the nose and pharynx), however, receive a dual autonomic supply from the sympathetic and parasympathetic divisions. The supply is mediated by the internal carotid plexus (postganglionic sympathetic innervation from the superior cervical plexus) and the visceral efferent fibers in 4 pairs of cranial nerves (parasympathetic innervation).

There are 4 pairs of autonomic ganglia—ciliary, pterygopalatine, otic, and submaxillary—in the head (Fig 19-3). Each ganglion receives a sympathetic, a parasympathetic, and a sensory root (a branch of the trigeminal nerve). Only the parasympathetic fibers make synaptic connections within these ganglia, which contain the cell bodies of the postganglionic parasympathetic fibers. The sympathetic and sensory fibers pass through these ganglia without interruption.

The **ciliary ganglion** is located between the optic nerve and the lateral rectus muscle in the posterior part of the orbit. Its parasympathetic root originates from cells in or near the Edinger-Westphal nucleus of the oculomotor nerve; its sympathetic root is composed of postganglionic fibers from the superior cervical sympathetic ganglion via the carotid plexus of the internal carotid artery. The sensory root comes from the nasociliary branch of the ophthalmic nerve. Distribution is through 10–12 short ciliary nerves that supply the ciliary muscle of the lens and the constrictor muscle of the iris. The dilator muscle of the iris is supplied by sympathetic nerves.

The **pterygopalatine ganglion,** located deep in the pterygopalatine fossa, is associated with the maxillary nerve. Its parasympathetic root arises from cells of the superior salivatory nucleus via the glossopalatine nerve and the great petrosal nerve. The ganglion's sympathetic root comes from the internal carotid plexus by way of the deep petrosal nerve, which joins the great superficial petrosal nerve to form the vidian nerve in the pterygoid (vidian) canal. Most of the sensory root fibers originate in the maxillary nerve, but a few arise in cranial nerves VII and IX via the tympanic plexus and vidian nerve. Distribution is through the **pharyngeal rami** to the mucous membranes of the roof of the pharynx; via the **nasal** and **palatine rami** to the mucous membranes of the nasal cavity, uvula, palatine tonsil, and hard and soft palates; and by way of the **orbital rami** to the periosteum of the orbit and the lacrimal glands.

The **otic ganglion** is located medial to the mandibular nerve just below the foramen ovale in the infratemporal fossa. Its parasympathetic root fibers arise in the inferior salivatory nucleus in the medulla and course via cranial nerve IX, the tympanic plexus, and the lesser superficial petrosal nerve; the sympathetic root comes from the superior cervical sympathetic ganglion via the plexus on the middle meningeal artery. Its sensory root probably includes fibers from cranial nerve IX and from the geniculate ganglion of cranial nerve VII via the tympanic plexus and the lesser superficial petrosal nerve. The otic ganglion supplies secretory and sensory fibers to the **parotid gland.** A few somatic motor fibers from the trigeminal nerve pass through the otic ganglion and supply the **tensor tympani** and **tensor veli palatini** muscles.

The **submaxillary ganglion** is located on the medial side of the mandible between the lingual nerve and the submaxillary duct. Its parasympathetic root fibers arise from the superior salivatory nucleus of nerve VII via the glossopalatine, chorda tympani, and lingual nerves, its sympathetic root from the plexus of the external maxillary artery, and its sensory root from the geniculate ganglion via the glossopalatine, chorda tympani, and lingual nerves. It is distributed to the **submaxillary** and **sublingual glands.**

VISCERAL AFFERENT PATHWAYS

Visceral afferent fibers have their cell bodies in **sensory ganglia** of some of the cranial and spinal nerves. Although a few of these fibers are myelinated, most are unmyelinated and have slow conduction velocities. The pain innervation of the viscera is summarized in Table 19–1.

Pathways to the Spinal Cord

Visceral afferent fibers to the spinal cord enter by way of the **middle sacral, thoracic,** and **upper lumbar nerves.** (Recent studies suggest that some fibers enter the spinal cord by way of the anterior spinal roots but that most travel with the posterior spinal roots.) The sacral nerves carry sensory stimuli from the pelvic organs, and the nerve fibers are involved in reflexes of the sacral parasympathetic outflow that control various sexual responses, micturition and defecation. Axons carrying visceral pain impulses from the heart, upper digestive tract, kidney, and gall bladder travel with the thoracic and upper lumbar nerves. These visceral afferent pathways are associated with sensations such as hunger, nausea, and poorly localized, dull visceral pain (Table 19–1). Pain impulses sometimes travel from a viscus to a particular region of the skin, causing referred pain. Typical examples of the phenomenon are the shoulder pains associated with gallstone attacks and the pains of the left arm or throat associated with myocardial ischemia (see also Chapter 13).

Pathways to the Brain Stem

Visceral afferent axons in the **glossopharyngeal nerve** and (especially) the **vagus nerve** carry a variety of sensations to the brain stem from the heart, great vessels, and respiratory and gastrointestinal tracts. The ganglia involved are the inferior glosso-

Table 19-1. Pain innervation of the viscera.

Division	Nerve(s) or segment(s)	Structures
Parasympathetic	Vagus	Esophagus, larynx, trachea
Sympathetic	Splanchnic (T7–L1)	Stomach, spleen, small viscera, colon, kidney, ureter, bladder, (upper part), uterus (fundus), ovaries, lungs
	Somatic (C7–L1)	Parietal pleura, diaphragm, parietal peritoneum
Parasympathetic	Pelvic (S2–S4)	Rectum, trigone of the bladder, prostate, urethra, cervix of the uterus, upper vagina

pharyngeal nerve ganglion and the inferior vagus nerve ganglion (formerly called the nodose ganglion). The afferent fibers are also involved in reflexes that regulate blood pressure, respiratory rate and depth, and heart rate through specialized receptors or receptor areas. These **baroreceptors,** which are stimulated by pressure, are located in the aortic arch and carotid sinus (Fig 19–7). The chemoreceptors are located in the aorta and carotid bodies, and the chemosensitive area is located in the medulla (Figs 19–7 and 19–8).

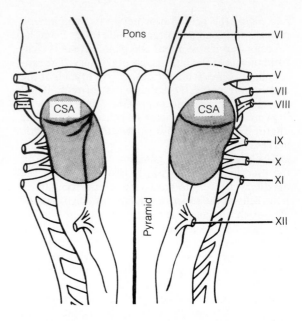

Figure 19–8. Chemosensitive areas (CSA) on the ventral surface of the medulla. (Modified and reproduced, with permission, from Mitchell RA, Severinghaus JW: Cerebrospinal fluid and regulation of respiration. *Physiol Physicians* 1965;**3**[3].)

ORGANIZATION OF THE AUTONOMIC NERVOUS SYSTEM

There is a functional hierarchy in certain regions of the brain and spinal cord; through a complex interplay of connections, this hierarchy exerts its influence on visceral reflexes.

Spinal Cord

Autonomic reflexes such as peristalsis and micturition are mediated by the spinal cord, but descending pathways from the brain modify, inhibit, or initiate the reflexes (Fig 19–9). This can be demonstrated in patients who have suffered a transection of the spinal cord. A state of spinal shock develops, with hypotension and loss of reflexes governing micturition and defecation. Although the reflexes return after a few days or weeks, they may be incomplete or abnormal. For example, often the bladder cannot be completely emptied, which may result in cystitis, and voluntary initiation of micturition may be absent (**autonomic,** or **neurogenic, bladder**). Depending on the level of the transection, the neurogenic bladder may be spastic or flaccid (Figs 19–10 and 19–11).

Medulla

Medullary connections to and from the spinal cord are lightly myelinated fibers of the **tractus**

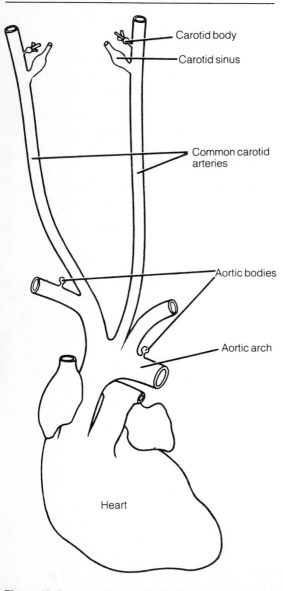

Figure 19–7. Location of carotid and aortic bodies. (Reproduced, with permission, from Ganong WF: *Review of Medical Physiology,* 14th ed. Appleton & Lange, 1989.)

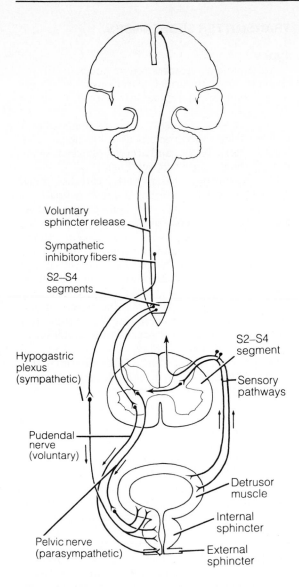

Voluntary
sphincter release

Sympathetic
inhibitory fibers

S2–S4
segments

Hypogastric
plexus
(sympathetic)

Pudendal
nerve
(voluntary)

Pelvic nerve
(parasympathetic)

S2–S4
segment

Sensory
pathways

Detrusor
muscle

Internal
sphincter

External
sphincter

Figure 19-9. Descending pathway and innervation of the urinary bladder.

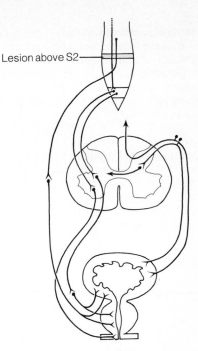

Lesion above S2

Figure 19-10. Spastic neurogenic bladder, caused by a more or less complete transection of the spinal cord above S2.

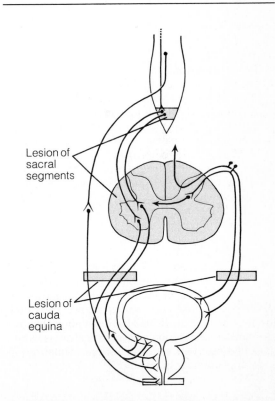

Lesion of
sacral
segments

Lesion of
cauda
equina

Figure 19-11. Flaccid neurogenic bladder, caused by a lesion of either the sacral portion of the spinal cord or the cauda equina.

proprius around the gray matter of the cord. Visceral afferent fibers of the glossopharyngeal and vagus nerves terminate in the solitary tract nucleus and are involved in control of respiratory, cardiovascular, and alimentary functions (see also Chapters 6 and 7). The major reflex actions have connections with visceral efferent nuclei of the medulla and areas of the reticular formation. These areas may contribute to the regulation of blood glucose levels and to other reflex functions, including salivation, micturition, vomiting, sneezing, coughing, and gagging. The medulla is therefore an important link in the hierarchic chain of autonomic function control.

Pons

The **nucleus parabrachialis** consists of a group of neurons that are located near the superior cerebellar peduncle and that modulate the medullary neurons responsible for rhythmic respiration. This **pneumotaxic center** continues to control periodic respiration if the brain stem is transected between the pons and the medulla.

Midbrain

Accommodation, pupillary reactions to light, and other reflexes are integrated in the midbrain, near the nuclear complex of nerve III. Pathways from the hypothalamus to the visceral efferent nuclei in the brain stem course through the dorsal longitudinal fasciculus in the periaqueductal and periventricular gray matter.

Hypothalamus

An important area of coordination, the hypothalamus integrates autonomic activities in response to changes in the internal and external environments (thermoregulatory mechanisms; see also Chapter 8). The posterior portion of the hypothalamus is involved with sympathetic function, and the anterior portion is involved with parasympathetic function. The descending pathway is the dorsal longitudinal fasciculus, and the connections with the hypophysis aid in the influence of the hypothalamus on visceral functions.

Limbic System

The limbic system (see also Chapter 18) has been called the visceral brain and has close anatomic and functional links with the hypothalamus. Various portions of the limbic system exert control over the visceral manifestations of emotion and drives such as sexual behavior, fear, rage, aggression, and eating behavior. Electrical stimulation of limbic system areas elicits such autonomic reactions as cardiovascular and gastrointestinal responses, micturition, defecation, piloerection, and pupillary changes. These reactions are probably channeled through the hypothalamus.

Cerebral Neocortex

The cerebral neocortex may initiate autonomic reactions such as blushing or blanching of the face in response to receiving unexpected information or bad or good news. These widely known anecdotal observations are confirmed by the findings that destruction or stimulation of neocortical areas in humans can interfere with the normal regulation of many autonomic responses.

TRANSMITTER SUBSTANCES

Types

Autonomic neurotransmitters mediate all visceral functions; the principal transmitter agents are acetylcholine and norepinephrine (see also Chapter 3).

Acetylcholine is liberated at all preganglionic endings. High concentrations of acetylcholine, choline acetyltransferase, and acetylcholinesterase are found in cholinergic nerve endings.

Norepinephrine (levarterenol), a catecholamine, is the chemical transmitter at most sympathetic postganglionic endings. Norepinephrine and its methyl derivative, **epinephrine,** are secreted by the adrenal medulla. Although many viscera contain both norepinephrine and epinephrine, the latter is not considered to be a mediator at sympathetic endings; only the norepinephrine content can be related to the number of sympathetic nerve endings in the organ. Drugs that block the effects of epinephrine but not norepinephrine have little effect on the response of most organs to stimulation of their adrenergic nerve supply.

Substance P, somatostatin, vasoactive intestinal peptide (VIP), adenosine, and **adenosine triphosphate (ATP)** may also function as visceral neurotransmitters.

Functions

The autonomic nervous system can be divided into **cholinergic** and **adrenergic** divisions, based on the chemical mediator released. Cholinergic neurons include preganglionic and parasympathetic postganglionic neurons, sympathetic postganglionic neurons to sweat glands, and sympathetic vasodilator neurons to blood vessels in skeletal muscle. There is usually no acetylcholine in circulating blood, and the effects of localized cholinergic discharge are generally discrete and short-lived because of high concentrations of cholinesterase at the cholinergic nerve endings (Figs 19–12 and 19–13; Table 19–2). In the adrenal medulla, the postganglionic cells have lost their axons and become specialized for secreting catecholamine directly into the blood; the cholinergic preganglionic neurons to these cells act as the secretomotor nerve supply to the adrenal gland. Sympathetic postganglionic neurons are generally considered adrenergic except for the sympathetic vasodilator neurons and sweat gland neurons. Note that norepinephrine has a more prolonged and wider action than does acetylcholine.

Receptors

The target tissues on which norepinephrine acts can be separated into 2 categories, based on their different sensitivities to certain drugs. This is related to the existence of 2 types of catecholamine

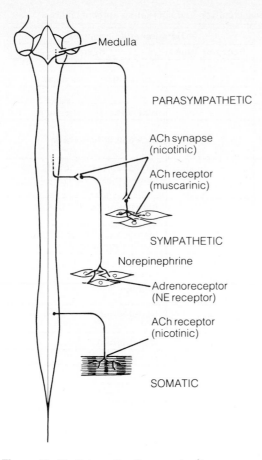

Figure 19–12. Schematic diagram showing some anatomic and pharmacologic features of autonomic and somatic motor nerves.

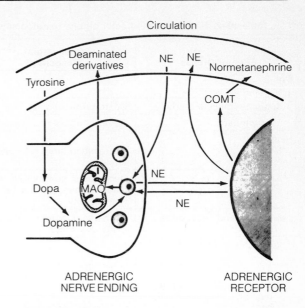

Figure 19–13. Formation, uptake, and metabolism of norepinephrine at adrenergic nerve endings. Norepinephrine in the granulated vesicles is released from the endings mainly by action potentials in the sympathetic nerves. Some of the norepinephrine constantly diffuses from the granules to the mitochondria, however, where it is oxidized to deaminated derivatives. Norepinephrine in the vesicles is formed from dopamine, taken up from the circulation, and taken up again after its release from the endings (reuptake). NE, norepinephrine; COMT, catechol-O-methyltransferase; MAO, monoamine oxidase. (Reproduced, with permission, from Ganong WF: *Review of Medical Physiology,* 14th ed. Appleton & Lange, 1989.)

receptors—α and β—in the target tissues. The α **receptors** mediate vasoconstriction, and the β **receptors** mediate such actions as the increase in cardiac rate and the strength of cardiac contraction. There are 2 subtypes of α receptors (α_1 and α_2) and 2 subtypes of β receptors (β_1 and β_2). The α and β receptors occur in both preganglionic endings and postganglionic membranes. The preganglionic β-adrenergic endings are of the β_1 type; the postganglionic receptors are of the β_2 type (see Fig 19–14 and Table 19–2).

Effects of Drugs on the Autonomic Nervous System

Certain drugs affect the autonomic nervous system by mimicking or blocking cholinergic or adrenergic discharges (Table 19–3; see also Fig 19–12). Drugs can also produce other effects such as synthesis, storage in nerve endings, release near

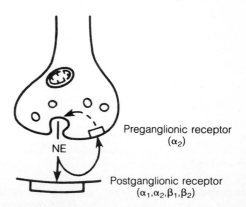

Figure 19–14. Preganglionic and postganglionic receptors at the ending of a noradrenergic neuron. The preganglionic receptor shown is α; the postganglionic receptors can be α_1, $9\alpha_2$, β_1, or β_2. (Reproduced, with permission, from Ganong, WF: *Review of Medical Physiology,* 14th ed. Appleton & Lange, 1989.)

Table 19-2. Responses of effector organs to autonomic nerve impulses and circulating catecholamines.*

Effector Organs	Cholinergic Response	Noradrenergic Impulses	
		Receptor Type	Response
Eye			
Radial muscle of iris	. . .	α	Contraction (mydriasis)
Sphincter muscle of iris	Contraction (miosis)	. . .	. . .
Ciliary muscle	Contraction for near vision	β	Relaxation for far vision
Heart			
S-A node	Decrease in heart rate; vagal arrest	β_1	Increase in heart rate
Atria	Decrease in contractility and (usually) increase in conduction velocity	β_1	Increase in contractility and conduction velocity
A-V node and conduction system	Decrease in conduction velocity; A-V block	β_1	Increase in conduction velocity
Ventricles	. . .	β_2	Increase in contractility and conduction velocity
Arterioles			
Coronary, skeletal muscle, pulmonary, abdominalviscera, renal	Dilation	α	Constriction
		β_2	Dilation
Skin and mucosa, cerebral, salivary glands	. . .	α	Constriction
Systemic veins	. . .	α	Constriction
		β_2	Dilation
Lung			
Bronchial muscle	Contraction	β_2	Relaxation
Bronchial glands	Stimulation	?	Inhibition(?)
Stomach			
Motility and tone	Increase	α,β_2	Decrease (usually)
Sphincters	Relaxation (usually)	α	Contraction (usually)
Secretion	Stimulation	. . .	Inhibition(?)
Intestine			
Motility and tone	Increase	α, β_2	Decrease
Sphincters	Rexalation (usually)	α	Contraction (usually)
Secretion	Stimulation	. . .	Inhibition(?)
Gallbladder and ducts	Contraction	. . .	Relaxation
Urinary bladder			
Detrusor	Contraction	β	Relaxation (usually)
Trigone and sphincter	Relaxation	α	Contraction
Ureter			
Motility and tone	Increase(?)	α	Increase (usually)
Uterus	Variable†	α, β_2	Variable†
Male sex organs	Erection	α	Ejaculation
Skin			
Pilomotor muscles	. . .	α	Contraction
Sweat glands	Generalized secretion	α	Slight localized secretion‡
Spleen capsule	. . .	α	Contraction
		β_2	Relaxation
Adrenal medulla	Secreation of epinephrine and norepinephrine	. . .	. . .
Liver	. . .	α, β_2	Glycogenolysis

(continued)

Table 19-2. (cont'd.) Responses of effector organs to autonomic nerve impulses and circulating catecholamines.*

Effector Organs	Cholinergic Response	Noradrenergic Impulses	
		Receptor Type	Response
Pancreas			
Acini	Increase secretion	α	Decreased secretion
		α	Decreased insulin and gluca-gon secretion
Islets	Increased insulin and gluca-gon secretion	β₂	Increased insulin and gluca-gon secretion
		α	Thick secretion
Salivary glands	Profuse watery secretion	β₂	Amylase secretion
Lacrimal glands	Secretion	...	...
Nasopharyngeal glands	Secretion	...	...
Adipose tissue	...	β₁	Lipolysis
Juxtaglomerular cells	...	β₁	Increased renin secretion
Pineal gland	...	β	Increased melatonin synthesis and secretion

*Modified from Gilman AG et al (editors): *Goodman and Gilman's The Pharmacological Basis of Therapeutics,* 7th ed. Macmillan, 1985. Reproduced, with permission, from Ganong WF: *Review of Medical Physiology,* 13th ed. Appleton & Lange, 1987.
†Depends on stage of menstrual cycle, amount of circulating estrogen and progesterone, pregnancy, and other factors.
‡On palms of hands and in some other locations (adrenergic sweating).

effector cells, action on effector cells, and destruction within the stages of transmitter activity. Sometimes, a drug action may release two mediators rather than one.

Despite apparent similarities in the transmitter chemistry of preganglionic and postganglionic cholinergic neurons, agents can act differently at these sites. **Muscarine** has little effect on autonomic ganglia, for example, but stimulates visceral cholinergic postganglionic neurons. Drugs with muscarine action include acetylcholine, acetylcholine-related substances, and inhibitors of cholinesterase (certain nerve gases, etc). Atropine, belladonna, and other natural and synthetic belladonna-like drugs block the muscarine effects of acetylcholine by preventing the mediator from acting on visceral effector organs.

Although small doses of acetylcholine stimulate postganglionic cells, large doses block the transmission of impulses from pre- to postganglionic neurons. These actions are not affected by atropine. Because **nicotine** produces the same actions, the actions of acetylcholine in the presence of atropine are called its nicotine effects.

Curariform agents, hexamethonium, and mecamylamine act principally by blocking transmission at the cholinergic motor neuron endings on skeletal muscle fibers; they are used in the treatment of hypertension.

Drugs that block the effects of norepinephrine on visceral effectors are often called adrenergic-neuron-blocking agents, adrenolytic agents, or sympatholytic agents.

Sensitization

Autonomic effectors (smooth muscle, cardiac muscle, and glands) that are partially or completely separated from their normal nerve connections become more sensitive to the action of chemical substances. Known as Cannon's law of denervation, the effect is more pronounced after postganglionic interruption than after preganglionic interruption.

CASE 26

A 55-year-old male clerk consulted his physician about drooling, difficulty in swallowing, and a "funny-sounding" voice. Indirect laryngoscopy showed decreased motility of the right vocal cord. Findings in all other examinations and tests were within normal limits. Drugs were given to control the patient's hypersalivation.

Eight months later, the patient returned with a 10-day history of lightheadedness and fainting. He was referred to a hospital for observation and examination. The only additional abnormal findings were fasciculations in the right side of the tongue and changes in blood pressure with postural changes (lying down, 140/90; sitting up, 100/70; and standing up, a rate that was too low to read).

Table 19-3. Some chemical agents that affect sympathetic activity, listing only the principal actions of the agents.*

Site of Action	Agents that Augment Sympathetic Activity	Agents That Depress Sympathetic Activity
Sympathetic ganglia	**Stimulate postganglionic neurons** Nicotine Dimethphenylpiperazinium **Inhibit acetylcholinesterase** Physostigmine (eserine) Neostigmine (Prostigmin) Parathion	**Block conduction** Chlorisondamine† Hexamethonium† Mecamylamine (Inversine) Pentolinium† Tetraethylammonium† Trimethaphan (Arfonad) Acetylcholine and anticholinesterase drugs in high concentrations
Endings of postganglionic neurons	**Release norepinephrine** Tyramine Ephedrine Amphetamine	**Block norepinephrine synthesis** Metyrosine **Interfere with norepinephrine storage** Reserpine Guanethidine (Ismelin) **Prevent norepinephrine release** Bretylium tosylate Guanethidine (Ismelin)‡ **Form false transmitters** Methyldopa (Aldomet)
α Receptors	**Stimulate α_1 receptors** Methoxamine (Vasoxyl) Phenylephrine (Neo-Synephrine) **Stimulate α_2 receptors** Clonidine§	**Block α receptors** Phenoxybenzamine (Dibenzyline) Phentolamine (Regitine) Prazosin (blocks α_1) Yohimbine (blocks α_2)
β Receptors	**Stimulate β receptors** Isoproterenol (Isuprel)	**Block β receptors** Propranolol (Inderal) and others (block β_1 and β_2) Metoprolol and others (block β_1) Butoxamine† (blocks β_2)

*Modified and reproduced, with permission, from Ganong WF: *Review of Medical Physiology,* 13th ed. Appleton & Lange, 1987.
†Not available in the USA.
‡Note that guanethidine is believed to have 2 principal actions.
§Clonidine stimulates α_2 receptors in the periphery, but along with others α_2 agonists that cross the blood-brain barrier, it also stimulates α_2 receptors in the brain which decrease sympathetic output. Therefore, the overall effect is decreased sympathetic discharge.

Lumbar puncture analysis showed a protein level of 95 mg/dL. While in the hospital, the patient had one episode of rotatory vertigo. After 4 days, he went back to work.

Three months later, the patient returned with complaints of dizziness, fainting, and increased problems in swallowing; his speech was difficult to understand. His drop in blood pressure with postural changes was still present. Neurologic examination showed a normal mental status; flat optic disks; visual fields full, with pupils normal and reactive to light; normal extraocular movements; bilateral neural hearing deficits; dysarthria; midline palate location with normal gag reflex; and a weak tongue that deviated to the right when protruded. The patient's gait was wide-based and unsteady. The heel-to-shin test showed ataxia on the right, and other cerebellar tests results were normal. The deep tendon reflexes were also normal. A CT scan showed moderate ventricular enlargement.

Where is the lesion? What is the nature of the lesion? What is the explanation for the autonomic dysfunctions?

Cases are discussed further in Chapter 24.

REFERENCES

Brooks CM, Koizumi K, Sato AY (editors): *Integrative Functions of the Autonomic Nervous System.* Elsevier, 1979.

Gershon MD: The enteric nervous system. *Annu Rev Neurosci* 1981;**4:**227.

McLeod JG, Tuck RR: Disorders of the autonomic nervous system. 1. Pathophysiology and clinical features. *Ann Neurol* 1987;**21**:419.

Newman PP: *Visceral Afferent Functions of the Nervous System.* Edward Arnold, 1974.

Pick J: *The Autonomic Nervous System: Morphological, Comparative, Clinical and Surgical Aspects.* Lippincott, 1970.

Swanson LW, Mogensen GJ: Neural mechanisms for the functional coupling of autonomic, endocrine and somatomotor responses in adaptive behavior. *Brain Res Rev* 1981;**3**:1.

The cerebral cortex contains components of the functional systems related to the initiation of movement and to sensation from the body and the special sensory organs. The cortex is also the substrate for functions that convey comprehension, cognition, and communication. Lesions of the cortex or of the diencephalon and brain stem structures can reduce consciousness or cause coma (see Chapter 17).

LANGUAGE & SPEECH

Language, the comprehension and communication of abstract ideas, is a cortical function that is separate from the neural mechanisms related to primary visual, auditory, and motor function.

The motor cortex (area 4), which is connected to the motor nuclei of the brain stem (cranial nerves V, VII, IX, X, and XII), is involved in the production of audible speech. The supplementary motor cortex (area 6) is involved in mechanisms for sequencing and coordinating sounds. The development of expressive language ability—speech—is dependent on cortical connections between areas 4 and 6, the auditory association areas in the temporal lobe (areas 3a and 22), and the frontal association cortex (Broca's areas 44 and 45) of the dominant hemisphere (see below). The pathways for these connections lie in the white matter of the frontal, parietal, and temporal lobes. The subcortical connection between temporal and frontal speech areas is the **arcuate fasciculus.** Note that lesions in one or more of these areas or their connections lead to speech disorders that differ from language disturbances caused by the impairment of mental processes.

Aphasia

Aphasia, as the term is generally used, refers to motor and sensory language disturbances caused by brain lesions (Figs 20–1 and 20–2; Table 20–1), but it does not include those caused by mental defects, disturbances in the sense organs, or dysfunction of the muscles and nerves essential for speech. The precise location of the cortical lesions may vary between individuals.

A. Expressive (Motor) Aphasia: Motor aphasia is usually caused by a lesion in the lower frontal gyrus in the dominant hemisphere (Broca's area) and is sometimes called **Broca's aphasia.** The speech of patients with Broca's aphasia is labored,

ungrammatical, telegraphic, sparse, and nonfluent. Comprehension of spoken language, however, is normal. Pronunciation of single words improves with repetition, but combinations of more than 3 words are extremely difficult. Patients are often hemiplegic, with the arm worse than the leg; they are concerned and appropriately depressed. In this type of aphasia, the capacity to program and coordinate the sequence of muscle contractions necessary to produce intelligible sounds is destroyed. This is in contrast to **dysarthria,** a speech disorder in which the mechanism for speech is damaged by lesions in the corticobulbar pathways; in one or more cranial nerve nuclei or nerves V, VII, IX, X, and XII; in the cerebellum; or in the muscles that produce speech sounds. Dysarthria is characterized by dysfunction of the phonation, articulation, resonance, or respiration aspects of speech.

A different form of impaired expression of language is **nominal aphasia,** or **anomia**—the inability to name objects or persons. This disorder is associated with lesions in the angular gyrus or nearby in the parietal lobe. One theory explaining this disorder is that patients with anomia do not really understand the questions when they are asked to name things.

Agraphia—an inability to write—is another type of expressive aphasia. Because writing involves the use of symbols for speech (symbolic sounds), it is therefore a more difficult and complex function than speech. Writing ability can be affected by lesions in various locations, including the descending motor pathways and the cerebral cortex. In primary agraphia, there is an inability to construct letters, but there are no disturbances in the spheres of speech and vision. The lesion causing primary agraphia is usually in the posterior frontal cortex, excluding Broca's area. Secondary agraphia may be due to defects in language.

B. Receptive (Sensory) Aphasia: This type of aphasia, also called **Wernicke's aphasia,** is caused by a lesion in or near the superior temporal gyrus of the temporal lobe cortex (Wernicke's area; see Figs 20–1 and 20–2). There is usually no hemiplegia. Patients have impaired language comprehension and sometimes use substitutions for words they do not fully understand (**paraphasia**). They usually have no expressive aphasia and are, in fact, often euphoric, with fluent speech. Patients with Wernicke's aphasia may be given a mistaken diagnosis of a psychiatric disorder.

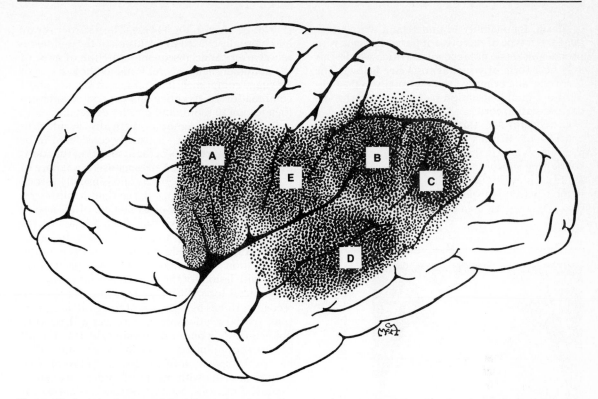

Figure 20-1. Aphasic zone of the left cerebral hemisphere showing areas and the associated neurologic deficits. *A:* Middle and inferior frontal gyri and lower precentral gyrus—dysarthria, alexia, contralateral facial weakness. *B:* Supramarginal gyrus—generalized aphasia, hemianesthesia, hemianopia. *C:* Angular gyrus—aphasia with reading disturbance, anomia quadrantanopia, hemianesthesia. *D:* Posterior superior and middle temporal gyri—sensory aphasia, paraphasia, jargon aphasia. *E:* Area including the insula—severe aphasia, dysarthria, right hemiplegia. (Modified, from Bailey P: *Intracranial Tumors.* Thomas, 1933.)

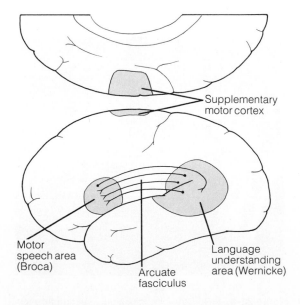

Figure 20-2. Central speech areas of the dominant cerebral hemisphere.

Table 20-1. Aphasia.

Expressive aphasia (motor)	Broca's aphasia—nonfluent speech; motor or speech aphasia Agraphia—loss of ability to write Anomia—loss of ability to name things or persons Paraphasia—substitution of words in motor speech aphasia
Receptive aphasia (sensory)	Wernicke's aphasia—incomprehension of language Visual agnosia—inability to recognize things or persons visually Alexia—inability to understand written language
Global aphasia	Loss of all language understanding and speech fluency

Alexia, the inability to understand written language, is a type of receptive aphasia. Patients with primary alexia do not recognize written words; this may be a form of visual agnosia (see below). The lesion causing primary alexia is usually in the temporo-occipital association pathways or in the visual association cortex.

C. Global Aphasia: The central speech area consists of Broca's area in the frontal lobe, Wernicke's area in the temporal lobe, and an interconnecting subcortical bundle of fibers, the arcuate fasciculus (Fig 20–2); this pathway is involved in the repetition of spoken words. A deep lesion in the central speech area can lead to global aphasia

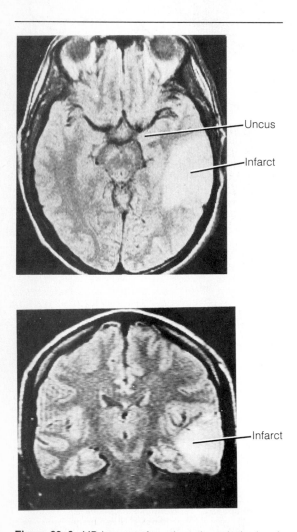

(Fig 20–3; see also Fig 11–12). The disorder is rare and is usually caused by occlusion of the middle cerebral artery and subsequent infarction of most of the dominant hemisphere. Patients show a loss of language comprehension and speech fluency and a combination of receptive and expressive aphasias (in addition to motor and sensory defects).

D. Agnosia: Agnosia—difficulty in identification or recognition—is usually considered to be caused by disturbances in the association functions of the cerebral cortex. **Astereognosis** is a failure of tactile recognition of objects and is usually associated with parietal lesions in the right hemisphere. **Anosognosia,** the lack of awareness of disease or denial of disease, may result from a lesion of the parietal lobe in the area of the supramarginal gyrus. **Autotopagnosia,** the impaired recognition (localization or orientation) of body parts, may occur with lesions of the posteroinferior portion of the parietal lobe. **Visual agnosia,** the inability to recognize things by sight (eg, objects, pictures, persons, spatial relationships), can occur with or without hemianopia on the dominant side. It is a result of parietooccipital lesions or the interruption of fibers in the splenium of the corpus callosum. (Although patients with mental disorders may show these dysfunctions, usually no gross cortical lesions are demonstrable.) Absence of the corpus callosum would also contribute to this type of agnosia; however, functional deficits in patients without a corpus callosum (usually an incidental finding; Fig 20–4) have been incompletely studied.

E. Apraxia: This is an inability to carry out a requested complex or skilled movement. The in-

Figure 20–3. MR images of sections through the head. *Top:* Horizontal section with a large high-intensity area in the temporal lobe, representing an infarct caused by occlusion of a middle cerebral artery branch. *Bottom:* Coronal section showing the same area of infarction. (Parallel lines on the periphery of the brain represent artifacts caused by patient motion.)

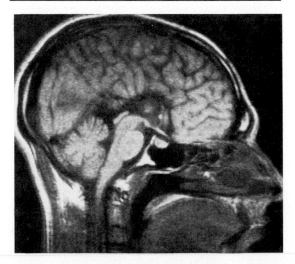

Figure 20–4. MR image of a midsagittal section through the head. There is no corpus callosum, and the gyral pattern is abnormal.

ability is caused, not by paralysis, ataxia, sensory changes, confusion, or deficiencies of understanding, but by lesions in the associative motor areas of the parietal lobe.

CEREBRAL DOMINANCE

Clinical findings and experimental work have established that the 2 cerebral hemispheres are not equal in certain functions. Although the projection systems of motor and sensory pathways are alike, left and right, each hemisphere is specialized and dominates the other in some specific functions. The left hemisphere controls language and speech in most people; the right hemisphere leads in interpreting 3-dimensional images and spaces. Other distinctions have been postulated, such as music understanding in the left hemisphere, arithmetic and design in the right.

Cerebral dominance is related to handedness. Most right-handed people are left-hemisphere dominant; so are 70% of left-handed people, while the remaining 30% are right-hemisphere dominant. This dominance is reflected in anatomic differences between the hemispheres. The slope of the left lateral fissure is less steep, and the upper aspect of the left superior temporal gyrus (the planum temporale) is broader in people with left-hemisphere dominance.

When neurosurgery is contemplated in a patient, it can be useful to establish which cerebral hemisphere is dominant for speech. Typically, amobarbital or thiopental sodium is injected into a carotid artery while the patient is counting aloud and making rapidly alternating movements of the fingers of both hands. When the carotid artery of the dominant side is injected, a much greater and longer interference with speech function occurs than with injection of the other side.

MEMORY & LEARNING

The 3 types of memory are immediate recall, short-term memory, and long-term (or remote) memory.

Immediate recall is the phenomenon that allows people to remember and repeat a small amount of information shortly after reading or hearing it. In tests, most people can repeat, parrotlike, a short series of words or numbers for up to 10 minutes. The anatomic substrate is thought to be the auditory association cortex.

Short-term memory can last up to an hour. Tests usually involve short lists of more complicated numbers (eg, telephone numbers) or sentences for a period of an hour or less. This type of memory is associated with intactness of the deep temporal lobe. If a patient's temporal lobe is stimulated during surgery or irritated by the presence of a lesion, he or she may experience **déjà vu,** characterized by sudden flashes of former events or by the feeling that new sensations are old and familiar ones. (Occasionally, the feeling of déjà vu occurs spontaneously in normal, healthy persons.)

Long-term memory allows people to remember words, numbers, other persons, events, and so forth for many years. The hippocampus and adjacent structures appear to be involved in the consolidation of short-term and long-term memory (see Chapter 18).

Clinical Correlations

If both temporal lobes are removed or bilateral temporal lobe lesions destroy the mechanism for consolidation, new events or information will not be remembered—but previous memories will remain intact. This unusual disorder, called **anterograde,** or **posttraumatic amnesia,** may also result from traumatic or electric shock. Extensive lesions of the brain may result in loss of long-term memory; **retrograde amnesia** is the loss of memory for events prior to the lesion. The loss of immediate recall and short-term memory is a characteristic of Alzheimer's disease (see Chapter 21); the mechanism for these types of memory loss in patients suffering from the disease is poorly understood, however.

Appropriate stimuli and repetition can aid learning in an intact brain. Reading a text twice or reading it aloud, for example, will retard forgetting. Other factors that influence learning include the desire to learn, interest in the subject matter, the ability to concentrate, and the goals of the learner. Some drugs or chemicals (eg, alcohol) depress learning. Although others, such as methionine, are said to improve learning, careful testing under experimental conditions has failed to confirm this theory.

EPILEPSY

Dysfunction of the cerebral cortex, alone or together with dysfunction of deeper structures, can lead to some forms of epilepsy (Table 20–2). Epilepsy is characterized by sudden, transient alterations of brain function, usually with motor, sensory, autonomic, or psychic symptoms; it is often accompanied by alterations in consciousness. Coincidental pronounced brain-wave alterations in the electroencephalogram may be detected during these episodes (see Chapter 23).

Classification

A. Absence (Petit Mal) Seizures: In petit mal seizures, the patient may have a minor or abor-

Table 20-2. Classification of epilepsies.*

Primary generalized epilepsies
  Absence (petit mal) seizures.
  Tonic-clonic (grand mal) seizures: Status epilepticus.
  Myoclonic seizures.
Partial epilepsies
  Simple partial (jacksonian) epilepsy.
  Complex partial epilepsy:
    Simple partial epilepsy at onset followed by impairment of consciousness and automatisms.
    Impairment of consciousness at onset:
      Motionless stare and impaired consciousness followed by automatisms (temporal lobe epilepsy).
      Complex motor automatisms at start of impaired consciousness (frontal lobe, somatosensory, or occipital lobe epilepsy).
      Akinetic (drop) attack with impaired consciousness and automatisms (temporal lobe syncope).
Secondary generalized epilepsies
  Simple partial epilepsy evolving to tonic-clonic (secondary tonic-clonic) seizures.
  Infantile febrile spasms (propulsive petit mal, infantile myoclonic encephalopathy).
  Myoclonic astatic or atonic epilepsies in children with mental retardation.
  Progressive myoclonic epilepsies in adolescents and adults with dementia.
Unclassified epilepsies

*Modified from the classification of the International League Against Epilepsy and the World Health Organization.

tive attack with no falling or convulsive movements of the body. Instead, there will be a momentary or transient loss of consciousness, so fleeting or camouflaged in ordinary activity that neither the patient nor anyone else may be entirely aware of it. The classic absence seizure is characterized by a sudden vacant expression (brief absence) and cessation of motor activity, sometimes with loss of muscle tone. This is followed by the abrupt return of consciousness and resumption of mental and physical activity. As many as 100 attacks may occur in a day.

Patients with petit mal seizures may appear to be day-dreaming, especially when attacks are frequent. Staring and blank spells often occur without the patient's knowledge. Impaired learning ability, short attention span, and restlessness are often associated with this type of epilepsy. Symptoms of the disorder may be mistaken for aimless wandering, erratic behavior, or incoherent speech.

B. Tonic-Clonic (Grand Mal) Seizures: An aura may signal an impending attack. The aura is usually specific for the individual patient and may consist of a sensation of nausea or numbness, an odor, a visual image, or a flash of memory. Loss of consciousness usually ensues, and the patient falls to the floor. The patient may cry out and frequently incurs some bodily injury. Convulsions usually follow, with the patient lying stiff and mildly rigid for as long as 1–2 minutes and the muscles of the body in a state of mild tonic contraction. A clonic stage follows in which rhythmic, severe, synchronous, convulsive movements of the body occur. Control of the bowel and bladder is frequently lost, and biting injuries to the tongue are common. More rarely, fractures of bones may occur. Following a grand mal episode or a series of brief seizures, patients may remain confused for several minutes (or hours). Disorientation, anxiety, hallucinations, paranoid delusions, excitement, and aggressive activity may be overwhelming. A variable period of sleep or stupor, usually lasting 1–4 hours, may follow this phase. Later, there is little recollection of events occurring during this period. Upon full recovery from the attack, the patient is frequently aware of painful muscles.

Children with epilepsy often appear to be restless, hyperactive, aggressive, and irritable. These traits as well as learning difficulties and apparent mental retardation are sometimes improved by adequate anticonvulsant therapy.

C. Status Epilepticus: This serious disorder consists of a train of severe seizures with relatively short—or no—intervals between. The patient becomes exhausted and, frequently, hyperthermic. Death is not uncommon during such attacks.

D. Myoclonic Seizures: This unusual form of epilepsy is characterized by sudden simple, bilateral jerking movements. Patients report that they are unaware of the attack itself and that they simply find themselves in an unusual position afterward, often on the floor. This disorder differs from hemiballismus and ballismus, which are caused by destruction of one or both subthalamic nuclei (see Chapter 12). Myoclonic seizures also differ from myoclonic jerks of the limbs or muscles. The latter are usually not considered epileptic and can occur either without evident alteration of consciousness or in association with a typical absence seizure. Myoclonic jerks tend to occur more frequently in the morning and on going to sleep; normal individuals may have rare myoclonic jerks in drowsiness or light sleep.

E. Simple Partial (Jacksonian) Epilepsy: Seizures resulting from focal irritation of a portion of the motor cortex may be confined to the appropriate peripheral area. Consciousness may be retained, and the seizure may spread over the rest of the adjacent motor cortex to involve adjacent peripheral parts. This type of seizure is most commonly associated with organic lesions such as brain tumor, cerebral edema, or glial scar. Electrical stimulation of the exposed cortex during neurosurgery has aided in mapping the cortex and in understanding localized, partial seizures (Fig 20–5; see also Figs 9–14 and 9–15).

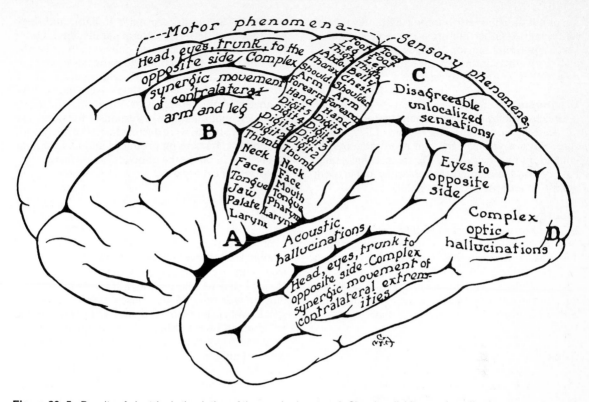

Figure 20–5. Results of electrical stimulation of the cerebral cortex. *A:* Chewing, licking, and swallowing movements. *B:* Eyes turned toward the opposite side, without visual aura. *C:* Sensory aura in the opposite leg, followed by complex synergistic movements. *D:* Unformed optical phenomena such as flames and lights. (After Foerster. Reproduced, with permission, from Bailey P: *Intracranial Tumors.* Thomas, 1933.)

F. Complex Partial Epilepsy: There are several types of complex partial epilepsy, as outlined in Table 20–2. In **temporal lobe epilepsy,** for example, there may be automatism, patterned movements, apparently purposeful movements, incoherent speech, turning of the head and eyes, smacking of the lips, twisting and writhing movements of the extremities, clouding of consciousness, and amnesia. Complex acts and movements such as walking, lipsmacking, and chewing may occur for periods of several seconds or as long as 10 minutes. An abnormal feeling of familiarity (déjà vu) may be present. Depersonalization, in which familiar things (eg, faces and places) become strange, may also appear occasionally as part of a seizure syndrome. It has been postulated that equivalent states exist in which the patient exhibits a behavioral disturbance rather than a classic convulsion. Temporal lobe foci (spikes, sharp waves, or combinations of these) are frequently associated with this type of epilepsy.

G. Akinetic (Drop) Attacks: These are partial seizures of sudden, brief loss of postural tone, with the patient slumping a little before realizing it

or recovering just after the body or knees touch the ground. These attacks differ from the paroxysmal sleep periods seen in patients suffering from narcolepsy.

H. Infantile Febrile Spasms: Fever and convulsions are commonly encountered in the very young. An infantile febrile spasm is apt to be the first convulsion of an epileptic child, and febrile convulsions are said to be about twice as common among children with a family history of epilepsy.

Causes

Epilepsy has been found in many cases to be caused by abnormal activity of the brain tissue that results from an injury, infection, or unknown agent; idiopathic epilepsy tends to run in families. Metabolic disorders such as uremia, hypoglycemia, hypocalcemia, and excessive hydration may also give rise to seizures.

The most common causes of symptomatic epilepsy in children are birth injury and anoxia, inflammatory brain lesions, cerebrovascular accidents, head injuries, and congenital brain malformations.

In susceptible individuals, physical stimuli such

as sound, touch, or stroboscopic light may precipitate seizures. Other factors—excessive alcohol intake, emotional tension, fatigue, or lack of food and sleep—may indirectly affect the susceptibility of a particular patient to seizures.

Diagnosis

Epilepsy can be diagnosed on the basis of a history of recurrent seizures and observation of a typical seizure. Physical, neurologic, and neuroradiologic examinations may be helpful. Electroencephalography has become a most important objective tool in the diagnosis of epilepsy (see Chapter 23).

Treatment

The objective of therapy is the complete suppression of symptoms. Most epileptic patients must continue to receive anticonvulsant therapy throughout life, and in a few patients neurosurgery is necessary. Epileptic patients should avoid hazardous occupations and driving. An epilepsy identification card should be carried at all times.

CASE 27

A 60-year-old right-handed widow had been experiencing intermittent brief episodes of blurred vision in the right eye for a year or so. One month prior to admission to the hospital, she had a 5-minute episode of numbness and tingling in the left arm and hand, accompanied by loss of movement in the left hand. Two days before admission, she fell to the floor while taking a shower and lost consciousness. She was found by a neighbor who put her to bed. The patient was unable to move her left arm and leg, and her speech—although slurred and slow—made sense.

Neurologic examination on admission showed a blood pressure of 180/100 with a regular heart rate of 84 beats per minute. The patient was slow to respond but roughly oriented with regard to person, place, and time. She ignored stimuli in the left visual field. The pupils responded to light, and there was slight but definite bilateral papilledema. Other findings included decreased pain sensation on the left side of the face, complete paralysis of the left central face, and complete flaccid paralysis of the left arm and left leg. Reflexes were more pronounced on the left than on the right, and there was a left plantar extensor response. Responses to all sensory stimuli were decreased on the left side of the body. CT scanning produced an image similar to Fig 11–12, but in the opposite hemisphere.

What is the diagnosis?

CASE 28

A 63-year-old clerk suddenly experienced a strange feeling over his body, which he characterized as an electric shock, with flashes of blue light. He said that he felt as though he were falling and that he was only partly conscious and could not speak. When he recovered shortly afterwards, he felt tired and went to bed. The next day he still felt tired and weak, and a day later, when he got up he inadvertently walked into the right doorjamb. He also did not notice his wife bringing him a cup of coffee as she approached from his right side. During the next 2 weeks, he continued to bump into people and objects on his right side. He said he thought that his eyesight was all right, but his wife urged him to see a doctor. When asked about his medical history, the patient indicated that he had rheumatic heart disease that had been completely under control for the past 3 years.

Neurologic examination showed normal visual acuity, and normal optic papillae, but there was right hemianopia. No other neurologic abnormality was found.

Where is the lesion? What further tests would be helpful in confirming the site? What is the most likely diagnosis?

Cases are discussed further in Chapter 24.

REFERENCES

Bloom FE, Lazerson A: *Brain, Mind, and Behavior.* Freeman, 1988.

Damasio AR, Geschwind N: The neural basis of language. *Annu Rev Neurosci* 1984;**7**:127.

Matthews WB, Glaser GH (editors): *Recent Advances in Clinical Neurology.* Vol 2. Churchill-Livingstone, 1978.

Roland PE et al: Different cortical areas in man in organization of voluntary movements in extrapersonal space. *J Neurophysiol* 1980;**43**:137.

Springer SP, Deutch G: *Left Brain, Right Brain.* Freeman, 1987.

Aging, Degeneration, & Regeneration

21

NEUROBIOLOGY OF AGING

Although the human life span has not increased significantly, average life expectancy has lengthened markedly in this century. This increase is mainly due to medical advances: antibiotics, vaccination, a reduction in infant mortality, and a decrease in the incidence of heart disease and stroke. The increase in life expectancy may well be paralleled by an increased incidence of dementia, however, and the deterioration of intellectual function in aged persons due to organic disease is often associated with a decrease in the quality of life. The elderly constitute a growing fraction of the population of the USA. The burgeoning development of research in this area, **gerontology,** and of the clinical specialty of **geriatrics** is recognized by scientists and medical practitioners alike.

Normal Aging

A. Gross Changes in the Brain: A number of anatomic differences between the brains of elderly people and those of young adults have been consistently noted (Figs 21-1 and 21-2).

By age 80, the brain has lost 15% of its weight. Many cortical gyri have decreased in bulk, and the sulci are wider. The spaces containing cerebrospinal fluid are enlarged. The finding of big ventricles, however, does not necessarily mean that the patient is demented. In addition, arterial disease affecting both large and small vessels is usually present in older people, with a concomitant reduction of blood flow and oxygen consumption.

B. Histologic Changes in the Brain: Some characteristics of the aging process are the reverse of growth changes in the young; others are present solely in elderly people. However, the significance of any of these findings and their cause and effect are not clear.

In normal older people, the number of **neurons** in various cortical regions is significantly lower than in young adults. One study reported that only 50% of the small neurons remained in the most severely affected regions. The **dendrites** of cortical

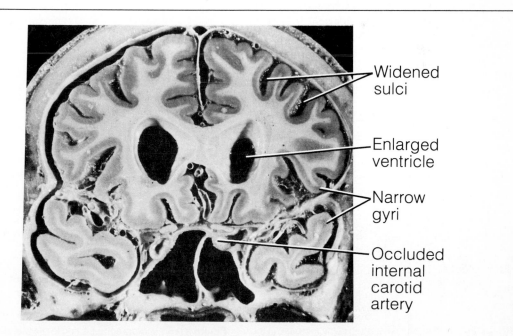

Figure 21-1. Coronal section through the head of a 78-year-old patient.

Widened sulci

Enlarged ventricle

Narrow gyri

Occluded internal carotid artery

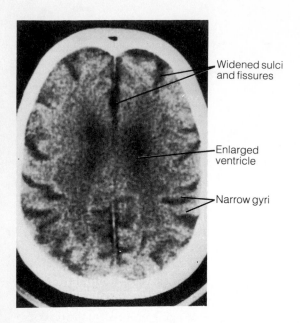

Figure 21–2. MR image of a horizontal section through the head of an 80-year-old patient.

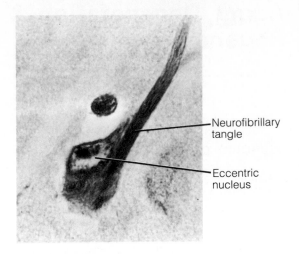

Figure 21–4. Micrograph of a nerve cell containing a neurofibrillary tangle. (Silver stain, × 800.)

pyramidal cells (demonstrated by Golgi stain) are also found to be much shorter, thicker, and fewer in old people than in young adults (Fig 21–3).

Synaptic density in the cortex decreases with age, and **neurofibrillary tangles** are found in the cerebral cortices (especially in the hippocampus) of elderly people (Fig 21–4). These tangles are neither the normal neurotubules nor neurofilaments (intermediate filaments). They consist of paired helical filaments that are similar in size to neurofilaments but that apparently share at least one antigenic determinant with neurotubules.

Neuritic (senile) plaques consist of amyloid deposits surrounded by a web of astrocytic processes, swollen neurites, and neuron rests in the cortex (Fig 21–5). Intracellular **eosinophilic inclusions (Hirano bodies)** are seen in the brain cells of older people, and **granulovascular organelles** are seen, especially in hippocampal neurons. **Lipofuscin,** a yellow, insoluble material in the cell bodies is more abundant in old people than in young adults; however, this substance is apparently harmless to the cells.

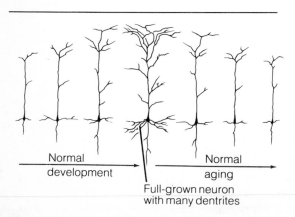

Figure 21–3. Schematic illustration of the increase in the size and number of dendrites and the decrease that occur with approaching age.

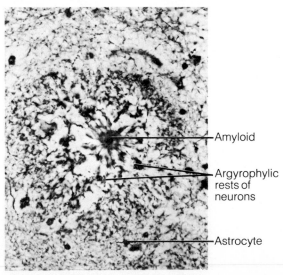

Figure 21–5. Micrograph of a senile plaque, showing an amyloid-containing center amid remnants of nerve processes and glial cells. (Silver stain, × 800.)

C. Biochemical and Physiologic Changes:

By age 80, there is a 30% reduction in the amount of total brain protein. There is a concomitant progressive increase in total DNA, presumably caused by proliferation of glial cells (gliosis). Lipid constituents (neural fats, cerebrosides, and phosphatides) show a minimal decrease with age, and there is only a slight increase in water content. A reduction in blood flow and oxygen consumption occurs with age.

Changes in neurotransmitter systems (enzymes, receptors, transmitters, and their metabolites) occur with aging. The synthesis and degradation of neurotransmitters are carried out by enzymes. Changes in the amount of these enzymes produced or a reduction in their efficacy could explain some of the characteristics of senescence: changes in sleep patterns, mood, appetite, neuroendocrine function, motor activity, and memory. There is, moreover, a drastic reduction in the total amount of those enzymes involved in the synthesis of dopamine and norepinephrine. There is often a reduction of the electroencephalographic variations in evoked potentials to auditory stimuli. In addition, recovery from brain damage is slower and less complete than in younger individuals.

D. Hypotheses for the Molecular Mechanism of Aging:

Several mechanisms of aging have been proposed.

1. There may be a specific gene that induces the changes of senility.

2. The genetic apparatus may not contain a specific program for changes leading to senility, but random or induced errors in duplication of DNA probably increase with age, so that abnormal RNA and protein molecules are formed.

3. Mutations and chromosomal anomalies may increase with age, so that as some genes cease to function, reserve sequences of genes begin to operate until they, too, are exhausted and senescence ensues.

4. Cells (eg, fibroblasts) may possess a biological clock that regulates their life span by limiting the number of cell divisions they can undergo. This theory would not apply to nerve cells, however, since the total complement of neurons is present shortly after birth, and no cell divisions occur after 6 months of age.

5. Reduction in the number of cells in the **nucleus basalis** of the brain has been associated with aging and dementia. The nucleus basalis has extensive cholinergic projections to large areas of the cerebral cortex; it lies in the basal forebrain below the anterior commissure (see Fig 8–7A).

DEMENTIA

The normal changes in form and function of the aged brain must be distinguished from those caused by diseases that abnormally intensify some of the aging processes. Such diseases are often characterized as an impairment of cognitive function or as dementia. There are 2 types of cognitive dysfunction: disturbance of the **level** of consciousness (see Chapter 17), and disturbance of the **content** of consciousness. The second type of cognitive dysfunction includes dementia as well as limited defects in memory and language (see Chapter 20).

Dementia is defined as a loss of intellectual functions, such as memory, learning, reasoning, problem solving, and abstract thinking, while vegetative (involuntary) functions remain intact.

Classification

Dementia is associated with several types of diseases.

A. Diseases Associated with Medical Syndromes: These include hypothyroidism, Cushing's disease, nutritional deficiencies, AIDS dementia complex, and so forth.

B. Diseases Associated with Neurologic Syndromes: This group includes Huntington's chorea, Schilder's disease, and other demyelinative processes; Creutzfeldt-Jakob disease; brain tumors; brain trauma; brain and meningeal infections; and the like.

C. Diseases with Dementia as the Only or Prominent Sign: Alzheimer's disease and Pick's disease are in this category.

Epidemiology

In the USA, of the individuals over 65 years of age (30 million and increasing) almost 15% show moderate mental impairment; about 5% of this age group is seriously demented, and about 70% or more of this 5% probably have Alzheimer's disease (1.5 million individuals). Another 13% (4 million) are mildly demented. About 25% of the over-80 age group show significant dementia. The economic burden imposed on society by dementia is heavy, both because of the cost of care and because of the decreased quality of life for every afflicted individual, who often becomes dependent on the immediate family (which exacts a further cost). Once dementia becomes fully developed, life expectancy is less than 5 years; this means that at least 200,000 demented patients die each year in the USA. While death may be the result of complicating diseases, the underlying disease, senile dementia of the Alzheimer's type (SDAT), contributes greatly to the high mortality rate (patients with the **presenile form** may survive for many years). In some studies, this combination of diseases is reported to be the fourth most common cause of death.

Senile Dementia of the Alzheimer Type

A. Characteristics: **Alzheimer's disease** is a common type of dementia whose cause is un-

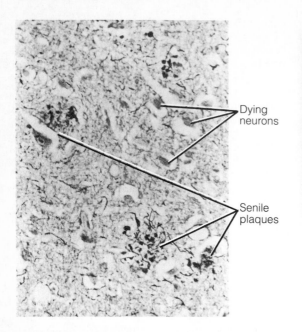

Figure 21-6. Micrograph of a small section of the cerebral cortex of a patient suffering from senile dementia; multiple plaques are seen amid dying neurons. (Silver stain, × 200.)

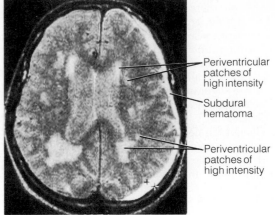

Figure 21-7. MR image of a horizontal section through the head of an 81-year-old patient suffering from dementia. The periventricular patches of demyelination and a left-sided subdural hematoma are clearly visible.

known. Autopsy studies reveal that more than half of patients who died of **senile dementia** had the Alzheimer-type disease (Fig 21–6). In most patients, gross brain weight at the time of autopsy is much lower and the ventricles and sulci are much larger than normal for that age. Demyelination and increased water content of brain tissue have been found adjacent to the lateral ventricles and in a few other areas deep in the cerebral hemispheres in elderly patients, especially those suffering from Alzheimer's disease (Fig 21–7). (This form of demyelination can be distinguished from that of multiple sclerosis on the basis of age and distribution: Patients with multiple sclerosis are much younger, and plaques are present in many areas other than the hemispheres.) In patients with senile dementia of the Alzheimer's type, there is a dramatic increase (in comparison with normal elderly patients) in the number of **neurofibrillary tangles** and **neuritic plaques** as well as a 60–90% decrease in cortical levels of **choline acetyltransferase** (the enzyme that brings about the synthesis of acetylcholine). Other gross or microscopic changes associated with age are often present in the brain. The presence of many **proteinaceous infectious particles (prions)** in the brains of demented persons suggests that Alzheimer's disease may be an infection caused by a slow virus.

B. Course and Treatment: Although the course of Alzheimer's disease is irreversible, therapeutic measures may delay the inevitable death or improve the patient's quality of life. Aggressive treatment of the associated depression, loving care by family members or spouses, and the use of memory crutches may delay institutionalization. Experimental causal therapy uses repeated oral doses of physostigmine or an acetylcholine pump implanted under the skin to try to remedy the acetylcholine deficiency associated with Alzheimer's disease. Successful results have been achieved in a dozen volunteers. In a few cases, implants of young brain cells have shown promising—but transient—improvement.

Other Diseases Associated with Dementia

Pick's disease is an often hereditary presenile dementia. Far less common than Alzheimer's disease, it is characterized grossly by circumscribed frontotemporal cerebral atrophy and associated ventricular enlargement.

Huntington's disease (Huntington's chorea) is a dominantly inherited disease of the basal ganglia and cerebral cortex that manifests itself in adulthood. The disease is characterized by progressive mental deterioration and **choreiform movements.** The head of the caudate nucleus may be clearly reduced in size, and greatly decreased levels of GABA and choline acetyltransferase activity are seen in patients with this disease.

DEGENERATION & REGENERATION

Nerve Degeneration

A. Effects of Peripheral Nerves Lesions:
The loss of a nerve's ability to conduct impulses results in impaired motor, sensory, and trophic function. Motor loss is manifested by paralysis or muscle weakness. Sensory involvement may be subjective or objective. Subjective sensory findings include pain and paresthesias (numbness, tingling, formication [sensation of something crawling over the skin], and so forth). These findings usually point to partial or irritative lesions; the pain of peripheral nerve lesions is frequently worse at night. Objective findings include the loss of various sensibilities (analgesia, anesthesia, etc). Trophic disturbances reflect impaired nutritional and metabolic activities in tissues that are partly under neurogenic control. Most marked in the cutaneous tissues, they are manifested in numerous ways, such as dryness, cyanosis, ulcerations, hair loss, brittleness of the nails, and slow wound healing.

B. Histologic Findings: The cell body maintains the functional and anatomic integrity of the axon (Fig 21-8). If the axon is cut, the part distal to the cut degenerates (**wallerian degeneration**), since materials for maintaining the axon, (mostly proteins), are formed in the cell body and can no longer be transported down the axon (**axoplasmic transport**).

Proteins associated with synaptic transmitters are also synthetized in the endoplasmic reticulum of the cell body and are transported to the axon terminals via fast (400 mm/d) and slow (1-4mm/d)

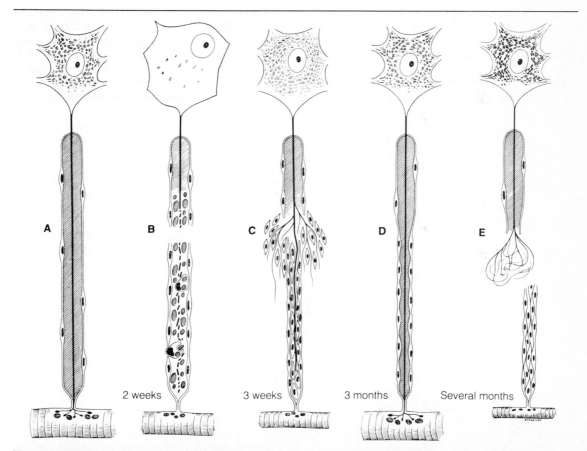

Figure 21-8. Main changes that take place in an injured nerve fiber. *A:* Normal nerve fiber, with its perikaryon and the effector cell (striated skeletal muscle). Note the position of the neuron nucleus and the amount and distribution of Nissl bodies. *B:* When the fiber is injured, the neuronal nucleus moves to the cell periphery, Nissl bodies become greatly reduced in number, and the nerve fiber distal to the injury degenerates along with its myelin sheath. Debris is phagocytized by macrophages. *C:* The muscle fiber shows pronounced disuse atrophy. Schwann cells proliferate, forming a compact cord that is penetrated by the growing axon. The axon grows at a rate of 0.5-3 mm/d. *D:* In this example, the nerve fiber regeneration was successful, and the muscle fiber was also regenerated after receiving nerve stimuli. *E:* When the axon does not penetrate the cord of Schwann cells, its growth is not organized. (Redrawn and reproduced, with permission, from Willis RA, Willis AT: *The Principles of Pathology and Bacteriology,* 3rd ed. Butterworth, 1972.)

transport (see Chapter 2). Fast transport relies on ATP and oxidative metabolism of the neuron and appears to depend on microtubules. Transported material may be attached to filaments formed in the cell body and slide along the microtubules to the axon.

Regeneration

A. Peripheral Nerves: Regeneration denotes a nerve's ability to repair itself, including the reestablishment of functionally useful connections (Figs 21–8 and 21–9). Shortly (1–3 days) after an axon is cut, the tips of the proximal stumps form enlargements, or growth cones, under the influence of nerve growth factor (NGF). The cones send out many exploratory pseudopodia that are similar to the axonal growth cones formed in normal development. Each axonal growth cone is capable of forming many branches that continue to advance away from the site of the original cut. If these branches can cross the scar tissue and enter Bungner's bands (rows of Schwann cells after degeneration), successful regeneration with restoration of function may occur.

Overproduction of branching axons occurs in the early stages of regeneration, and it is possible to see as many as 20 fine axons lying within a single Bungner's band. This number does become reduced, however. Maturation of nerve fibers and the development of a normal axon diameter and myelin sheath are dependent upon reinnervation. Myelination occurs *only* if an axon successfully re-

innervates an end organ, and the new myelin segments are thinner and shorter. Regrowth of regenerating axons occurs at the rate of about 1–4mm/d—the same rate as slow axonal transport.

In mammals, peripheral system axons will reinnervate both muscle and sensory targets; however, motor axons will not connect to sensory structures, or sensory axons to muscle. While a motor axon will reinnervate any denervated muscle, it will preferentially connect to its original muscle.

B. Central Nervous System: Axonal regeneration is typically abortive in the central nervous system. The reasons for the failure of regeneration are not clear, but the glial scar, which is largely formed by astrocytic processes, may be responsible. It may instead be the properties of the oligodendroglial cells (in contrast to those of the Schwann cells of peripheral nerves) that account for the difference in regenerative capacity: no Bungner's bands are formed. Some experimental work in animals indicates that the mechanical barrier of a scar is not the key deterrent to regeneration; rather, the key is the inability of nerve fibers to grow out and seek their original connections. Recent experiments observed through the electron microscope have shown that regrowing fibers form new, inappropriate synapses.

Axonal regrowth in the central nervous system is more successful when vascular damage and scarring are minimal or absent, but even in such situations, the regrowth of axons is not followed by successful reconnection with target neurons. When an axon undergoes demyelination without being severed itself, the myelin may reform—as can happen during the remission phases of multiple sclerosis.

C. Collateral Sprouting: This phenomenon has been demonstrated in the central nervous system as well as in the peripheral nervous system (see Fig 21–9). It occurs when an innervated structure has been partially denervated. The remaining axons then form new collaterals that reinnervate the denervated part of the end-organ. This kind of regeneration demonstrates that there is considerable plasticity in the nervous system and that one axon can take over the synaptic sites formerly occupied by another.

NEURAL PLASTICITY

Neural plasticity is a property of the nervous system that elicits structural changes in response to experience and adaptation to changing conditions and repeated stimuli. Plasticity is clearly evident in developing organisms. The final definitive pattern of neural connections in the adult, for example, does not form all at once. Instead, in many parts of the central and peripheral nervous system, connections are formed more abundantly and more dif-

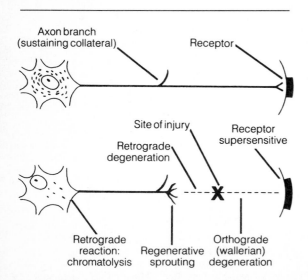

Figure 21–9. Summary of changes occurring in a neuron and the structure it innervates when its axon is crushed or cut at the point marked *X*. (Modified from D. Ries. Reproduced, with permission, from Ganong WF: *Review of Medical Physiology,* 14th ed. Appleton & Lange, 1989.)

fusely at first than is ultimately required. During development, these connections somehow rearrange and refine themselves, and the amount of motor innervation matches the amount of muscle to be innervated.

The projection from the lateral geniculate nucleus to the visual cortex (see Chapter 14) is refined and made more precise during development; the ocular dominance columns in layer IV of the calcarine cortex are formed by progressive segregation of the afferents from both eyes. There is a critical period in this segregation process, as shown experimentally: If one eye is forced to remain closed during the period of ocular dominance formation (but not before or after), the precise pattern of the dominance columns is disrupted and remains unrecognizable for life.

Neural plasticity is evident in the ongoing fine-tuning and adjustment of our reflexes and perception. For example, a new pair of prescription eyeglasses may make the wearer dizzy at first; after the new glasses are worn for a while, however, the dizziness disappears—and putting on the old eyeglasses will cause dizziness. This particular example of plasticity is well illustrated in a neurophysiologic experiment showing that it is possible for a person to adapt to prismatic spectacles that displace the image laterally on the retina. It is not yet clear, however, how the wearer can compensate completely, within hours, for the initially distorted sense of localization caused by the prism.

Neural plasticity is also evident in some examples of neural regeneration in animals. Cells in the septal complex receive afferent fibers from 2 distinct sources: the fibers of hippocampal origin that reach the septal nuclei via the fornix, and the axons that arise in the hypothalamus and travel to the septal nuclei in the medial forebrain bundle. The hippocampal fibers terminate almost exclusively on the dendrites of septal cells. The hypothalamic axons, on the other hand, make axosomatic as well as axodendritic synapses with septal neurons. If one of these pathways to the septum is cut and allowed to degenerate, analysis (with an electron microscope) of the remaining pathway indicates enlargement of its terminal distribution to include the postsynaptic sites previously occupied by the now-degenerate pathway. Quantitative studies indicate that the rate of new synapse formation by one pathway is closely linked to the rate of degeneration in the other.

Demonstration of anatomic plasticity in the brain have so far been limited to rather artificial experimental situations; however, it is likely that similar organizational modifications and the tendency to form connections underlie such natural phenomena as learning and memory.

CASE 29

A 67-year-old single woman who lived alone had been reasonably well until some 3 years previously, when her friends noted changes in her behavior and mental ability: She began to be unable to carry out simple tasks (writing, telephoning, cooking), and she was depressed and sometimes confused. The patient complained of forgetfulness and of inability to find the right words. Her worried friends urged her to see a physician and brought her to the hospital.

Physical examination showed a thin, listless woman with a dry, thin skin with pigment-deficient areas. She also showed a yellow arc in the cornea and had hardened arteries.

Neurologic examination demonstrated marked confusion and disorientation with regard to person and place, memory defects (especially for recent events), nominal aphasia, and a tendency toward perseveration. Generalized muscular weakness and atrophy were present, and there was apraxia for washing and dressing.

A provisional diagnosis was made, and the patient was referred to a nursing home. Three years later she developed severe bronchopneumonia, and upon readmission to the hospital, seemed totally forgetful and apathetic.

Which neuroradiologic procedure would aid in the diagnosis? What is the differential diagnosis? What is the most likely diagnosis?

Cases are discussed further in Chapter 24. Questions and answers pertaining to Section IV (Chapters 12 through 21) can be found in Appendix D.

REFERENCES

Algeri S, Gershon S, Grimm VE, Toffano G: Aging of the brain. In: *Aging,* Vol 22, Samuel D (editor). Raven, 1983.

Bach-y-Rita P (editor): *Recovery of Function. Theoretical Considerations for Brain Injury Rehabilitation.* Huber, 1980.

Bennett R (editor): *Aging, Isolation and Resocialization.* Van Nostrand Reinhold, 1980.

Berry M: Regeneration in the central nervous system. In: *Recent Advances in Neuropathology.* Smith WT, Cavanagh JB (editors). Churchill-Livingstone, 1979.

Cotman C: *Neuronal Plasticity.* Raven, 1978.

Kierman JA: Hypotheses concerned with axonal regeneration in the mammalian nervous system. *Biol Rev* 1979;**54**:155.

Lund RD: *Development and Plasticity of the Brain.* Oxford Univ Press, 1978.

Robbins AS et al: *Geriatric Medicine: An Education Resource Guide.* Ballinger Publishing, 1981.

Rosenblum ML, Levy RM, Bredesen DE: *AIDS and the Nervous System.* Raven, 1988.

Terry RD: Alzheimer's disease. In: *Textbook of Neuropathology,* 2nd ed. Davis DL, Robertson DM (editors). Williams & Wilkins, 1990.

Van Horn G: Dementia. *Am J Med* 1987;**83**:101.

Section V.
Diagnostic Aids

Imaging of the Brain

22

Scientists have tried for many decades to obtain an image of the skull and brain. The first successful effort was in 1895, when Wilhelm C. Roentgen produced an image (a roentgenogram, or x-ray film) of the skull. In 1927, Egas Moniz injected contrast material into the cerebral arteries of a patient before making a roentgenogram; this was the first cerebral arteriogram. It is only with the modern computer-aided techniques developed by G.N. Hounsfield and A.M. Cormack in the 1960s (and first used in the United States in 1973) that success was achieved in obtaining an image of the brain itself.

Images of the skull, the brain and its vessels, and spaces in the brain containing cerebrospinal fluid can aid immeasurably in the localization of lesions, especially after a complete history taking and physical examination. In emergency cases, images of unconscious patients may be the only diagnostic information available. Traditionally, the views shown in most images have been lateral, anteroposterior (frontal), or oblique. Since the introduction of computed tomography, magnetic resonance imaging, and other methods that display sections of the head, the sagittal, coronal (frontal) and horizontal (axial) planes are commonly used. These are shown in Fig 22–1.

ROENTGENOGRAPHY

Although now limited in its general use, skull radiography with x-rays remains an excellent means of imaging calcium and its distribution in and around the brain when more precise methods are unavailable. Plain films of the skull, taken in various planes, can be used to define the extent of a skull fracture and a possible depression or determine the presence of calcified brain lesions, foreign bodies, or tumors involving the skull. They can also detect asymmetry of brain volume, found by locating the calcified pineal body in an anteroposterior view; chronically increased intracranial

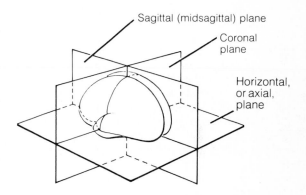

Figure 22-1. Planes used in modern imaging procedures.

pressure, accompanied by thinning of the dorsum sellae; and abnormalities in the size and shape of sella turcica, which suggest large pituitary tumors. Skull films are sometimes used to screen for metal objects before beginning magnetic resonance imaging of the head.

When modern imaging methods are not available, **pneumoencephalography** has been useful in studying patients with epilepsy, cerebral atrophies, congenital brain lesions, and posttraumatic cerebral disorders. The technique involves replacing measured quantities of cerebrospinal fluid with air or some other suitable gas introduced by means of lumbar puncture (or, more rarely, by cisternal or C1–C2 puncture). Most air is absorbed in 48 hours.

Headache, nausea, and vomiting are common complications that may occur after pneumoencephalography; they usually respond well to symptomatic therapy and resting flat in bed. Disturbances of intracranial pressure and beginning tentorial or medullary pressure cones may lead to grave consequences, and immediate ventricular tap and prompt decompression may be necessary. Note that pneumoencephalography is hazardous in the presence of elevated cerebrospinal fluid pressure.

ANGIOGRAPHY

Cerebral Angiography

Angiography (arteriography) of the head and neck is a neurodiagnostic procedure used especially in cases in which a vessel abnormality such as occlusion, malformation, or aneurysm is suspected (Figs 22–2 to 22–12; see also Chapter 11). Angiography can also be used to determine whether the position of the vessels in relation to intracranial structures is normal or pathologically changed. Arteriovenous fistulas or vascular malformations can be treated by interventional angiography using balloons, a quickly coagulating solution known as glue, or small, inert pellets that act like emboli.

A standard set of angiograms, usually in at least 2 projections, or views (anteroposterior, oblique, or lateral), consists of a series of x-ray films showing contrast material introduced into a major artery (eg, via a catheter in the femoral) under fluoroscopic guidance. Arterial-phase films are followed by capillary and venous-phase films (see Figs 22–6 to 22–10). Right and left internal carotid and vertebral angiograms may be complemented by other films, eg, by an external carotid series in cases of meningioma or arteriovenous malformation. The films are often presented as subtracted, ie, as reversal prints superimposed on a plain film of the skull.

Digital Subtraction Angiography

Since the introduction of computed tomography of the head, angiography has been used less frequently as a diagnostic tool. A modern form of angiography, digital subtraction angiography (extraneous tissue in the image is erased, or subtracted), makes use of selective venous or arterial injections of contrast material (Fig 22–12). The digitally enhanced x-ray images are slightly less detailed than traditional angiograms. This method is

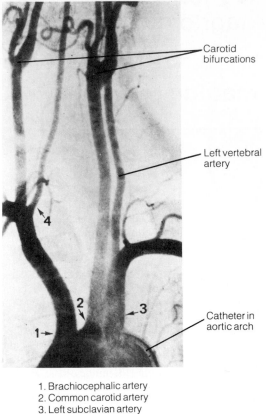

1. Brachiocephalic artery
2. Common carotid artery
3. Left subclavian artery
4. Right vertebral artery

Figure 22–2. Angiogram of the aortic arch and stem vessels. Normal image. *1:* Brachiocephalic artery; *2:* common carotid artery; *3:* left subclavian artery; *4:* right vertebral artery. (Reproduced, with permission, from Peele TL: *The Neuroanatomical Basis for Clinical Neurology.* Blakiston, 1954.)

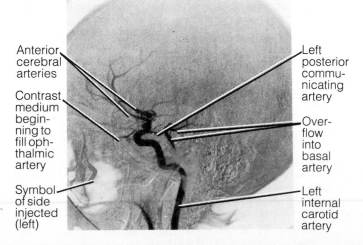

Figure 22–3. Left internal carotid angiogram, early arterial phase, lateral view. Normal image (compare with Fig 22–4).

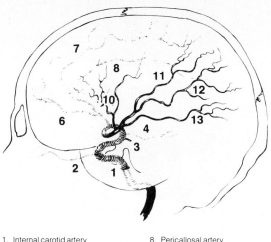

1. Internal carotid artery
2. Ophthalmic artery
3. Posterior communicating artery
4. Anterior choroidal artery
5. Anterior cerebral artery
6. Frontopolar artery
7. Callosomarginal artery
8. Pericallosal artery
9. Middle cerebral artery
10. Ascending frontoparietal artery
11. Posterior parietal artery
12. Angular artery
13. Posterior temporal artery
14. Lenticulostriate arteries

Figure 22-4. Schematic drawing of a normal angiogram of the internal carotid artery, arterial phase, lateral projection. (Redrawn and reproduced, with permission, from List, Burge, Hodges: Intracranial angiography. *Radiology* 1945;**45**:1.)

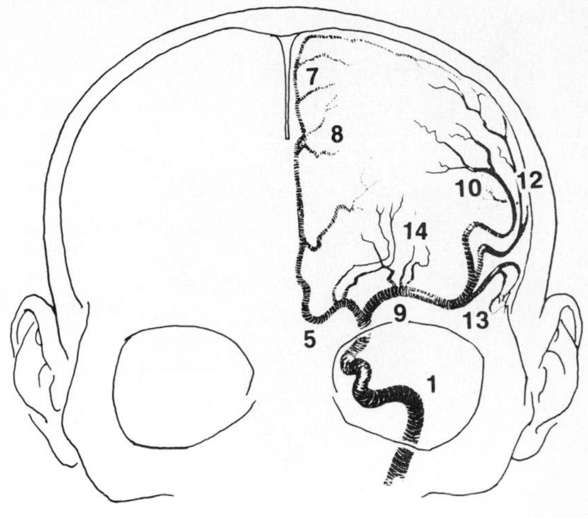

Figure 22-6. Schematic drawing of a normal angiogram of the internal carotid artery, arterial phase, frontal projection. (For significance of numbers see Fig 22-4. Redrawn and reproduced, with permission, from List, Burge, Hodges: Intracranial angiography. *Radiology* 1945;**45**:1.)

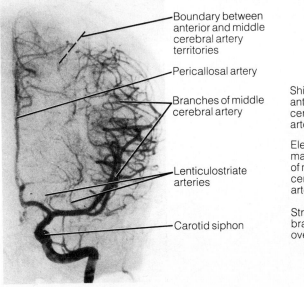

Boundary between anterior and middle cerebral artery territories

Pericallosal artery

Branches of middle cerebral artery

Lenticulostriate arteries

Carotid siphon

Figure 22-5. Left internal carotid angiogram, arterial phase, lateral view. Normal image (compare with Fig 22-6).

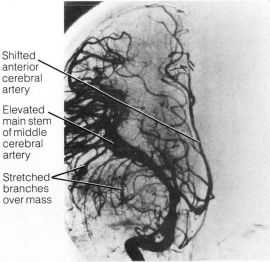

Shifted anterior cerebral artery

Elevated main stem of middle cerebral artery

Stretched branches over mass

Figure 22-7. Right internal carotid angiogram, arterial phase, anteroposterior view. Abnormal image.

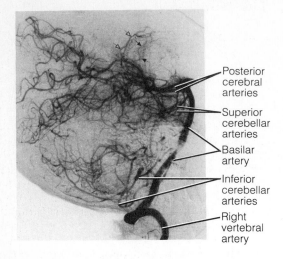

Figure 22-8. Vertebral angiogram, arterial phase, right lateral view. Normal image. Arrows indicate posterior choroidal arteries.

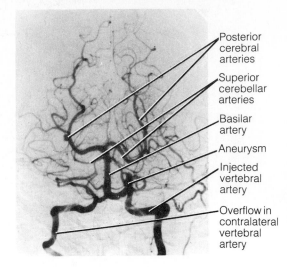

Figure 22-9. Vertebral angiogram, arterial phase, anteroposterior view, with head flexed (Towne position). An aneurysm is present, but the pattern of the vessels is normal.

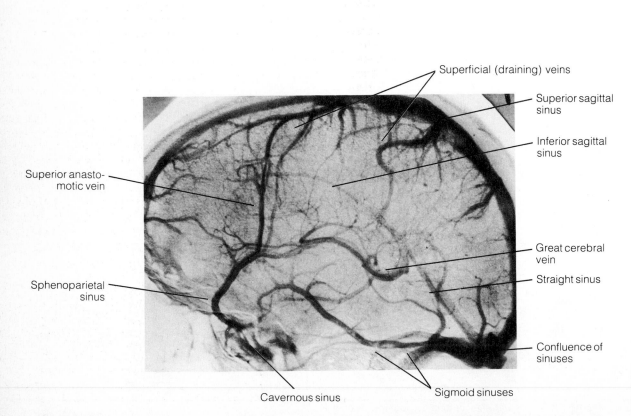

Figure 22-10. Left internal carotid angiogram, venous phase, lateral view. Normal image. (Compare with Figs 22-11 and 11-9.)

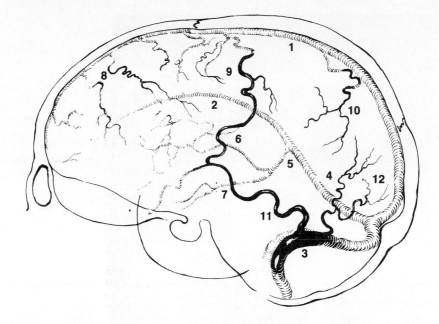

1. Superior sagittal sinus
2. Inferior sagittal sinus
3. Transverse sinus
4. Straight sinus
5. Great cerebral vein of Galen
6. Internal cerebral vein
7. Basal vein of Rosenthal
8. Frontal ascending vein
9. Rolandic vein of Trolard
10. Parietal ascending vein
11. Communicating temporal vein of Labbé
12. Descending temporo-occipital vein

Figure 22–11. Schematic drawing of normal venogram in lateral projection, obtained by carotid injection. Superficial veins are shaded more darkly than the sinuses and deep veins. (Redrawn and reproduced, with permission, from List, Burge, Hodges: Intracranial angiography. *Radiology* 1945;**45**:1.)

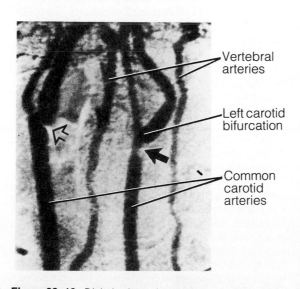

Vertebral arteries

Left carotid bifurcation

Common carotid arteries

Figure 22–12. Digital subtraction angiogram of the neck vessels, oblique anterior view. Open arrow shows small sclerotic plaque; closed arrow shows large plaque.

frequently used to inspect large vessels in the neck or at the base of the skull.

ULTRASONOGRAPHY

In contrast to x-ray equipment, ultrasonic imaging equipment produces no tissue ionization. In addition to being harmless and fast, ultrasonography is relatively simple and requires no elaborate machinery; newer systems use computers to clean up the pictures obtained.

In ultrasonography, information about structures is obtained by analyzing the time and intensity of echoes from mechanical waves directed into the tissues. The clinical use of ultrasonography for depicting brain structures is severely limited by the dense echoes of the surrounding skull. This method may be used, however, in a young child (up to 18 months) who has open fontanelles (Figs 22–13 and 22–14), in a patient who has had a craniotomy in preparation for brain surgery, and

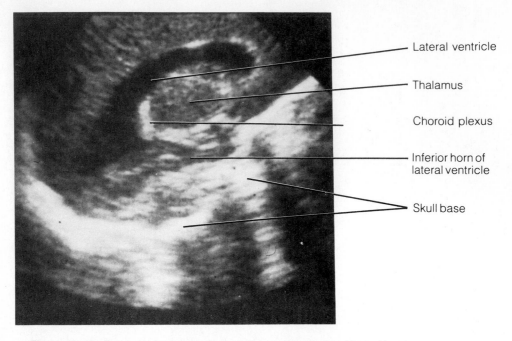

Figure 22–13. Cerebral ultrasonogram of a newborn, lateral view. Normal image.

in the rare patient whose skull flap has not healed. Ultrasonography is also used for evaluation of the carotid bifurcation, where changes caused by plaque formation and stenosis are most commonly found.

COMPUTED TOMOGRAPHY

Computed tomography (also called computed axial tomography) affords the possibility of in-

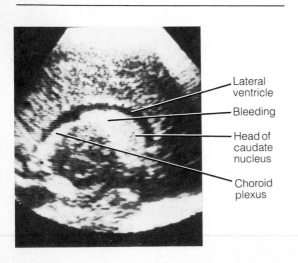

Figure 22–14. Cerebral ultrasonogram of a newborn, lateral view. Abnormal image.

specting cross sections of the skull, brain, ventricles, cisterns, large vessels, falx, and tentorium. Since its development in the 1960s, the CT scan has become a primary tool for demonstrating the presence of abnormal calcifications, brain edema, hydrocephalus, many types of tumors and cysts, hemorrhages, large aneurysms, vascular malformations, and other disorders.

CT scanning is noninvasive, fast, and safe. Although it has a high degree of sensitivity, its specificity is relatively limited. Therefore, in the presence of an abnormality, correlation with the clinical history and physical examination is an absolute requirement. Often, angiography or another neurodiagnostic procedure is required later to define and characterize a lesion better. In the case of a subarachnoid hemorrhage, for example, while a CT scan may quickly localize the areas containing blood, angiography is often required to determine whether the cause was an aneurysm or an arteriovenous malformation.

The CT scanning apparatus rotates a narrow x-ray beam around the head, and the amount of x-ray transmitted is precisely measured. Using an algorithm that consists of a series of simultaneous equations, the quantity of x-ray absorbed in small volumes (voxels [volume elements, or units]) of brain—measuring approximately 0.5 mm square by 1.5 or more millimeters in length—is computed. The exact amount of x-ray absorbed in any slice of the head can be thus determined and depicted in various ways as pixels (picture elements) in a ma-

Table 22-1. CT coefficients of absorption (density).

Substance	Coefficients (in Hounsfield units)
Air	−1000
Fat	−80
Water	0
Cerebrospinal fluid	0 to 16
Edematous tissue	8 to 20
White matter	24 to 36
Gray matter	30 to 50
Flowing blood	25 to 40
Clotted blood	40 to 90
Glioma (various types)	10, 60, and 400
Calcified tissue and bone	80 to 1000

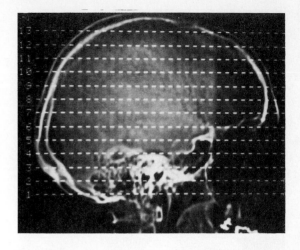

Figure 22-16. Lateral "scout view" used in CT procedure. Superimposed lines represent the levels of the images (sections). Line 1 is at the level of the foramen magnum; line 4 is at the level of the infraorbitomeatal plane.

trix. In most cases, absorption is proportional to the density of the tissue. A digital-analog converter translates the numeric value of each pixel to a gray scale. Black and white pictures of head slices are then displayed, with black representing low-density structures and white representing high-density structures (Table 22–1). The thickness of the slices can be varied, from 1.5 mm to 1 cm. The range of numerical absorption values that the gray scale represents can also be varied; although a setting at which brain tissue is distinguished best is commonly used, in some cases bone, fat, or air needs to be defined in great detail.

A series of 10–20 scans, each reconstructing a slice of brain, is usually required for a complete study. The plane of these sections is the orbitomeatal plane, which is parallel to both Reid's base plane and the intercommissural line used in stereotactic neurosurgery (Fig 22–15). Usually, a "scout view" similar to a lateral skull roentgeno-

gram is taken with a CT scanner to align the planes of section (Fig 22–16). With the modern technology now available, each scan takes only a few seconds. Examples of normal and abnormal CT scans are shown in Figs 22–17 and 22–18 (see the figures in Chapter 5 also).

CT scanning of the posterior fossa is often unsatisfactory because of the many artifacts caused by dense bone. Injecting contrast material into the cisterns improves the image in some cases. This

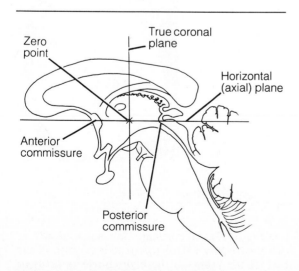

Figure 22-15. Schematic image of the zero horizontal and coronal planes. The line between anterior and posterior commissures parallels Reid's base line.

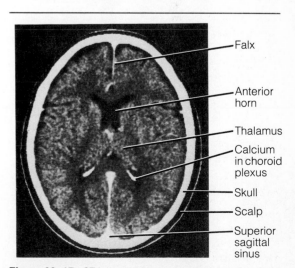

Figure 22-17. CT image, with contrast enhancement, of a horizontal section at the level of the thalamus. Normal image. Compare with Fig 12–4.

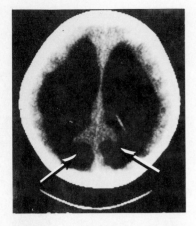

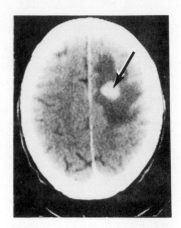

Top left: Hydrocephalus. Dilated ventricles in a 7-year-old boy who had undergone a shunting operation at age 1 year.

Top right: Brain tumor. Cerebral metastasis from carcinoma of lung in a 65-year-old man.

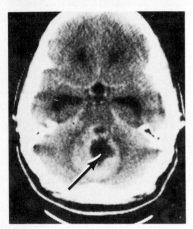

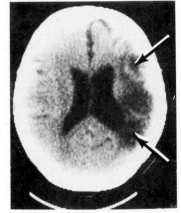

Center left: Brain tumor. Cerebellar medulloblastoma in a 16-year-old male.

Center right: Cerebral hemiatrophy History of subarachnoid hemorrhage 5 years previously in a 48-year-old woman.

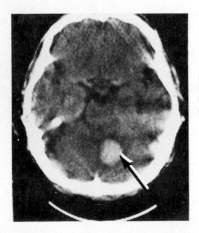

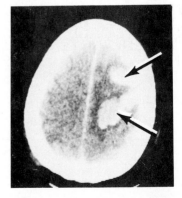

Lower left: Cerebellar hemorrhage. Eighty-one-year-old hypertensive man with acute onset of coma and quadriparesis.

Lower right: Traumatic intracerebral hemorrhage. History of a fall by an intoxicated 78-year-old man followed by confusion and hemiplegia.

Figure 22–18. Representative examples of CT images. (Courtesy of GP Ballweg.)

procedure of contrast enhancement has essentially replaced the pneumoencephalographic studies in which ventricles, cisterns, or both were filled with air prior to taking skull films. Images reformed by a computer from a series of thin sections allow visualization in any desired plane, eg, midsagittal (see Fig 5–17), or coronal. Coronal sections are often extremely useful for structures lying at the base of the brain, in the high convexity area, or close to the incisura. Detailed examination of orbital contents requires planes at right angles to the orbital axis.

Tissue density can change pathologically (see Figs 11–12 and 11–17). Areas of hyperemia or freshly clotted hemorrhage appear more dense; edematous tissue appears less dense. In such cases, the diagnostic sensitivity of CT scanning is increased by intravenous injection of iodinated contrast agents. When there are brain abnormalities, these agents will often pass into the abnormal tissue through defects in the blood-brain barrier. Iodine in the contrast agent absorbs a large quantity of the x-rays, making the lesion highly visible (see Fig 11–20A).

MAGNETIC RESONANCE IMAGING

Nuclear magnetic resonance (NMR) has been used in physical chemistry since the 1950s. In medicine, the magnetic resonance imaging method (MRI, or MR imaging) depicts certain nucleides (protons and neutrons) in a strong external magnetic field shielded from extraneous radio signals; no radiation is used.

The spatial distribution of elements with an odd number of protons (such as hydrogen) within slices of the body or brain can be determined by their reaction to an external radio frequency signal; gradient coils are used to localize the signal (Fig 22–19). The signal of every voxel is shown as a pixel in a matrix, similar to the CT technique. The resolution of the images is comparable to that of current CT scans, and with MR imaging, an image of any plane can be obtained directly: no reformation is required. Because bone is poorly imaged, axial spine scans are not often performed; however, sagittal images of the spine and spinal cord are informative.

With MR imaging, the flow of blood within medium and larger arteries and veins can be evaluated directly, with no need for intravenous injection of a contrast agent. This makes MR imaging particularly useful in coronary, renal, and cerebral vascular studies. Fast-flowing blood produces no signal; slow-flowing or turbulent blood produces a high-intensity signal (see Figs 11–4 and 11–9). Blurred images caused by heart contractions and pulse beat can be prevented by making MR images only at certain times of the heart cycle and using a gating technique with simultaneous electrocardiographic recording.

The sequence of radio frequency excitation followed by recording of tissue disturbance (echo signals) can be varied, in both duration of excitation and sampling time. The images obtained with short time sequences differ from those obtained with longer time sequences (Fig 22–20). Normal MR images are shown in Figs 22–20 and 22–21; other MR images, both normal and abnormal, are found in

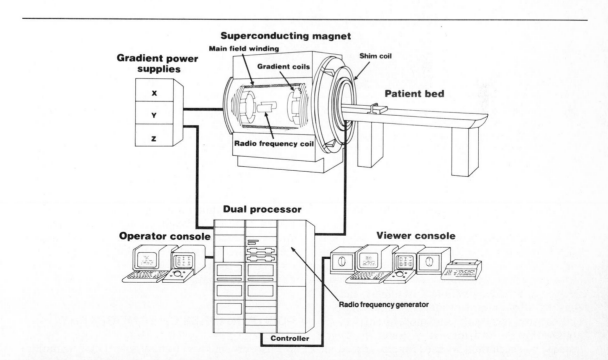

Figure 22–19. Schematic representation of MR imager and its components. (Courtesy L. Kaufmann. Reproduced, with permission, from de Groot J: *Correlative Neuroanatomy of Computed Tomography and Magnetic Resonance Imaging.* Lea & Febiger, 1984.)

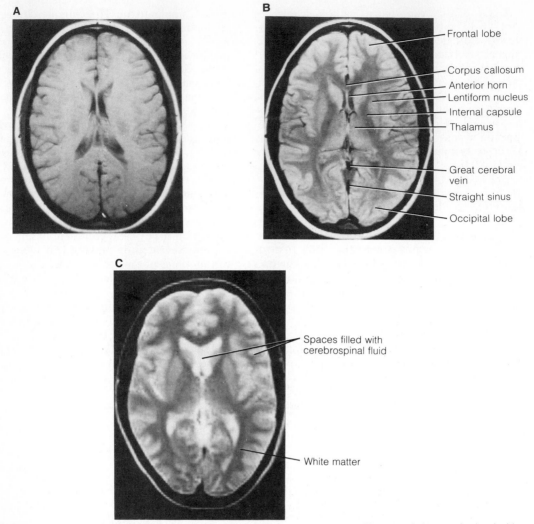

Figure 22–20. MR images of horizontal sections through the lateral ventricles. Normal images. *A:* Image obtained with a short time sequence; the gray-white boundaries are poorly defined, and the spaces filled with cerebrospinal fluid are dark. *B:* Image obtained with an intermediate time sequence. *C:* Image obtained with a long time sequence; the white matter is clearly differentiated from gray matter, and the spaces filled with cerebrospinal fluid are white.

Chapters 5 and 11 and elsewhere throughout this text.

The MR imaging process is relatively slow; it is safe for patients who have no ferromagnetic implants. The increasing sophistication of MR imaging technique (eg, with the use of contrast agents) is expected to broaden its clinical usefulness, and it is likely that further improvements will make the procedure faster, less costly, and more often used. Although only the distribution of water (hydrogen protons) has been thus far used for diagnostic purposes in patients, experimental work with phosphorus, nitrogen, and sodium is under way. In some major medical centers, MRI is now a primary method of examination, especially in cases of suspected tumors, demyelination, and infarcts. As with CT scanning, successful use of MR imaging for accurate diagnosis of an abnormality requires correlating the results with the clinical history and physical examination.

POSITRON EMISSION TOMOGRAPHY

Positron emission tomography (PET scanning) has become a major clinical research tool for the imaging of cerebral blood flow, brain metabolism, and other chemical processes (Fig 22–22). Radio-

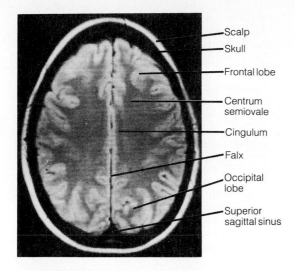

Figure 22-21. MR image of a horizontal high section through the head. Normal image.

Scalp
Skull
Frontal lobe
Centrum semiovale
Cingulum
Falx
Occipital lobe
Superior sagittal sinus

isotopes are inhaled or injected, and emissions are measured with a gamma-ray-detector system. One disadvantage is the lack of detailed resolution; another is that most positron-emitting nucleides decay so rapidly that their transportation from the cyclotron (the site of production) becomes a problem. Some isotopes, such as fluorine 18 (^{18}F) and gamma-aminobutyric acid, have a sufficiently long half-life that they can be shipped by air. A few,

such as ruthenium derivatives, can be made at the site of examination.

SINGLE PHOTON EMISSION COMPUTED TOMOGRAPHY

Recent advances in nuclear medicine instrumentation and radiopharmaceuticals have opened renewed interest in single photon emission computed tomography (SPECT) of the brain. The increasing use of investigative agents in conjunction with PET imaging has stimulated the development of diagnostic radiopharmaceuticals for SPECT; these are routinely available to clinical nuclear medicine laboratories. The first of these was 1-123-iodoamphetamine (1-123-IMP). A more recent Tc-99m-based compound—Tc-99m-HMPAO (Tc-99m-hexamethylpropyleneamineoxime)—is gaining even wider use. Both chemicals are sufficiently lipophilic to diffuse readily across the blood-brain-barrier and into nerve cells along the blood flow. They remain in brain tissue long enough to permit assessment of the relative distribution of brain blood by SPECT in 1.0–1.5 cm coronal, sagittal, and horizontal tomographic slices. SPECT studies

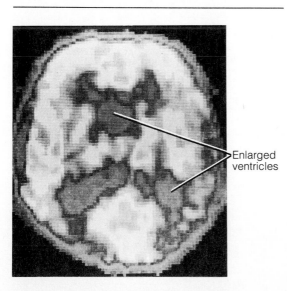

Enlarged ventricles

Figure 22-22. PET scan of a horizontal section at the level of the lateral ventricles. The various shades of gray indicate different levels of glucose utilization.

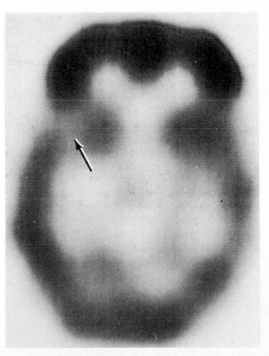

Figure 22-23. SPECT image of a horizontal section through the head at the level of the temporal lobe. An infarct (arrow) is shown as an interruption of the cortical ribbon. (Courtesy of D Price.)

include identifying epileptogenic foci, differentiating Alzheimer's disease from other types of dementia such as multi-infarct (Fig 22–23), determining brain tissue damage in patients with a recent stroke, and identifying and locating brain lesions in patients with repeated small strokes or TIAs.

REFERENCES

Brant-Zawadski M, Norman D (editors): *Magnetic Resonance Imaging of the Central Nervous System.* Raven, 1987.

deGroot J: *Correlative Neuroanatomy of Computed Tomography and Magnetic Resonance Imaging.* Lea and Febiger, 1984.

Ell PJ et al: Functional imaging of the brain. Pages 211–229 in *Seminars in Nuclear Medicine 17,* 1987.

Margulis AR (editor): *Clinical Magnetic Resonance Imaging.* Univ of Calif Press, 1983.

Mills CM, DeGroot J, Posin JP: *Magnetic Resonance Imaging: Atlas of the Head, Neck, and Spine.* Lea & Febiger, 1988.

Newton TH, Potts DG (editors): *Advanced Imaging Techniques.* Clavadel Press, 1983.

Oldendorf WH: *The Quest for an Image of the Brain.* Raven, 1980.

Osborn AG: *Introduction to Cerebral Angiography.* Harper & Row, 1980.

Ramsey RG: *Neuroradiology,* 2nd ed. Saunders, 1987.

Electrodiagnostic Tests 23

ELECTROENCEPHALOGRAPHY

Electroencephalography is the study of the electrical activity of the brain. The potentials of the brain are recorded in an electroencephalogram (EEG); they appear in wave form, with the dominant frequency ranging from 1 to 100 cycles per second (cps or hertz [Hz]) and an amplitude from 5 to several hundred microvolts. Because the average amplitude of electrical activity in the brain is only about 1% of that obtained from the heart in an electrocardiogram (ECG), sensitive (but stable) amplification is necessary to produce an undistorted record of brain activity.

Clinical Applications

Electroencephalography can provide useful information in patients with organic brain disease, especially when epileptiform attacks occur or are suspected. Because the localizing value of an EEG is limited to gross regions of the brain, electroencephalography is seldom performed when other tests, such as CT scanning or MR imaging, are available. When other tests are not available, an EEG can furnish considerable help in determining the area of cerebral damage. Electroencephalography has its limitations, however, and normal-appearing records can be obtained in spite of clinical evidence of severe organic brain disease. The use of **depth electrography**—the localization of a focus by recording from within the brain—may be advisable in certain cases.

Physiology

The activity recorded in the EEG originates mainly from the superficial layers of the cerebral cortex (see Chapter 9). Current is believed to flow between cortical cell dendrites and cell bodies (the dendrites are similarly oriented, densely packed units of the cerebral cortex). As excitatory and inhibitory endings on the cell dendrites become active, current flows into and out of these areas from the rest of the dendritic process and the cell body. The relationship between the dendrite and cell body is that of a constantly shifting dipole. When the sum of the dendritic activity is negative relative to that of the cell body, the cell as a whole becomes hypopolarized and hyperexcitable (see Chapter 3).

Technique

To detect changes in activity that may be of diagnostic importance, simultaneous recordings are obtained (when possible) from multiple analogous areas on both the left and right sides of the brain. Electrodes covered with electrolyte paste or jelly are ordinarily attached to the scalp over the frontal, parietal, occipital, and temporal areas; they are also attached to the ears (Fig 23–1).

With the subject recumbent or seated in a grounded, wire-shielded cage, a recording at least 20 minutes long is obtained; the eyes should be closed. Hyperventilation, during which the patient takes 40–50 deep breaths per minute for 3 minutes, is routinely employed during this time, since it frequently accentuates abnormal findings (epileptiform attacks) and may disclose latent abnormalities. Rhythmic light-flash stimulation (1–30 Hz) is carried out for 2 or more minutes as part of the recording routine.

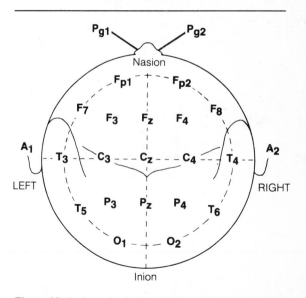

Figure 23-1. A single-plane projection of the head, showing all standard positions of electrode placement and the locations of the central sulcus (fissure of Rolando) and the lateral cerebral fissure (fissure of Sylvius). The outer circle is drawn at the level of the nasion and inion; the inner circle represents the temporal line of electrodes. This diagram provides a useful guide for electrode placement in routine recording. A, ear; C, central; C_z, central at zero, or midline; F, frontal; F_p, frontal pole; F_z, frontal at zero, or midline; O, occipital; P, parietal; P_g, nasopharyngeal; P_z, parietal at zero, or midline; T, temporal. (Courtesy of Grass Medical Instruments Co, Quincy, Mass.)

R = right   F = frontal   P = parietal   AT = anterior temporal   T = temporal
L = left   O = occipital   Pc = precentral   Pf = posterior frontal   E = ear

Calibration: 50 μV (vertical) and 1 s (horizontal).

LF–LAT

RF–RAT

LAT–LT

RAT–RT

LT–LO

RT–RO

LT–LPc

RT–RPc

Normal Adult

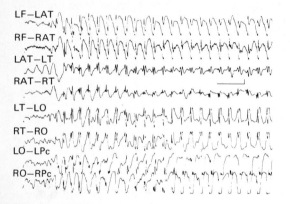

Petit Mal Epilepsy. Record of a 6-year-old boy during one of his "blank spells," in which he was transiently unaware of surroundings and blinked his eyelids during the recording.

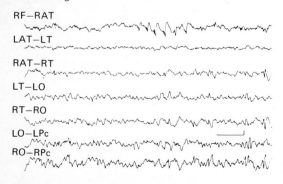

Epilepsy. EEG of a 6-year-old child who had suffered 3 major convulsions, 2 of which appeared to start in the left extremities.

LF–LAT

RF–RAT

LAT–LT

RAT–RT

LT–LO

RT–RO

LO–LPc

RO–RPc

Focal Motor Epilepsy. EEG of a 47-year-old man with focal motor seizures beginning in the left hand. He stated his seizures began 20 years previously, approximately one year after a severe head injury.

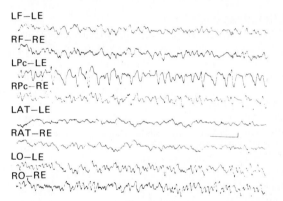

Epilepsy. Record of a 6-year-old girl with frequent nocturnal major convulsions as well as daily seizures in which she became stiff, started, and shook slightly.

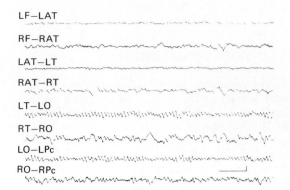

Psychomotor Epilepsy. Record of a 20-year-old man who had had monthly episodes for the previous 6 years characterized by motor automatisms and frequently followed by generalized tonic-clonic convulsions.

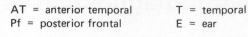

Figure 23–2. Representative EEGs.

Types of Wave Forms

The **synchronized** activity of many of the dendritic units forms the wave pattern associated with alpha rhythm when the patient is awake, but at rest, with the eyes closed. **Desynchronization**—replacement of a rhythmic pattern with irregular low-voltage activity—is produced by stimulation of specific projection systems from the spinal cord and brain stem up to the level of the thalamus.

When the eyes are opened, the alpha rhythm is replaced by an **alpha block,** a fast, irregular, low-voltage activity. Other forms of sensory stimulation or mental concentration can also break up the alpha pattern. Desynchronization is sometimes termed the **arousal,** or **alerting, response,** since this breakup of the alpha pattern may be produced by sensory stimulation and is correlated with an aroused or alert state.

Epilepsy is an expression of various groups of cortical diseases; all types are characterized by transient disturbances of brain function manifested by intermittent high-voltage waves (**spike** and **wave complexes**) in the EEG (Fig 23–2).

VISUALLY EVOKED RESPONSE

Flashing a light into a subject's eyes causes a massive synchronous depolarization of cells in the cortex: the visually evoked potentials (VEP) or response (VER). These are recorded over the left and right occipital poles (Fig 23–3). This reaction is clinically useful in detecting slight abnormalities in the visual pathways; eg, optic nerve lesions can be recognized by stimulating each eye separately since the response to stimulation of an affected optic nerve is absent or impaired. With visual pathway lesions behind the optic chiasm, a difference in response of the 2 cerebral hemispheres may occur. There might be a normal response in the occipital cerebral cortex of the normal cerebral hemisphere and an absent or abnormal response in the affected cerebral hemisphere (see also Chapter 14).

BRAIN STEM AUDITORY EVOKED RESPONSE

A standard brain stem auditory evoked response (BAER) consists of 7 potentials that are recorded from the human scalp within 10 ms of a single appropriate acoustic stimulus. Abnormalities in the response may provide evidence suggesting clinical neurologic disorders involving the brain stem. The test has some clinical value and is useful in demonstrating structural brain stem damage caused by various disorders (see also Chapter 15).

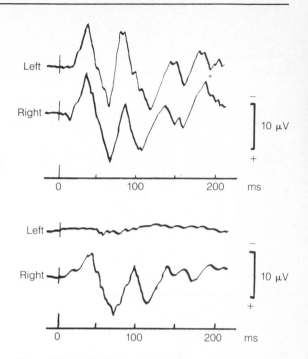

Figure 23-3. Visually evoked responses recorded from over the left and right occipital poles. *Top:* normal responses. *Bottom:* responses in a case of right homonymous hemianopia. No response is recorded over the left hemisphere. (Courtesy of M Feinsod. Reproduced, with permission, from Vaughan D, Asbury T, Tabbara KF: *General Ophthalmology,* 12th ed. Appleton & Lange, 1989.)

Technique

Short-latency brain stem auditory evoked potentials can be averaged and analyzed with the aid of computer techniques (Fig 23–4). In a normal human subject with scalp electrodes placed on the vertex, a click stimulus presented to the ear may evoke typical responses with 7 wave components that are believed to come from the region of the auditory nerve (wave I), dorsal cochlear nucleus (wave II), superior olive (wave III), lateral lemniscus (wave IV), and inferior colliculus (wave V). Wave VI may indicate activity of the rostral midbrain or caudal thalamus or thalamocortical projection, and wave VII originates in the auditory cortex. Peak-to-peak amplitudes and the latencies from the stimulus to each peak are all measured. At least 2 separate trials and averages of 2000–4000 responses are recorded for each ear.

ELECTROMYOGRAPHY

Electromyography is concerned with the study of the electrical activity arising from muscles at rest and those that are actively contracted.

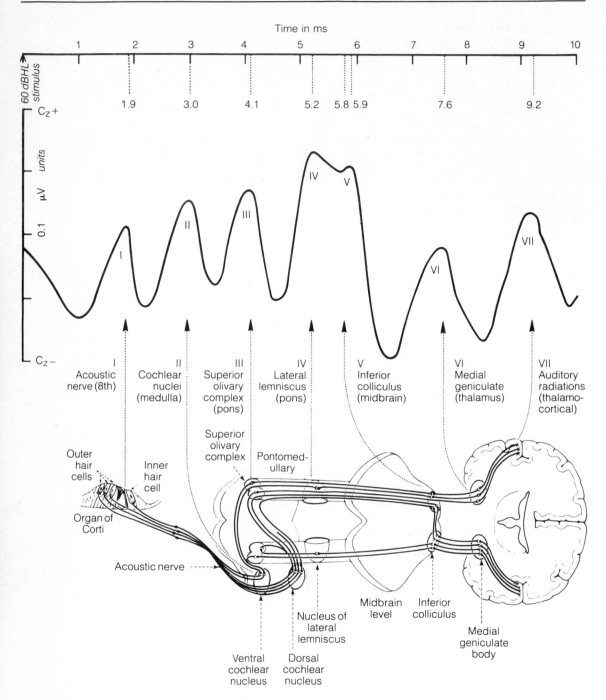

Figure 23-4. Far-field recording of brain stem auditory response latencies in humans showing proposed functional-anatomic correlations. Diagram shows normal latencies for vertex-positive brain stem auditory evoked potentials (waves I–IV) evoked by clicks of 60 dBHL (60 dB above normal hearing threshold) at a rate of 10/s. Lesions at different levels of the auditory pathway tend to produce response abnormalities beginning with the indicated components. Intermediate latency (5.8 ms) between latencies of waves IV and V is the mean peak latency of fused wave IV/V when present. C_z^+, vertex positivity, represented by an upward pen deflection, C_z^-, vertex negativity, represented by a downward pen deflection. (Reproduced, with permission, from Stockard JJ, Stockard JE, Sharbrough FW: Detection and localization of occult lesions with brain stem auditory responses. *Mayo Clin Proc* 1977;**52**:761.)

Clinical Applications

Electromyography is a particularly useful aid in diagnosing lower-motor-neuron disease or primary muscle disease and in detecting defects in transmission at the neuromuscular junction. Although it is helpful, the test does not give a specific clinical diagnosis; information from the electromyogram (EMG) must be integrated with results of other tests, muscle biopsy if necessary, clinical features, and so forth to arrive at a final diagnosis.

Physiology

Human striated muscle is composed functionally of motor units in which the axons of single motor cells in the anterior horn innervate many muscle fibers (hundreds of muscle fibers may be innervated by a single axon). All the fibers innervated by a single motor unit respond immediately to stimulation in an all-or-none pattern, and the interaction of many motor units can produce relatively smooth motor performance. Increased motor power results from the repeated activation of a given number of motor units or the single activation of a greater number of such units.

The action potential of a muscle consists of the sum of the action potentials of many motor units; in normal muscle fibers, it originates at the motor end-plates and is triggered by an incoming nerve impulse at the myoneural junction. Clinical studies indicate that normal muscle at rest shows no action potential. In simple movements, the contracting muscle gives rise to action potentials, while its antagonist relaxes and exhibits no potentials. During contraction, different portions of the same muscle may discharge at different rates, and parts may appear to be transiently inactive. In strong contractions, many motor units are active, producing numerous action potentials.

Technique

Stimulation is usually applied over the course of the nerve or at the motor point of the muscle being tested. Muscles should always be tested at the motor point, which is normally the most excitable point of a muscle in that it represents the greatest concentration of nerve endings. It is located on the skin over the muscle and corresponds approximately to the level at which the nerve enters the muscle belly.

A concentric (coaxial) needle, usually 24 gauge by 3–4 cm long, or a monopolar solid steel needle coated almost to the tip with insulating plastic or varnish is inserted at the motor point of a muscle and advanced by steps to several depths. Variations in electrical potential between the needle tip and a reference electrode (a metal plate) on the skin surface are amplified and displayed. The electrical activity can be displayed on a cathode-ray oscilloscope and played on a loudspeaker for simulta-

neous visual and auditory analysis. Observations are made in each area of the electrical activity evoked in the muscle by insertion and movement of the needle, the electrical activity of the resting muscle with the needle undisturbed, and the electrical activity of the motor units during voluntary contraction (Fig 23–5). Since various muscle fibers may respond differently, several insertions of the needle into different parts of a muscle may be necessary for adequate analysis.

Types of Activity

The term **fibrillation** is reserved for spontaneous independent contractions of individual muscle fibers that are so minute that they cannot be observed through the intact skin. Denervated muscle may still show electromyographic evidence of fibrillations 1–3 weeks after losing its nerve supply (see below). **Fasciculations,** or twitches, on the other hand, can be seen and palpated, and they can be heard with the aid of a stethoscope; they represent contractions of muscle fibers of a motor unit. Spontaneous fasciculations can vary because of the length and number of muscle fibers involved; they may result from disorders of the lower motor neuron. Benign fasciculations, such as those from exposure to cold or temporary ischemia (crossed legs), are unassociated with other clinical or electrical signs of denervation (see Fig 23–5).

In a complete nerve lesion, fibrillation potentials occur without motor unit potentials, while partial nerve lesions show both fibrillation and motor unit activity from voluntary muscle contraction. Diminution or cessation of fibrillation potentials and the appearance of small, disintegrated motor unit action potentials occur with nerve regeneration. Fibrillations in a paretic muscle are increased by warmth, activity, and neostigmine; they are decreased by cold or immobilization.

After complete section of a nerve, denervation fibrillation potentials are evident (after about 18 days) in all areas of the muscles supplied by a peripheral nerve. Some motor unit discharges persist in partial nerve injuries, despite the clinical appearance of complete paralysis. Mapping the areas of denervation fibrillation potentials aids in the diagnosis of single nerve root disorders and spinal nerve root compression.

The response to single or repeated nerve stimulation can be studied in pathologic states and under modifications produced by therapy. These studies help estimate the conduction velocities of motor nerves and evaluate the effectiveness of medication in modifying the reaction of muscles in such conditions as myasthenia gravis.

Normal Formula of Response

Two electrodes are needed to use galvanic current in electrical stimulation. The broad indifferent

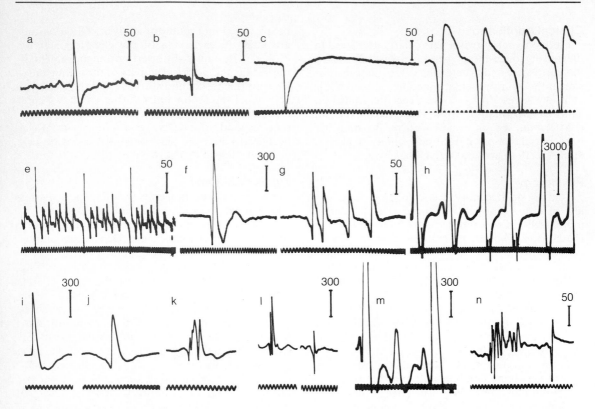

Figure 23–5. Action potentials in electromyography. *a:* Nerve potential from normal muscle; *b:* fibrillation potential and *c:* positive wave from denervated muscle; *d:* high-frequency discharge in myotonia; *e:* bizarre high-frequency discharge; *f:* fasciculation potential, single discharge; *g:* fasciculation potential, repetitive or grouped discharge; *h:* synchronized repetitive discharge in muscle cramp; *i:* diphasic, *j:* triphasic, and *k:* polyphasic motor unit action potentials from normal muscle; *l:* short-duration motor unit action potentials in progressive muscular dystrophy; *m:* large motor unit action potentials in progressive muscular dystrophy; *n:* highly polyphasic motor unit action potential and short-duration motor unit action potential during reinnervation. Calibration scale (vertical) in microvolts. The horizontal scale shows 1000 Hz waveforms. An upward deflection indicates a change of potential in the negative direction at the needle electrode. (Reproduced, with permission, from *Clinical Examinations in Neurology,* 3rd ed. Members of the Section of Neurology and Section of Physiology, Mayo Clinic and Mayo Foundation for Medical Education and Research, Graduate School, University of Minnesota, Rochester, Minnesota. Saunders, 1971.)

electrode must be placed against a large flat surface, eg, the patient's back, to afford good contact. The stimulating electrode is small and is placed over the nerve or motor point of the muscle being tested. Either electrode may be used as the anode (A) and the other as the cathode (C). Ordinarily, only closing, or "make" (those that "make" the circuit), shocks are used, since opening, or "break," shocks usually require a painful amount of current to produce a response. Using the cathode as the stimulating electrode requires less current than does using the anode. In other words, the cathode closing contraction (CCC) exceeds the anode closing contraction (ACC); the normal formula of response (NFR) can thus be written as CCC > ACC (Fig 23–6).

Degeneration of motor neurons may cause denervated muscles to fail to contract upon stimula-

tion with interrupted current of electrical pulses of short duration (less than 0.5 ms). This change, which occurs after 2–3 weeks, compares in significance with the fibrillation denervation potentials shown in the EMG.

MEASUREMENT OF NERVE-CONDUCTION VELOCITY

Reaction of Degeneration

The characteristic electrical changes caused by lower-motor-neuron lesions are known as the reaction of degeneration (RD). This reaction may be partial or complete, depending upon the severity of the injury. It is always necessary to wait 10–14 days after the injury before testing the reaction, since that much time is required for the degeneration of

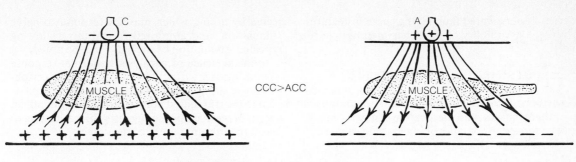

Figure 23-6. The normal formula for response.

an injured nerve. Both galvanic and faradic currents are used to test the degree of the reaction of degeneration (Fig 23-7; see also Chapter 3). In mild partial RD, faradic stimulation of the nerve requires more current than normal, and galvanic stimulation of the nerve and muscle produces a normal response. In severe partial RD, faradic stimulation of the nerve produces no contraction, while galvanic stimulation of the nerve and muscle produces a normal response. In complete RD, neither faradic nor galvanic stimulation of the nerve produces a response, and galvanic stimulation of the muscle produces vermicular contractions.

Diagnostic significance. This reaction is absent in upper-motor-neuron lesions and functional paralysis; it is present in lower-motor-neuron lesions and true organic lower-motor-neuron paralysis. The reaction of degeneration is not present when motor loss results from cut tendons; it is therefore useful in differentiating such lesions from motor loss caused by changes in lower motor neurons.

Electrical resistance of the skin may be greatly increased in disorders that impair peripheral or autonomic nerve function with an associated increase in sweat secretion. Although changes in the reaction of degeneration were at one time thought to aid in predicting recovery of functions, this has not proved to be the case.

Strength-Duration Curves

The excitability of nerve and muscle can be measured with the help of stimulators that provide interrupted current with pulses varying in length from 0.0001 to 1 second. In general, the shorter the pulse, the greater the current required to reach the threshold of excitation. A strength-duration curve can be plotted to show the excitation time characteristics of a particular locus. Although this method is not as sensitive as electromyography, the curves may show evidence of denervation following nerve injury or chronic lower-motor-neuron disease at times when spontaneous fibrillations are difficult to detect. In normal muscle, where the nerves remain the most excitable component, the curve reflects the excitability characteristic of

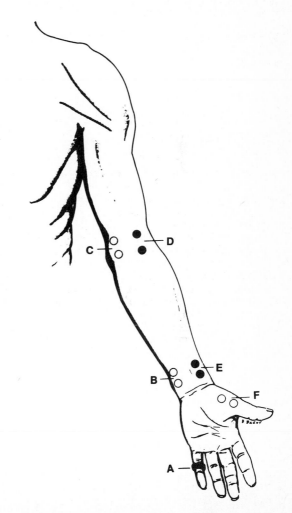

Figure 23-7. Nerve-conduction-velocity studies. A, B, and C are electrode placements for ulnar-nerve evoked potentials. A is a ring-shaped stimulating electrode; B and C are recording electrodes. D, E, and F are electrode placements for median-nerve motor-conduction-velocity study. D and E are points where the nerve is stimulated; F is the recording electrode. (Reproduced, with permission, from Samaha FJ: Electrodiagnostic studies in neuromuscular disease. *N Engl J Med* 1972;**285**:1244.)

nerve. In denervated muscle, the curve instead reflects the excitability of the denervated muscle fibers.

Electrical Stimulation of Nerve Trunks

The presence, absence, or reduction of innervation can be determined by electrical stimulation of peripheral nerves, and the location of a nerve block can be shown. Anomalies of innervation can be detected by noting which muscles respond to nerve stimulation, and abnormal fatigability following repeated stimulation of the nerve can be noted.

In the presence of paralysis, a normal response of innervated muscles to stimulation of the peripheral nerve shows that the cause of paralysis is proximal to the stimulated point. On the other hand, an absent or weak response suggests further testing to detect the site and nature of the defect.

REFERENCES

Aminoff MJ (editor): *Electrodiagnosis in Clinical Neurology,* 2nd ed. Churchill-Livingstone, 1986.

Aminoff MJ: *Electromyography in Clinical Practice,* 2nd ed. Churchill-Livingstone, 1987.

Chiappa KH: *Evoked Potentials in Clinical Medicine.* Raven, 1985.

Moore EJ (editor): *Bases of Auditory Brain-Stem Evoked Responses.* Grune & Stratton, 1983.

Porter RJ, Morselli PL (editors): *The Epilepsies.* Butterworth, 1985.

Section VI.
Discussion of Cases

Discussion of Cases 24

The important question, where is the lesion? (what is the precise location of the deficit?), must be followed by the equally important question, what is the lesion? (what is the nature of the disease?). The answers should lead to the differential diagnosis, correct diagnosis, and prognosis, and the **patient** (the person, not the case) should benefit from appropriate treatment.

THE LOCATION OF LESIONS

Lesions can be located in one or more of the following anatomic sites:
- **Muscles.**
- **Motor end-plates and transmitter processes.**
- **Peripheral nerves.** Peripheral nerve lesions can be differentiated from lesions of the muscle or motor end-plate and transmitter process by electrical tests or biopsy. Both lower-motor-neuron and sensory deficits are present in peripheral nerve or cord lesions.
- **Roots.** A motor root lesion results in a precise segmental motor deficit, which in some cases (eg, plexus lesions) is mediated through several nerves. A single sensory root deficit is difficult to diagnose because of the adjacent overlapping dermatomes (Fig 4–9). Sensory root symptoms include increased pain associated with laughing, sneezing, and coughing, which cause a sudden increase in abdominal pressure.
- **Spinal cord.**
- **Brain stem.** Functional deficits in the long tracts that pass from the brain to the spinal cord or vice versa, together with cranial nerve signs and symptoms, suggest a lesion in the brain stem. Lesions in the medulla involve the last few cranial nerves, while lesions in the midbrain involve nerve III and possibly nerve IV.
- **Cerebellum.** Lesions in the cerebellum or its peduncles result in characteristic motor disorders.
- **Diencephalon.** Hypothalamic lesions are often complex, with visual and endocrinologic disturbances. Thalamic and subthalamic lesions may cause sensory and motor dysfunction. Epithalamic lesions are most frequently pineal region tumors, which can compress the cerebral aqueduct.
- **Subcortical white matter.** The presence of abnormal myelin (leukodystrophy, which is more common in children than in adults) or the destruction of normal myelin (a finding in several disorders) results in abnormal nerve conduction and deficits of function.
- **Subcortical gray matter (basal ganglia).**
- **Cerebral cortex.** Specific functional deficits may be caused by lesions in the cortical projection areas; some syndromes are less well localized. Irritation or compression of the cerebral cortex may result in seizures.
- **Meninges.** Hemorrhages in the subarachnoid, subdural, and epidural spaces have characteristic clinical and neuroradiologic features. The diagnosis of infection (meningitis) can often be confirmed by lumbar puncture.
- **Skull, vertebral column, and associated structures.** Associated structures include the intervertebral disks, ligaments, and articulations. Lesions may also involve adjacent neural structures; often the result of trauma, they can be found by neuroradiologic procedures.

THE NATURE OF LESIONS

The following is a common neuropathologic classification of disorders:
- **Vascular disorders.** Sudden events, often associated with trauma or hypertension, suggest the occlusion or rupture of vessels. Vessel wall disease, which tends to be chronic, can lead to sudden occlusion unless an anastomosis masks the deficit.
- **Trauma.** Injuries to the skull and meninges or to the spine can destroy neural tissue or cause vascular lesions.
- **Tumors.** As neoplasms grow, they produce progressively more signs and symptoms. Sudden

deterioration of the patient's condition may be caused by bleeding in a tumor, by obstruction of cerebrospinal fluid circulation, or by herniation of brain parts, often with compression of the brain stem.

• **Infections and inflammations.** These disorders (eg, meningitis, abscess formation, encephalitis, and granulomas) may be accompanied by fever, especially if the onset is acute. Most infections and inflammations have characteristic signs, symptoms, and causes.

• **Toxic, deficiency, and metabolic disorders.** Poisoning, vitamin deficiency, and enzyme defects leading to abnormal lipid storage in neurons are examples of this heterogeneous group. Various substances in different amounts (too much or too little) can cause selective lesions or deficits.

• **Demyelinating diseases.** Multiple sclerosis and leukodystrophy are representative of this group. There is often a characteristic pattern of absent or abnormal myelin; other features such as age and geography aid in the diagnosis.

• **Degenerative diseases.** This heterogeneous group of diseases for which the cause has not yet been determined includes spinal, cerebellar, subcortical, and cortical degenerative disorders that are often characterized by specific functional deficits.

• **Congenital malformations and perinatal disorders.** Exogenous factors (eg, infection or radiation of the motor cortex) or genetic and chromosomal factors can cause abnormalities of the brain or spinal cord in newborn infants. Hydrocephalus, Chiari malformation, cortical lesions, cerebral palsy, neural tumors, vascular abnormalities, and other syndromes may persist after birth.

• **Neuromuscular disorders.** This group includes muscular dystrophies, congenital myopathies, neuromuscular junction disorders, transmitter deficiencies, and nerve lesions or neuropathies (inflammation, degeneration, and demyelination).

ADDITIONAL CONSIDERATIONS

While some disorders occur only at specific anatomic locations, in other cases the site and nature of the nervous system lesion can be determined by careful analysis of the following aspects of history and examination:

• **Age.** Some tumors occur in childhood, while others occur in advanced age.

• **Gender.** Some diseases are more frequent in one gender than the other.

• **Geography.** Some diseases, such as multiple sclerosis, tend to occur in colder climates; others, such as protozoan infections, are more common in warmer regions.

• **Course of disease.** Lesions occur suddenly in

vascular disorders; tumors and degenerative diseases have a longer course of development.

• **Other factors.** The nature of the lesion can also be determined by checking vital signs and body temperature and by performing blood and cerebrospinal fluid analyses (Table 24–1), radiologic examinations, biopsies, and special tests (see Appendixes A, B, and C).

CASES

Case 1, Chapter 3

Abnormal, gradual tiring of the muscles for eye movement and chewing is suggestive of a neuromuscular disorder. Nerves and muscles normally do not fatigue quickly in adults; transient motor end-plate dysfunction is more likely. This was confirmed by the absence of sensory deficits. The patient's disorder was characterized by the transient nature of the fatigue; rest seemed to cure the problem. All the signs suggest **myasthenia gravis,** a disease in which the neurotransmitter acetylcholine becomes exhausted because of a lack of cholinesterase. Electromyography is a useful procedure to confirm the diagnosis. In addition, skeletal muscle antibodies are often present, especially when the patient has a tumor of the thymus gland. Injection of anticholinesterase drugs such as neostigmine or edrophonium chloride may cure the fatigue and prevent further attacks.

Comment: This disease should not be confused with **myasthenic syndrome,** an autoimmune disease that affects neuromuscular junctions (except in the extraocular muscles).

Case 2, Chapter 4

The shoulder pain radiating into the left arm suggests involvement of the left C6 dorsal root, since the early signs were purely sensory. (This finding determines the general area of the lesion.) The recent weakness in the left extremities, abnormal reflexes in the legs, and decreased reflexes in the left arm all suggest a lower-motor-neuron-type lesion in the left C6 ventral root and an upper motor lesion in the corticospinal tract (probably on both sides). The sensory deficits indicate a level of C6, or perhaps C7, bilaterally. The course of the disease shows a slow progression and recent deterioration, a series of events typical of a slowly expanding mass that rather suddenly compresses the spinal cord against the hard wall of the vertebral canal. This was confirmed by myelography, which showed a left-sided, intradural, extramedullary mass compressing and displacing the spinal cord at the C6–C7 level.

The differential diagnosis includes a mass associated with spinal roots, meninges and nerves; a tumor from the arachnoid (**meningioma**); and a

Table 24–1. Cerebrospinal fluid findings in various diseases.

Condition	Appearance	Pressure (in mm of water)	Cells (per μL)	Protein	Miscellaneous Findings
Tap Normal lumbar	Clear and colorless	70–180	0–5	15–45 mg/dL	Glucose 50–75 mg/dL
Normal ventricular	Clear and colorless	70–190	0–5 (lymphocytes)	5–15 mg/dL	Nonprotein nitrogen mg/dL 10–35 mg/dL Kahn, Wasserman, and VDRL tests negative
Traumatic	Bloody; supernatant fluid clear	Normal	Red blood cells	4 mg/dL rise per 5000 red cells	. . .
Cerebral hemorrhage (ventricular or subarachnoid)	Bloody; supernatant fluid yellow	Slightly increased	Red blood cells	4 mg/dL rise per 5000 red cells	Blood equal in each specimen obtained
Meningitis Acute purulent	Clear, cloudy, milky, or xanthochromic; occasional clot formation	Moderately or greatly increased (250–700)	Polymorphonuclear cells, usually over 1000	Increased	Glucose decreased early; chlorides decreased late; organisms on smear and culture
Acute tuberculous	Opalescent to turbid; faint fibrin web or pellicle formation	Moderately increased (200–450)	10–500 (lymphocyctes)	Increased	Chlorides decreased early, often before decrease of glucose. Smear, culture, and guinea pig inoculation for organisms
Acute syphilitic	Clear to turbid; fibrin clot	Moderately increased (200–350)	100–1000 (mostly lymphocytes)	Slightly increased	Wassermann test positive
Brain tumor	Usually clear and colorless	Increased	Normal or increased	Increased	Findings depend on location and type of tumor
Brain abscess	Clear and colorless	Greatly increased (up to 700)	Polymorphonuclear cells normal or increased	Increased	. . .
Subdural hematoma	Classically yellow, but often clear and colorless	Usually increased	Normal	Normal or slightly increased	. . .
Encephalitis	Clear and colorless	Normal	Normal or increased (mostly lymphocytes)	Normal or slightly increased	Serologic tests of value in virus infections
Arterial hypertension	Clear	Normal or decreased	Normal	Normal or slightly increased	Choked disk may suggest brain tumor
Epilepsy (idiopathic)	Normal fluid	Normal	Normal	Normal	. . .
Multiple sclerosis	Normal fluid	Normal or low	Normal or increased	Normal or increased (increased gamma globulin)	Negative serology

(continued)

Table 24-1 (cont'd). Cerebrospinal fluid findings in various diseases.

Condition	Appearance	Pressure (in mm of water)	Cells (per μL)	Protein	Miscellaneous Findings
Spinal cord tumor Partial block	Clear and color-less	Normal	Normal	Slightly in-creased	. . .
Complete block	Yellow	Normal or low	Slightly in-creased	Marked rise (200–600 mg/dL)	Coagulation may occur
Uremia	Clear and color-less	Slightly in-creased	Normal	Normal or slightly in-creased	Nonprotein ni-trogen
Lead encepha-lopathy	Clear or slightly cloudy	Increased	Lymphocytes	Normal or slightly in-creased	Lead in CSF
Diabetic coma	Clear and color-less	Decreased	Normal	Normal or slightly in-creased	Glucose elevated; may reach 200–300 mg/dL
Acute alcoholic coma	Clear and color-less	Slightly in-creased	May be slightly increased	Normal	Alcohol content of CSF parallels that of blood

nerve tumor (sometimes called a **neuroma**). Abscesses may form a mass, but the patient's history does not suggest an infection.

The diagnosis is a **nerve root tumor** of the left C6 nerve. During neurosurgery, the tumor was completely removed, and the C6 sensory root was sacrificed. Pathologic studies showed a schwannoma. The patient's recovery was complete and uneventful; 6 months later, she danced at the junior prom.

Comment: MR imaging can now be used instead of myelography to demonstrate such root tumors (Figs 24–1 and 24–2).

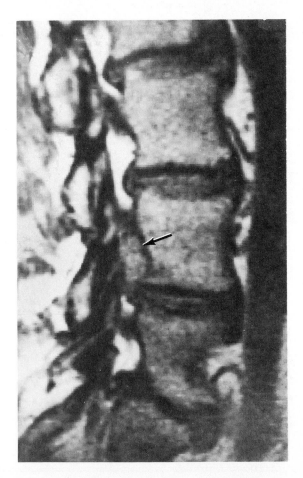

Figure 24-2. MR image (surface coil technique) of a parasagittal section through the lumbar spine in a patient with a root tumor (arrow).

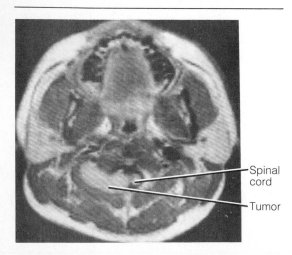

Spinal cord

Tumor

Figure 24-1. MR image of horizontal section through the neck and lower face (a different patient). The image shows a dumbbell-shaped tumor growing out of the spinal canal.

Case 3, Chapter 4

The following features in the history and examination indicate extensive involvement of the motor system: weakness, atrophy, cranial motor nerve deficits (difficulty in swallowing and speech), and fasciculations (see Appendix A). The distribution of deficits over all the extremities suggests an extensive, generalized motor disorder. The abnormal reflexes suggest both lower- and upper-motor-neuron-type lesions. The absence of any sensory deficit strengthens a diagnosis of a pure motor disorder, and the results of the muscle biopsy confirm this.

The diagnosis is **motor neuron disease,** also known as **amyotrophic lateral sclerosis** and popularly called **Lou Gehrig's disease.** All motor neurons in the spinal cord, brain stem and motor cortex are gradually destroyed; there is no cure (Fig 24–3).

Case 4, Chapter 5

The cause—trauma—and the location—lower cervical spine—of the lesion are clear in this case. In the acute phase, traumatic involvement of the spinal cord usually produces spinal shock with flaccid paralysis, loss of temperature control, and hypotension. Precise neurologic localization of the extent of the lesion must therefore be delayed for several weeks. Plain films of the spine in several projections can be used to demonstrate the location and extent of the trauma to the bony spine. Because there may be a traumatic tear in the dura, myelography is contraindicated.

The later neurologic examination showed lesions in the left corticospinal and spinothalamic tracts. There was a left lower-motor-neuron lesion around the C7 area. The lack of sensory deficit in the C7 segment can be explained by the segmental overlapping of dermatomes.

Brown-Sequard syndrome was incompletely represented in this case, because the dorsal column tract on the affected side was spared (see Figs 4–22B and E and 4–23).

The diagnosis is a **traumatic lesion of the spinal cord** at C7. Neurosurgical decompression of the bone fragments prevented further damage to the spinal cord, but the functional deficits caused by local cord destruction could not be corrected. (Physical therapy in such cases may be useful.)

Case 5, Chapter 5

Mild trauma to the lower back, followed by pain down the sciatic region, is suggestive of **sciatica.** One of the underlying causes is herniation of the nucleus pulposus (the soft center of the intervertebral disk). The aggravation of pain by coughing, sneezing, straining, and bending backward (movements that increase abdominal pressure), and the stretching of dural root sleeves by leg raising, are highly suggestive of root involvement (right L5 nerve). The location is confirmed by the presence of paresthesia in the patient's right calf together with the absence of the Achilles tendon reflex (L5, S1). Spasm of the paravertebral muscles and tenderness along the course of the sciatic nerve are common in this disorder.

Plain radiographs are useful only for showing a decrease in the height of the intervertebral disk space; myelography may show an extradural defect and root amputation. The precise location of the lesion can best be shown by CT scanning or MR imaging (Figs 24–4 and 24–5).

The diagnosis is **herniation of the nucleus pulposus** at **L5–S1.** Three weeks after the MRI study was performed, the patient underwent laminectomy with removal of the protruding disk fragment. His recovery was uneventful, with minimal sequelae.

Case 6, Chapter 6

Careful analysis of the signs and symptoms shows that the following systems were involved: the vestibular system (dizziness and nystagmus); the trigeminal system, including the descending

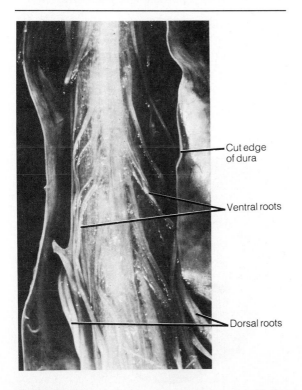

Cut edge of dura

Ventral roots

Dorsal roots

Figure 24–3. Ventral view of the spinal cord (with the dura opened) of a patient with motor neuron disease (amyotrophic lateral sclerosis). Note the reduction in size of the ventral roots compared with the normal dorsal roots.

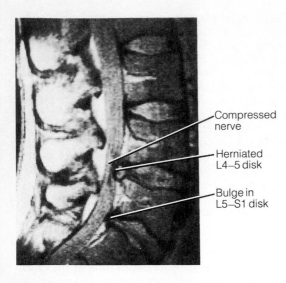

Figure 24-4. MR image (surface coil technique) of a sagittal section through the lower lumbar spine of a patient with low back pain. Note the herniation of the nucleus pulposus at L4–5 compressing the cauda equina.

Compressed nerve

Herniated L4–5 disk

Bulge in L5–S1 disk

spinal tract of V (loss of pain sensation in the right half of the face); the spinothalamic system (contralateral pain deficit); the cerebellum (the inability to execute the right finger-to-nose test or to make rapid alternating movements and the presence of intention tremor and ataxia in the right lower extremity; see Appendix A); and the vagus nerve and ambiguous nucleus (hoarseness). The combination of these findings suggests a location in the posterior cranial fossa, probably in the brain stem. The combination of miosis, ptosis, enophthalmus, and decreased sweating on one side of the face suggests Horner's syndrome, caused by interruption of the sympathetic pathway. This pathway can be interrupted in the lateral brain stem fibers that descend from higher centers in the lateral column of the upper thoracic cord, the upper sympathetic ganglia, or the postsynaptic fibers of the carotid plexus (see Fig 19–6).

Because the patient's disorder had a sudden onset and rapid course, a tumor was unlikely. The most frequent sudden neurologic deficits in the patient's age group have a vascular basis: occlusion or bleeding. Of these, occlusion (ischemic infarct) is the more common (see Chapter 11).

The only anatomic region where all these systems are contiguous is the lateral portion of the medulla; this is the site of the lesion: **lateral medullary syndrome (Wallenberg's syndrome).** Damage to the lateral medulla results from occlusion of small branches of either the posterior inferior cerebellar or the vertebral artery. In 1895 Wallenberg described 6 patients with similar signs and symptoms and recognized the vascular basis of the disorder (Figs 24–6 and 24–7). There is no adequate therapy; symptoms are treated and anticoagulants are sometimes given to prevent additional infarcts.

Case 7, Chapter 6

The patient's signs and symptoms during his first admission to the hospital suggest lesions in the

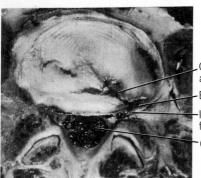

Crack in annulus

Bulging disk

Intervertebral foramen

Cauda equina

Figure 24-5. Photograph of a horizontal section through L4–5 intervertebral disk in a patient with low back pain. Note the lateral herniation of the nucleus pulposus. (Reproduced, with permission, from de Groot J: Correlative Neuroanatomy of *Computed Tomography and Magnetic Resonance Imaging.* Lea & Febiger, 1984.)

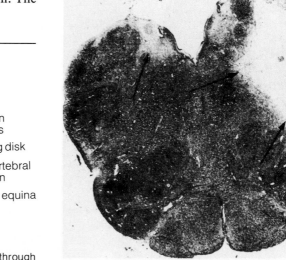

Figure 24-6. Photograph of a section through the open medulla (from Wallenberg's original publication). A large infarct is visible on the right, a smaller one on the left (arrows).

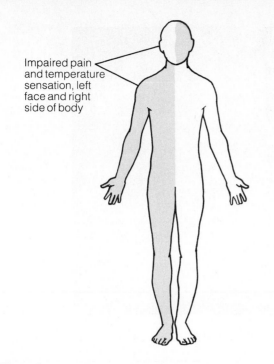

Impaired pain and temperature sensation, left face and right side of body

Figure 24–7. Left posterior inferior cerebellar artery occlusion (Wallenberg's syndrome).

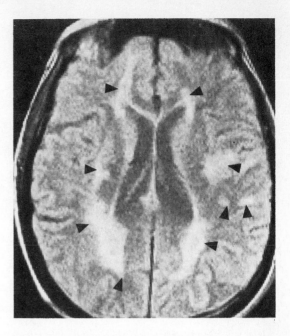

Figure 24–8. MR image of a horizontal section through the head of a 28-year-old patient, showing the lesions (arrow heads) of multiple sclerosis.

left side of the visual system, nerve III or its nucleus, the vestibular system, the portion of the corticobulbar pathway that supplies the face, and the corticospinal tract. It would be difficult for one lesion to involve all these areas. Findings on the second admission 3 weeks later showed additional deficits in the cerebellum or cerebellar peduncles as well as in the lower cranial nerves (VII, X, and XII, the nerves of articulation); once again, the lesions appeared in several systems or sites.

Signs and symptoms of multiple lesions at different times are characteristic of a disseminated infectious disease, multiple infarcts, or a multifocal demyelinating disorder. Disseminated infection was unlikely in this patient because he had no fever and was not a drug user. A CT image did not show multiple infarcts. The lumbar puncture findings were within normal limits, with a slightly increased gamma globulin level (see Table 24–1). The age of the patient (third decade), the repeated attacks, and the multifocal nature of the deficits are indicative of **multiple sclerosis,** a disease for which there is no specific cure (Figs 24–8 and 24–9). Physical therapy and administration of corticosteroids or corticotropin (adrenocorticotropic hormone) or other drugs may be helpful in some cases.

Comment: The risk of multiple sclerosis in populations living between latitudes 40 °N and 40 °S is low. The time course of the disease varies, with

some patients remaining relatively healthy after the first episode, other patients (like the one in this case) continuing to have worsening episodes and relatively few symptom-free intervals, and yet others experiencing a course that falls between these types. The disease is usually most active in people between 10 and 45 years of age. CT scans may show the lesions if they are large enough or in the acute phase. The procedure of choice, however, is MR imaging, which readily demonstrates patches of demyelination as areas with a high-intensity signal.

Case 8, Chapter 7

All signs and symptoms are related to a lesion in the functional components of nerve VII (see Appendix A). Because there were no long-tract signs and no other cranial nerve deficits, it is unlikely that the lesion was in the brain stem, where the nuclei of nerve VII occupy small, dispersed areas. Although the sudden onset of the problem may point to a vascular cause, this is unlikely because only one nerve was involved; the history suggests an infectious (viral) origin of the disorder, and the patient was otherwise in excellent health.

The most probable diagnosis is **peripheral facial paralysis (Bell's palsy)** (Fig 7–14). As in this case, the paralysis is almost always unilateral. The syndrome always includes dysfunction of the brachial efferent fibers of the facial nerve, but visceral ef-

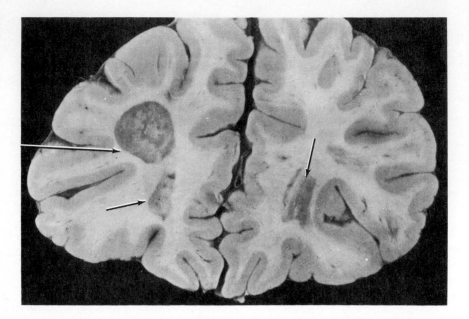

Figure 24–9. Areas of demyelination of the white matter (arrows) in the frontal lobe of a 54-year-old man with multiple sclerosis.

ferent and afferent fiber functions may also be lost. In most cases, the patient recovers spontaneously. A viral cause (possibly the herpes group of viruses) has been suggested.

Case 9, Chapter 7

Several causes of facial pain must be considered: pain from dental causes, neurotic pain, sinusitis, migraine, tumors of the maxilla or nasopharynx, and other, rarer causes. These could be ruled out by careful and complete examination, including a CT scan or MR imaging of the face.

The description of brief attacks of very severe pain, triggered from a localized area in the face, in a patient who is otherwise found healthy, points to a diagnosis of **trigeminal neuralgia (tic douloureux)**. Medical treatment (with carbamazepine or phenotoin) may be effective. In cases where the pain attacks persist, neurosurgical treatment is indicated.

Case 10, Chapter 8

The finding of bitemporal hemianopia is indicative of an abnormal mass located in or near the base of the brain and impinging on the optic chiasm. This may explain the complaint of worsening eyesight; the beginning papilledema does not. The other signs and symptoms point to pituitary dysfunction, probably of considerable duration. Additional tests could confirm this, showing lowered levels of gonadotrophic and thyrotropic hor-

mones. The combination of headache and incipient papilledema indicated increased intracranial pressure, probably caused by a growing mass.

Differential diagnosis includes pituitary adenoma with pressure on the optic chiasm; a craniopharyngioma, a congenital tumor that can compress the pituitary gland, the optic chiasm, or both, and which usually causes symptoms either before the age of 20 years or in old age; a tumor of the hypothalamus and pituitary stalk, which is unlikely, because there were no other hypothalamic dysfunctions; and a gradually enlarging aneurysm of the anterior communicating artery, which is unlikely because there were endocrine dysfunctions.

Radiologic examination (CT or MR imaging) is helpful in determining the precise location, characteristics, and extent of the neoplasm (Fig 24–10). The most likely diagnosis is **pituitary adenoma.** Treatment is neurosurgical removal of the tumor and hormone-substitution therapy.

Case 11, Chapter 9

The mental impairment (disorientation, confusion, and partial loss of memory) of this patient suggests a lesion in one or both frontal lobes. The right facial signs made a left-sided lesion probable, and this was confirmed by the electroencephalogram and skull film. The seizure also suggested an irritative lesion in or near the motor cortex.

The differential diagnosis based on the above must include a slow-growing tumor, progressive

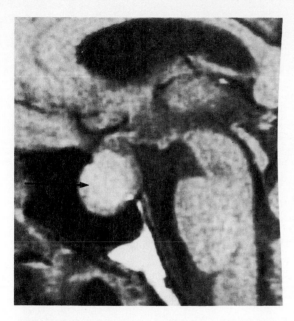

Figure 24–10. MR image through the base of the brain in a patient with a pituitary adenoma (arrow). The tumor has grown downward into the sphenoid sinus and upward to the optic chiasm.

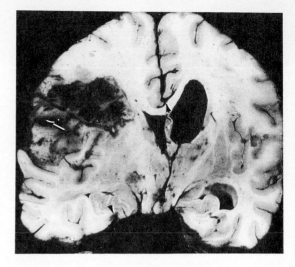

Figure 24–11. Coronal section through the brain of a patient with a hemispheric glial tumor. Histopathologic examination showed this to be a glioblastoma. Note the uncal and subfalcial herniations (arrow heads). A biopsy track is visible on the left (arrow).

bleeding from a large aneurysm or a gradual thrombosis, an unusual type of chronic infection with no history of fever, and a degenerative disorder. In the absence of a high-quality CT or MR image, the diagnosis was difficult to make, and a brain biopsy was performed. The pathologic diagnosis was **malignant glioma.** It was unfortunate and unusual that the biopsy procedure contributed to a progressive intracranial hemorrhage, which led to brain herniation and death (Fig 24–11).

The tumor was shown to be a glioblastoma with calcifications and bleedings. The small hemorrhages found in the brain stem at autopsy were indicative of rapid herniation and were probably caused by tearing of small vessels in the midbrain and pons (Duret hemorrhages).

Comment: Gliomas are a frequent type of brain tumor in most age groups (Tables 24–2 and 24–3). Astrocytoma is considered histologically to be the most benign glioma, and glioblastoma multiforme is considered the most malignant. Modern imaging techniques are useful in determining the site, and often the type, of a mass (Figs 24–12 and 24–13).

Case 12, Chapter 9

The history of ear pain, draining ear, and fever suggests acute middle-ear infection. The subsequent worsening of the patient's condition indicates that complications had occurred: involvement of

the left facial nerve (in the middle ear), headache, dysphasia, and mental deterioration. All this shows that the infection had penetrated the cranial cavity, and electroencephalographic findings confirmed that it had reached the left frontotemporal region.

The differential diagnosis includes otitis media with meningitis, which is unlikely because there was no stiffness of the neck; encephalitis caused by an intercurrent infection, which seems too coincidental to be likely; and cerebritis as a complication of a pyogenic infection.

Table 24–2. Frequency of major types of intracranial tumors.*

Types of Tumors†		Frequency of Occurrence
Gliomas		50%
Glioblastoma multiforme	50%	
Astrocytoma	20%	
Ependymoma	10%	
Medulloblastoma	10%	
Oligodendroglioma	5%	
Mixed	5%	
Meningiomas		20%
Nerve sheath tumors		10%
Metastatic tumors		10%
Cogenital tumors		5%
Miscellaneous tumors		5%

*Reproduced, with permission, from Way LW (editor): *Current Surgical Diagnosis & Treatment,* 6th ed. Lange, 1983.
†Exclusive of pituitary tumors.

Table 24–3. Brain tumor types according
to age and site.*

Age	Cerebral Hemisphere	Intrasellar and Parasellar	Posterior Fossa
Childhood and adolescence	Ependymomas; less commonly, astrocytomas.	Astrocytomas, mixed gliomas, ependymomas.	Astrocytomas, medulloblastomas, ependymomas.
Age 20–40	Meningiomas, astrocytomas; less commonly, metastatic tumors.	Pituitary adenomas; less commonly, meningiomas.	Acoustic neuromas, meningiomas, hemangioblastomas; less commonly, metastatic tumors.
Over age 40	Glioblastoma multiforme, meningiomas, metastatic tumors.	Pituitary adenomas; less commonly, meningiomas.	Metastatic tumors, acoustic neuromas, meningiomas.

*Reproduced, with permission, from Dunphy JE, Way LW (editors): *Current Surgical Diagnosis & Treatment,* 3rd ed. Lange, 1977.

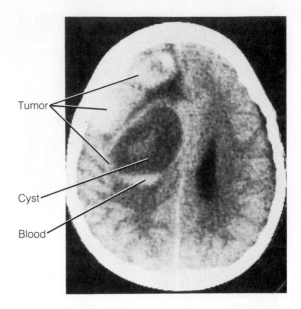

Figure 24–13. CT image of a horizontal section through the head at the level of the lateral ventricles in a patient with glioblastoma multiforma. A small amount of blood lies in the bottom of a cystic portion of the tumor.

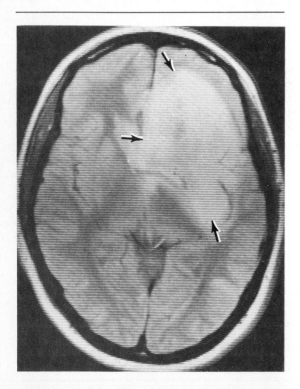

Figure 24–12. MR image of a horizontal section through the head at the level of the lentiform nucleus in a patient with a glioma surrounded by edema (arrows).

A CT image was useful for confirming the diagnosis of **cerebral abscess** (Fig 24–14; see also Table 24–1).

Comment: The high mortality rate in patients with this severe condition has been reduced by repeating the CT scan every 2 or 3 days to monitor the effects of antibiotics and to monitor the ripening of the abscess so that surgical drainage can be performed at the right time. Patients with an impaired immune system can develop an infection in any part of the body; in the brain, the agent is often **Toxoplasma gondii** (Fig 24–15).

Case 13, Chapter 10

The history, temperature, and blood count suggest this to be an infection with weight loss, malaise, and generally poor health. Fever, poor appetite, and cough suggest a severe respiratory infection, and the neck stiffness points to meningeal irritation. It is likely that the initial infection had developed into septicemia and spread to the central nervous system. The lumbar puncture findings are consistent with meningitis (see Table 24–1). The low level of glucose in the cerebrospinal fluid, especially with a normal level of glucose in the blood, is characteristic of bacterial infection, and a gram-stained smear showed pneumococci. The differential diagnosis is extremely limited.

The diagnosis is **pneumococcal meningitis** (Fig 24–16) as a complication of pneumonia. Treatment

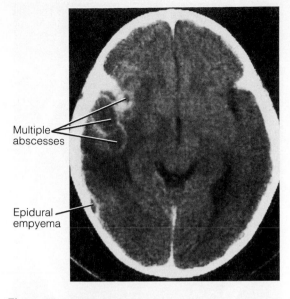

Figure 24–14. CT image of a horizontal section through the temporal lobes, showing an epidural lesion and multiple rounded confluent masses in the right lobe. Note similarity of this lesion to that in Fig 24–13.

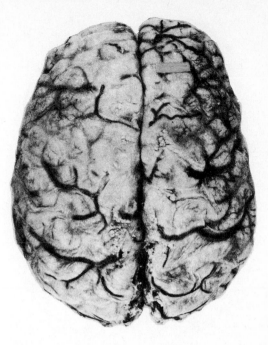

Figure 24–16. Pneumococcal meningitis. The convexity of the brain is covered by thick, yellow-green exudate in the subarachnoidal space.

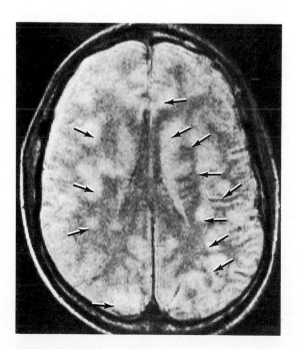

Figure 24–15. MR image of a horizontal section through the lateral ventricles in a patient with acquired immunodeficiency syndrome (AIDS). Note the multiple high-intensity regions throughout both hemispheres, representing cerebral abscesses (arrows).

consists of injecting the appropriate antibiotics intravenously. In addition, intrathecal injection may be considered.

Comment: Pneumococcal meningitis and other forms of purulent meningitis usually extend over the hemispheres, while tuberculous meningitis is more caseous and is often located in the basal cisterns (Fig 24–17). In both types, the circulation of cerebrospinal fluid may become impaired, leading to communicating hydrocephalus.

Case 14, Chapter 10

The history indicates trauma on the right side of the head and temporary loss of consciousness. Findings on early neurologic examination were unremarkable. At this stage, the differential diagnosis should include concussion, in which there is usually little or no loss of consciousness; contusion of the brain, which usually produces no deficits at first; and some type of intracranial hemorrhage. An immediate CT scan or MR image would have been useful to show intracranial blood. A skull film might have shown a fracture of the temporal squama but would not have shown the intracranial changes. In the absence of neuroradiologic procedures, a period of observation was indicated.

The vital signs were within normal limits at first but changed appreciably after a few hours. The combination of increasing blood pressure and de-

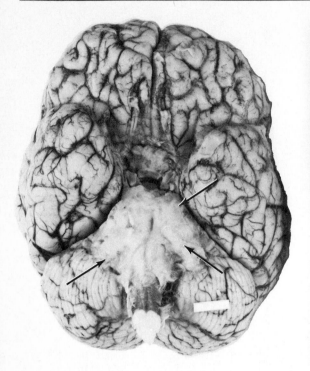

Figure 24–17. Basal view of the brain, showing tuberculous meningitis (arrows) in a 26-year-old man.

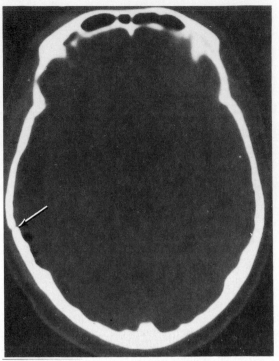

Figure 24–18. CT image through the head at the level of the external ears (bone window) in a patient with epidural hemorrhage. Note fracture site (arrow) and nearby air bubbles.

creasing pulse and respiratory rates is often indicative of increasing intracranial pressure (Cushing's phenomenon).

The repeat examination showed loss of consciousness again after a lucid interval. Together with the increased intracranial pressure, this suggested a rapidly growing mass on the right side and within the skull. The loss of right-sided functions of nerve III is indicative of beginning brain herniation.

The most likely diagnosis is **epidural hemorrhage,** perhaps with some intracerebral bleeding (contusion). Subdural hemorrhage is unlikely because of the rapid deterioration of the patient's condition. Intracerebral hemorrhage can be ruled out by radiologic studies (Fig 24–18; see also Figs 11–25 and 11–26). CT or MR imaging, when available, is superior to lumbar puncture.

Neurosurgical treatment of the bleeding and removal of the epidural blood should be done quickly and may indeed be lifesaving.

Case 15, Chapter 11

The headache and painful stiff neck indicate a process irritating the basal meninges. This could be infectious, the result of bleeding in the subarachnoid space, or the result of meningeal spread from a primary tumor. The suddenness of the disease makes a vascular cause more likely. Intracranial

hypertensive bleeding was unlikely in this normotensive patient, and there was no history of trauma. The severity of the disease, the slightly increased white blood count, and the increased erythrocyte sedimentation rate all pointed to a major abnormal vascular event, most likely a hemorrhage.

Blood in the subarachnoid space can irritate the meninges, cause neck stiffness and pain and vessel spasms, and affect the function of the cranial nerves. The motor deficits must be explained by involvement of the corticospinal tract. The most likely site is the left cerebral peduncle, where dysfunction of the cranial nerve III explains the eye findings. Severe bleeding in the subarachnoidal space can also trigger displacement of the cerebrum, followed by transtentorial herniation. Compression of the cerebral peduncle and nerve III between the posterior cerebral and superior cerebellar arteries is often seen as a complication of a supratentorial mass.

A lumbar puncture might have aggravated the beginning brain herniation, but if performed, it would have demonstrated frank blood in the cerebrospinal fluid (see Table 24–1) and established the diagnosis of acute **subarachnoid hemorrhage.** In this case, a CT image showed a high-density area in the cisterns, particularly on the right side (see Fig 11–19). In such cases, cerebral angiography can be performed a few days later, when a clot has sealed off the bleeding site.

The treatment of subarachnoid hemorrhage consists of neurosurgical removal or containment of the cause of the bleeding—an aneurysm or a vascular malformation.

Case 16, Chapter 11

The history shows the patient to be a belligerent alcoholic who had possibly received trauma to the head when he fell. His level of consciousness had become lowered, and he seemed to have had a seizure (incontinence and a bitten lip), both findings suggesting cerebral involvement. Results of the neurologic examination suggested a lesion in or near the right motor cortex, and the lumbar puncture showed xanthochromia (fresh and old blood) in the cerebrospinal fluid (see Table 24–1). All these findings indicated a hemorrhage; the time course favored subdural bleeding. Subarachnoid bleeding from a leaking aneurysm was less likely, since trauma initiated the process in this patient. An arachnoid tear could have produced the bloody cerebrospinal fluid, and subdural bleeding could occur repeatedly with additional (mild) trauma. The CT image demonstrated this (see Fig 11–22). The worsening of the patient's condition was caused by imminent herniation of the brain, triggered by the blood mass, the drop in cerebrospinal fluid pressure associated with lumbar puncture, or both.

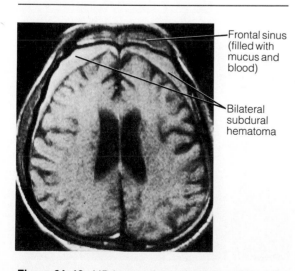

Figure 24–19. MR image of a horizontal section at the level of the lateral ventricles of a patient with bilateral subdural hematoma and congested frontal sinuses. The patient had fallen down a flight of stairs.

The diagnosis is repeated subacute right-sided **subdural hemorrhage.** Treatment consists of neurosurgical removal of the blood and closure of the bleeding veins.

Comment: Most subdural hematomas cover the upper part of the hemispheres, while epidural hematomas are often more circumscribed and located lower (compare Figs 11–25 and 11–26). Bilateral hematoma is not uncommon (Fig 24–19). When bilateral hematoma is found in a youngster, child abuse may be suspected.

Case 17, Chapter 12

The history indicates a motor disorder. In the absence of cerebellar signs and of corticospinal tract deficits, an abnormality in basal ganglia system function must be suspected. This is consistent with the findings of akinesia and unilateral tremor. All observations and test results were compatible with a dysfunction of the substantia nigra or its pathways (see Chapter 11).

The most likely diagnosis was **Parkinson's disease (paralysis agitans),** and neuroradiologic examinations served only to exclude other disorders. Treatment consisted of physical therapy and appropriate administration of drugs such as levodopa and dopamine agonists.

Comment: Neuropathology may confirm the diagnosis at autopsy by the finding of depigmentation of the substantia nigra (see Fig 12–8). Neuromelanin is normally absent in the midbrain and other brain stem sites up to the age of about 8 years.

Case 18, Chapter 12

The suddenness of the severe neurologic deficits in a hypertensive patient most likely indicates a vascular event, probably an intracerebral hemorrhage. In cases such as this, the hematoma may be (in order of frequency) in the putamen, thalamus, pons, or cerebellum. The bleeding in this patient involved the motor system (face, tongue, and corticospinal tract dysfunction). The most likely site of bleeding was either in the putamen, with spread to the globus pallidus and internal capsule (see Fig 11–17) or in the pons, with involvement of the corticospinal and corticopontine systems. However, the unilaterality of the motor deficits pointed to bleeding in the basal ganglia and internal capsule, rather than in the compact pons.

A lumbar puncture could be useful in ruling out a subarachnoid hemorrhage (see case 15 and Table 24–1). Normal cerebrospinal fluid findings would not help in differentiating other types of bleeding, however, and the procedure might even contribute to herniation of the brain. The neuroradiologic procedure of choice, CT imaging, is shown in Fig 11–17. MR imaging, if available, would also be helpful.

The diagnosis is hypertensive **intracerebral hemorrhage** in the left basal ganglia and adjacent structures. Treatment includes antihypertensive therapy, intensive care, and measures to relieve symptoms.

Comment: If bleeding occurs in the putamen, the amount of blood may be small, and the blood may later be reabsorbed (Fig 24–20). When the amount of blood is large, the blood may break through into the ventricles or subarachnoid space.

Case 19, Chapter 13

In the absence of cranial nerve signs and symptoms and cerebellar signs, the lesion must be in the spinal cord, on the right side, at the level of the lower-motor-neuron deficit, C6–C8. The numbness and tingling suggested involvement of the dorsal column system on the right side. Weakness in the right hand indicated additional motor deficits of the lower-motor-neuron type. Absence of acute pain sensation was based on a lesion in the spinothalamic (ventrolateral) system. The weakness and abnormal reflexes of the extremities indicated additional involvement of the corticospinal tracts. Peripheral nerve involvement could be ruled out because the patient had upper motor neuron signs (an extensor plantar response and stronger reflexes on the right side) and a dissociated sensory deficit (the areas of loss of touch were different from those of loss of pain sensation).

The differential diagnosis includes traumatic degeneration of the spinal cord, which is unlikely because there was no history of trauma in this case; myelitis, unlikely because there was no history of fever; and bleeding or thrombosis, unlikely because of the distribution of the deficits.

A plain film of the spine is not helpful in demonstrating intrinsic cord lesions; therefore, myelogra-

phy followed by CT imaging or magnetic resonance imaging is preferable. An MRI study was performed (Fig 24–21) and showed enlargement of the spinal cord by cavitation, or cyst formation, especially in the lower cervical segments.

The diagnosis is **syringomyelia.** The cavity extended from C4 to C7 and involved the right cuneate tract as well as portions of the ventral horns, causing atrophy of the hand muscles (Fig 4–25). Abnormal enlargement of the central canal is called **hydromyelia,** and draining the cavity neurosurgically can provide relief.

Comment: MRI findings in syringomyelia must be distinguished from those in the Arnold-Chiari malformation (Fig 24–22). The latter is a congenital disorder characterized by downward displacement of a small cerebellum, cavitation of the spinal cord, and other abnormalities.

Case 20, Chapter 13

The patient was an alcoholic, as the history indicates. The motor deficits (lower motor neuron type) in all extremities and the sensory irritation or

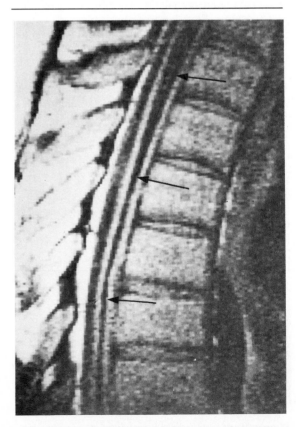

Figure 24–21. MR image (surface coil technique) of a sagittal section through the thoracic spine of a patient with syringomyelia (arrows).

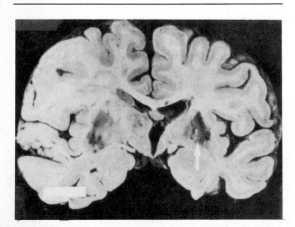

Figure 24–20. Lacunar cystic degeneration involving principally the left caudate and lenticular nuclei.

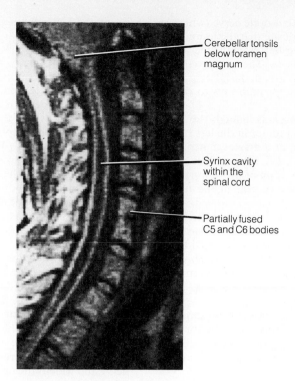

Cerebellar tonsils below foramen magnum

Syrinx cavity within the spinal cord

Partially fused C5 and C6 bodies

Figure 24–22. MR image (surface coil technique) of a midsagittal section through the upper spine of a patient with Chiari and other malformations. (Compare with Fig 6–24.)

loss of sensation, especially in the distal portions, are highly suggestive of peripheral nerve involvement (Fig 24–23). The differential diagnosis should include spinal cord disease, but the distribution of the lesions is not compatible with the somatotropic organization of pathways in the cord.

The diagnosis is **polyneuropathy,** which in this case is caused by thiamine deficiency secondary to alcohol abuse. Hyperalgesia of the soles and calf muscles is characteristic of this type of nerve disease. (There are many other causes of polyneuropathy, and hyperalgesia is not always present.) The treatment in this case should include injections of vitamin B1 (thiamine hydrochloride), daily ingestion of oral multivitamin pills, and institution of both a vitamin-rich diet and a therapy program for alcoholic addiction.

Case 21, Chapter 14

The history of an epileptiform attack in a 50-year-old woman indicates irritation of the cerebral cortex, and the results of examination (chronic papilledema) suggest a slow-growing space-occupying lesion. The mental status is compatible with involvement of one or both frontal lobes. The repeated occurrence of petit mal seizures indicates continued irritation (compression) of the cerebral cortex. The loss of olfaction on the left side and the

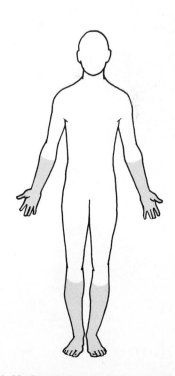

Figure 24–23. Distribution of sensory and lower-motor-neuron deficits in a patient with peripheral polyneuropathy.

atrophy of the adjacent left optic nerve (which resulted in a pale disk) indicate that the lesion is located in the base of the left frontal lobe and is compressing the optic nerve. The associated cerebral edema explains the loss of facial expression and the effect on the motor pathways to the extremities.

The differential diagnosis is limited: the lesion may be an intrinsic brain tumor in the left frontal lobe or olfactory region, or it may be a meningeal tumor in that region. A CT scan or MR image would show the exact location of the tumor; however, if calcification were present in the tumor, plain skull films could suffice.

Neurosurgical removal and pathologic studies of the abnormal tissue resulted in the diagnosis of **olfactory groove meningioma** with associated **Foster Kennedy's syndrome** on the left side. This syndrome consists of contralateral papilledema and ipsilateral optic atrophy caused by a mass in the low frontal region (Fig 24–24).

Comment: Meningiomas arise from abnormal arachnoid cells; therefore, this type of tumor often occurs in many intracranial locations as well as in the spinal region. Frequent sites are on the convex-ity of the hemisphere (Fig 24–25) and along the falx.

Case 22, Chapter 15

The key to determining the site of the lesion in this case is the long-standing impairment of cranial nerve VIII, evident first in the cochlear division and more recently in the vestibular division. The ensuing signs and symptoms all related to the adjacent cranial nerves (V, VI, and VII) or their nuclei and to the brain stem (corticospinal tracts and cerebellar peduncles). The initial complaints pointed to a lesion in the pontocerebellar angle, where nerves VII and VIII lie close to the brain stem. The long period of progressive worsening and the presence of papilledema made a slow-growing tumor likely.

Differential diagnosis includes a cranial nerve tumor, a tumor of the brain stem (eg, a glioma) or the adjacent arachnoid (eg, a meningioma), or another rare neoplasm. The lesion occurring most frequently in this region is a **nerve VIII tumor.** This type of tumor usually originates just inside the proximal end of the internal auditory meatus, where it later compresses the adjacent seventh nerve and widens the meatus. The tumor (usually a schwannoma) may grow to compress adjacent structures in the pontocerebellar angle (Fig 24–26). Treatment consists of surgical removal of the tumor. Function of nerve VIII may be permanently lost.

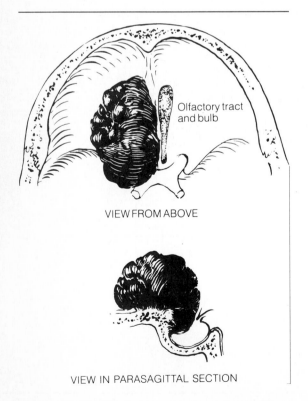

VIEW FROM ABOVE

VIEW IN PARASAGITTAL SECTION

Figure 24-24. Olfactory groove meningioma. (From Scarff: *Classic Syndromes of Brain Tumor.* Annual Clinical Conference of the Chicago Medical Society, 1953.)

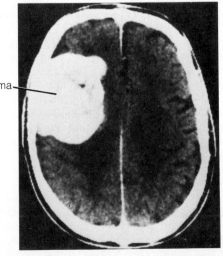

Figure 24-25. CT image, with contrast enhancement, of a horizontal section through the cerebral hemispheres. The absence of surrounding edema suggests a slow-growing tumor, in this case a meningioma.

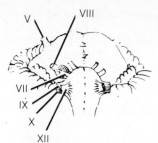

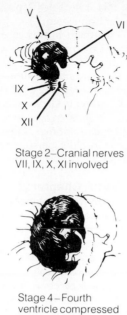

Stage 1—Only nerve
VIII involved

Stage 2—Cranial nerves
VII, IX, X, XI involved

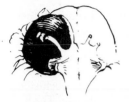

Stage 3—
Cerebellum involved

Stage 4—Fourth
ventricle compressed

First stage: Tinnitus; later, deafness and disturbances of
equilibrium.
Second stage: Weakness of facial muscles, pain in face,
dysphagia, and dysarthria.
Third stage: Ataxia and incoordination.
Fourth stage: Ventricles compressed. Evidence of increased intracranial pressure.

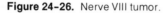

Figure 24–26. Nerve VIII tumor.

Case 23, Chapter 16

The syndrome of recurrent vertigo with tinnitus,
nausea, and progressive deafness suggests an abnormality in the inner ear. Spontaneous nystagmus
(horizontal or rotatory) is often present during an
attack. The most likely diagnosis is **Meniere's disease** (transient ischemic attacks caused by basilar
artery stenosis must first be ruled out). It is probably caused by an increase in the volume of labyrinthine fluid (endolymphatic hydrops). Bilateral
involvement occurs in 50% of the patients. Caloric
testing usually shows impaired vestibular function.
The patient should be referred to an ENT special-
ist.

Medical treatment of this disease may be effective (nicotinic acid every half hour during an attack; oral betahistamine between attacks), and
modern surgical treatment is available.

Case 24, Chapter 17

Transient ischemic attacks are clear signals of incipient occlusive cerebrovascular disease, especially in older patients, who have a higher
incidence of arteriosclerosis. The findings on neu-

rologic examination indicated the involvement of
several cranial nerves, some on the left and some
on the right side: nerves III, V, VI, VII, IX, and X
and the vestibular division of VIII (see Appendix
A). This locates the lesion in the brain stem, which
is supplied by the vertebrobasilar system of arteries. The involvement of the corticospinal system
(especially on the right) and the cerebellar deficits
are all compatible with a lesion in the brain stem.
The absence of visual field defects is in keeping
with a lesion below the diencephalon.

The most likely diagnosis is **stenosis (narrowing)
of the basilar artery,** a very serious condition that
can rapidly deteriorate to complete occlusion, resulting in coma or death. If stenosis occurs rather
suddenly and if the posterior communicating arteries are thin on both sides, the blood supply from
anastomoses may not be adequate to prevent infarction of the brain stem, a condition that is associated with a high mortality rate. The diagnosis of
stenosis may be confirmed by angiography. Treatment consists of symptomatic relief and anticoagu-
lant therapy to prevent thrombosis and total
occlusion.

Case 25, Chapter 18

Fever, malaise, and headache may suggest a subacute intracranial infection. The patient's "fits"
indicate irritation of the cortex, possibly caused by
edematous swelling of the brain. The lumbar puncture results confirmed the presence of infection
and increased intracranial pressure; however, the
basal meninges did not appear to be involved, since
there was no neck stiffness.

The dysphasia, the blood-brain barrier defects
seen on an isotope scan, and the electroencephalographic findings all indicated temporal lobe involvement on both sides. The CT scan findings
were compatible with swelling of these sites and
probably some bleeding.

The differential diagnosis includes encephalitis,
cerebritis, meningitis, and subarachnoid hemorrhage. Subarachnoid hemorrhage may be associated with a moderate rise in temperature and with
seizures and loss of consciousness; however, the
absence of blood in the cerebrospinal fluid, the absence of neck stiffness, the presence of dysphasia,
and the electroencephalographic findings make
this diagnosis unlikely. Meningitis is unlikely because there was no neck stiffness and because the
lumbar puncture specimen showed a white blood
cell count with mostly lymphocytes rather than
polymorphonuclear leukocytes (see Table 24–1).
Although cerebritis associated with abscess formation is a possible diagnosis, it is unlikely because
both temporal lobes were simultaneously involved,
there was no primary infection such as otitis
media, sinusitis, or endocarditis, and the predomi-
nance of lymphocytes suggests otherwise.

The most likely diagnosis is **encephalitis** caused by a virus. Localization in both temporal lobes is typical, as are the cerebrospinal fluid results and the findings on the MR image (see Fig 18–14). The diagnosis of **herpes simplex encephalitis** was confirmed at autopsy when the herpes virus could be demonstrated in the trigeminal ganglion. Organisms often enter via the cornea and ophthalmic division of nerve V; medical treatment is possible. This type of encephalitis is one of the central nervous system complications of AIDS.

Case 26, Chapter 19

The history indicates a slowly progressive process involving the lower cranial nerves (VIII, X, and XII), the brain stem nuclei of these nerves, and the cerebellar pathways, all predominantly on the right side. The ataxia and the increased level of protein in the cerebrospinal fluid pointed to an intracranial location of the lesion. The hypersalivation, postural hypertension, and the cranial nerve (or nuclei) signs can be explained by involvement of the lower brain stem, where the salivatory nuclei, vasomotor center, and pertinent cranial nerve nuclei are located.

The lesion is probably a **brain stem tumor** involving the right side of the stem more than the left and characterized by a slow progression over a period of 8 months, beginning papilledema (suggested by the finding of a flat disk), and localizing signs. The ventricular enlargement seen on CT scan is compatible with a posterior fossa block of the cerebrospinal fluid circulation. (CT images of this region are often suboptimal because of bone artifacts; the radiologist's report

in this case said, "possible enlargement of the lower brain stem.")

Treatment in this case consisted of subtotal removal of a mass that was located in the fourth ventricle and attached to the brain stem. Histopathologic studies showed that the tumor was an **ependymoma** (Fig 24–27).

Comment: The most common posterior fossa tumors in children are astrocytoms, medulloblastomas, and ependymomas. Different types of tumors may occur in older persons (Table 24–3; Figs 24–28 to 24–30).

Case 27, Chapter 20

The history indicates a series of transient ischemic attacks, which are highly suggestive of cerebrovascular occlusive disease. The most common cause in elderly persons is arteriosclerosis. The sudden deterioration of the patient's status may have been caused by bleeding or thrombotic occlusion of a major cerebral vessel on the right side. The bilateral papilledema indicated an intracranial mass effect, possibly swelling of the brain associated with an ischemic infarct. The flaccid paralysis and the sensory deficits showed involvement of the blood supply to the sensory motor cortex or the underlying white matter. The left incomplete hemianopia was most likely the result of ischemia of the optic radiation.

The distribution of the deficits indicates an occlusion of an artery (not a vein or sinus). The sudden nature of the disorder and the absence of a previous history of tumors or infections tend to eliminate neoplasm and infectious mass from the differential diagnosis. The neuroradiologic exami-

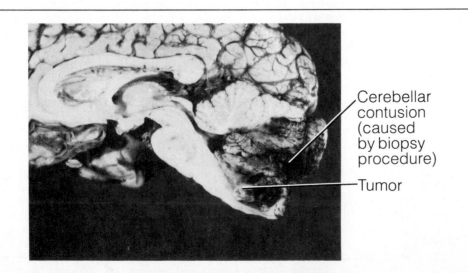

Figure 24–27. Midsagittal section through the brain of a patient with a brain stem tumor. Histologic findings showed the tumor to be an ependymoma. The biopsy track is visible (arrow).

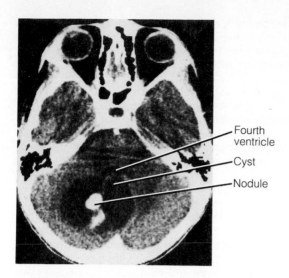

Figure 24–28. CT image, with contrast enhancement, of a horizontal section through the head. Note the low-density cystic astrocytoma with a high-density nodule in the posterior fossa, representing a glioma of the cerebellum.

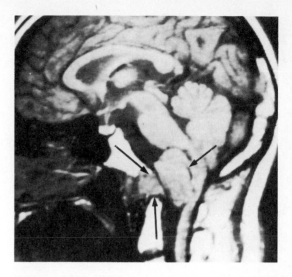

Figure 24–30. MR image of a midsagittal section through the head. The large mass that originates in the clivus and displaces the brain stem backward is a chordoma (arrows).

nation clarified the extent of the ischemia as well as its vascular origin (Fig 24–31; see also Figs 11–12 and 11–13).

The diagnosis is **thrombosis of the right middle cerebral artery.** Treatment sometimes consists of anticoagulants and symptomatic relief. Physical therapy may be helpful in later stages.

Case 28, Chapter 20

The patient described a type of sensory seizure with predominantly visual symptoms; this suggests involvement of the occipital lobe cortex. The sudden development of a right homonymous hemi-

anopia was probably caused by a vascular event that involved the left visual pathway behind the optic chiasm. The history of heart disease suggests embolism, in which small thrombi detach from the heart and pass into the major cerebral vessels. There was no headache, so migraine could be ruled out.

CT (or MR) imaging was helpful in confirming the diagnosis of **embolic infarction** of part of the left occipital lobe. Emboli passing to the brain often lodge in the largest vessels, the middle cerebral arteries. In this case, the infarct occurred in

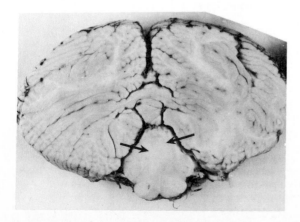

Figure 24–29. Astrocytoma of the medulla oblongata.

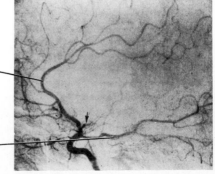

Anterior cerebral artery

Posterior cerebral artery

Figure 24–31. Left internal carotid angiogram, arterial phase, lateral view, showing occlusion of the middle cerebral artery (arrow). The posterior artery is well filled (compare with Fig 22–5).

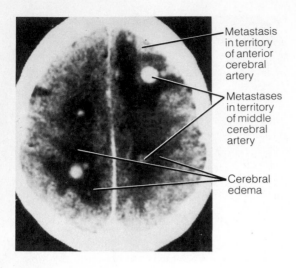

Metastasis
in territory
of anterior
cerebral
artery

Metastases
in territory
of middle
cerebral
artery

Cerebral
edema

Figure 24–32. CT image of a horizontal section through the upper hemispheres of a patient with a known bronchial carcinoma.

the territory of the posterior cerebral artery, which it may have reached by passage through a large (embryonic type) posterior communicating artery or by way of the vertebrobasilar system. Although angiography would help to determine this, it is seldom done shortly after an infarct has occurred.

Treatment of embolic infarction consists of controlled anticoagulation to prevent further emboli.

Comment: Emboli, such as blood-borne metastases to the brain, most frequently lodge in the territory of the middle cerebral artery (Fig 24–32).

Case 29, Chapter 21

The progressively worsening mental status, the absence of clear localizing signs, and the age of the patient suggest **senile dementia of the Alzheimer type.** Other diseases with dementia (Huntington's, Creutzfeld-Jacob, and Pick's diseases) have characteristic courses and epidemiologic findings but are also difficult to diagnose without further tests.

A CT image showed widening of the sulci and dilatation of the spaces containing cerebrospinal fluid (see Fig 21–2). This finding reinforced the most likely diagnosis. A definitive diagnosis, however, can be made only by pathologic examination of the brain.

There is no specific treatment for senile dementia of the Alzheimer type.

REFERENCES

Corey L, Spear PG: Infections with herpes simplex viruses. *N Engl J Med* 1986;**314:**686.

Davis RL, Robertson DM (editors): *Textbook of Neuropathology,* 2nd ed. Williams & Wilkins, 1990.

Escourolle R, Poirier J: *Manual of Basic Neuropathology,* 2nd ed. Saunders, 1978.

Okazaki H: *Fundamentals of Neuropathology.* Igaku-Shoin, 1983.

Pryse-Phillips W, Murray TJ: *Essential Neurology.* Med Exam Pub, 1982.

Raskin NH: *Headache,* 2nd ed. Churchill-Livingstone, 1988.

Rosenblum ML, Levy RM, Bredesen DE: *AIDS and the Nervous System.* Raven, 1988.

Rowland LP (editor): *Merritt's Textbook of Neurology,* 7th ed. Lea and Febiger, 1984.

Simon RP, Aminoff MJ, Greenberg DA: *Clinical Neurology.* Appleton & Lange, 1989.

Van Allen MW: *Pictorial Manual of Neurologic Tests.* Year Book, 1969.

Appendix A:
The Neurologic Examination

EXAMINING CHILDREN & ADULTS

HISTORY

A complete history of the nature, onset, extent, and duration of the chief complaint and associated complaints must be taken. This should include previous diseases, personal and family history, occupational data, and social history. It may be desirable—or necessary—to interview relatives and friends.

Detailed information is particularly important in regard to the following:

A. Headache: Note the duration, time of onset, location, frequency, severity, progression, precipitating circumstances, associated symptoms, and response to analgesics.

B. Seizures and Episodic Loss of Consciousness: Record the character of the individual episode, age at onset, frequency, duration, mental status during and after episodes, associated signs and symptoms, aura, and the type and effectiveness of previous treatment.

C. Visual Disturbances: The frequency, progression or remissions, scotomas, acuity changes, diplopia, field changes, and associated phenomena should be noted.

D. Pain: The onset, progression, frequency, characteristics, effect of physical measures, associated complaints, and type and effectiveness of previous treatment should be included.

THE PHYSICAL EXAMINATION

A general physical examination should always be made. In particular, the circulatory, respiratory, genitourinary, gastrointestinal, and skeletal systems should be studied and a record of the temperature, pulse rate, respiratory rate, and blood pressure routinely made. Note especially any deformity or limitation of the head, neck, vertebral column, or joints. Inspect and carefully palpate the scalp and skull for localized thickening of the skull, clusters of abnormal scalp vessels, depressed areas, abnormal contours or asymmetry of the skull, and craniotomy and other operative scars. Percussion may disclose local scalp or skull tenderness over diseased areas and, in hydrocephalic children, a tympanic cracked-pot sound. Auscultate the skull and neck for bruits; if bruits are present, the effect of separate carotid artery compression is also noted.

THE NEUROLOGIC EXAMINATION

Mental State

Mental changes are frequently encountered in clinical neurology, and an understanding of them is helpful for diagnosis and treatment. Although impaired intellectual functioning is quite common in cerebral disease, the type of mental disturbance is not specific for any given neurologic disorder. With some neurologic disorders (eg, brain tumor, multiple sclerosis, paralysis agitans), the insidious onset and the course of remissions and exacerbations frequently result in the misdiagnosis of psychogenic illness. Early neurologic disease may occur without significant physical, laboratory, radiologic, or other special diagnostic findings, and drugs used in treatment may further complicate the clinical picture.

A. General Behavior: Evaluate the patient's speech, appearance, concentration, cooperation, posture, general attitude, characteristic mannerisms, and movement.

B. Mood: Look for anxiety, depression, apathy, fear, suspicion, irritability, elation, and aggression.

C. Level of Consciousness: Assess the patient's ability to retain information, and check the level of alertness, denseness (obtundation), stupor, or coma. When possible, check for orientation with respect to time, place, person, and situation.

D. Level of Intelligence: Measures of intelligence include vocabulary, judgment, cultural outlook, and general information. Intellectual performance tests, such as the following, should be performed.

1. Memory—Details and dates of recent and remote events should be elicited, including such items as birth date, marriage date, names and ages of children and relatives, specific details of the past few days, and educational history with dates and names of schools attended.

2. General information—These questions should be adapted to the patient's background. Examples are the names of prominent political and world figures, the capitals of countries and states, and current events in politics, sports, and performing arts.

3. Similarities and differences—Have the patient compare wood and coal; iron and silver; book, teacher, and newspaper; president and king; dwarf and child; and lie and mistake.

4. Calculations—The patient should count backward from 100 by 7s; ie, subtract 7s from 100 $(100 - 7 = 93; 93 - 7 = 86; 86 - 7 = 79;$ etc). Add, multiply, or divide single numbers (eg, 3×5, 4×3, 16×3). Count from 1 to 20 and backward from 20 to 1. Calculate interest at 6% for 18 months. The examiner should make the calculations easier or more difficult depending upon the patient's background.

5. Retention—Ask the patient to repeat digits in natural or reverse order. (Normally, an adult can retain 7 forward and 5 backward.) After instruction, ask the patient to repeat a list of 3 cities and 3 two-digit numbers after a pause of 3 minutes.

6. Judgment—Ask the patient for the symbolic or specific meaning of simple proverbs such as the following: "A stitch in time saves nine." "A rolling stone gathers no moss." "People who live in glass houses should not throw stones." The content of a simple story or paragraph from a newspaper or magazine can be read and the patient's retention, comprehension, and formulation observed.

7. Memory and comprehension—The examiner tells a story, which is then retold in the patient's own words. The patient is also asked to explain the meaning of the story. The following stories are commonly used.

a. Cowboy story—A cowboy went to San Francisco with his dog, which he left at a friend's house while he went to buy a new suit of clothes. Dressed in his brand-new clothing, he came back to the dog, whistled to it, called it by name, and patted it. But the dog would have nothing to do with him in his new coat and hat. Coaxing was to no avail, so the cowboy went away and put on his old suit, and the dog immediately showed its wild joy in seeing its master as it thought he ought to be.

b. Gilded-boy story—At the coronation of one of the popes, about 300 years ago, a little boy was chosen to play the part of an angel. In order that his appearance might be as magnificent as possible, he was covered from head to foot with a coating of gold foil. The little boy fell ill, and although everything possible was done for his recovery except the removal of the fatal golden covering, he died within a few hours.

E. Content of Thought: Thought content may include obsessions, phobias, delusions, compulsions, recurrent dreams or nightmares, depersonalization, or hallucinations. Check special preoccupations and disorders of content, with attention to special topics of concern to the patient and the form they take.

F. Language: Evaluate the patient's comprehension of spoken language, ability to read and write, ability to recognize and name familiar objects, capacity for verbal and nonverbal means of expression, and ability to recognize errors. Look for spontaneous or automatic speech.

G. Insight: The patient's own evaluation and explanation of the illness may indicate his or her level of insight.

Cranial Nerves

A. Olfactory Nerve (I): Use familiar odors such as peppermint, coffee, menthol, or vanilla, and avoid use of irritants such as ammonia and vinegar. A test substance is rapidly passed toward the subject from a distance of about 1 meter, and the patient must then identify the substance with eyes shut and one nostril held closed. Complete or unilateral anosmia may be significant in the absence of intranasal disorders.

B. Optic Nerve (II):

1. Visual acuity test—A Snellen chart can be used to measure visual acuity and determine whether improvement is obtained with correction. For individuals with severe defects, cruder tests may be employed, eg, the ability to count fingers and detect hand movements and changes from dark to light.

2. Ophthalmoscopic examination—Each optic fundus must be examined as part of the neurologic examination. If necessary, the pupils may be dilated with drugs after the pupillary reflexes have been noted. Details of the ophthalmoscopic examination should include the color, size, and shape of the optic disk; the presence or absence of a physiologic cup; the distinctness of the optic disk edges; the size, shape, and configuration of the vessels; and the presence of hemorrhage, exudate, or pigment.

3. Visual field test—The visual fields can be roughly tested by confrontation, with the patient seated about 1 meter from the examiner. With the left eye covered, the patient looks at the examiner's left eye. The examiner slowly raises both hands upward from a position where they can barely be seen in the lower 2 quadrants, and the patient signifies when the examiner's moving hands first become visible. The upper quadrants are similarly tested, with the examiner's hands moving downward. The left eye of the patient is then tested against the right eye of the examiner.

More accurate visual field determination requires the use of a perimeter or tangent screen.

C. Oculomotor (III), Trochlear (IV), and Ab-

ducens (VI) Nerves: Strabismus, nystagmus, ptosis, exophthalmos, and pupillary abnormalities can be detected on initial examination. Test ocular movements by having the patient follow the movement of an object (eg, a finger or a light) to the extremes of the lateral and vertical planes.

The size and shape of each pupil are noted. The reactions of both pupils to a bright light flashed into one eye in a darkened room while the patient gazes into the distance are noted. The direct light reaction is the response of the pupil of the illuminated eye; the consensual light reaction is the reaction of the opposite pupil, which is carefully shielded from the stimulating light.

In testing the accommodation-convergence response, the examiner asks the patient to focus alternately on 2 objects, one distant and the other 15 cm (6 inches) from the patient's face.

D. Trigeminal Nerve (V): The ability to perceive a pinprick or the touch of a bit of cotton is tested over the face and anterior half of the scalp. The oronasal cavity sensation is tested by approaching the cornea from the side and touching it with a strand of cotton as the patient looks upward. Care must be taken not to touch the eyelashes or conjuctiva. Test the motor function of the trigeminal nerve by palpating the contraction of the masseter and temporalis muscles induced by a biting movement of the jaws.

E. Facial Nerve (VII): Note facial expression, mobility, and symmetry. Assess the voluntary movements of the lower facial musculature by having the patient smile, whistle, bare the teeth, and pucker his or her lips. Maneuvers such as closing the eyes or wrinkling the forehead are ways of testing the upper facial musculature.

Test taste sensation of the anterior two-thirds of the tongue by applying small quantities of test solutions to the protruded tongue with cotton applicators. The test solutions used are sweet (sugar), bitter (quinine), salt (saline), and sour (vinegar). As each taste is perceived, the patient responds by pointing to a labeled card. Between tests, the tongue should be irrigated with water.

F. Vestibulocochlear Nerve (VIII):

1. Cochlear nerve—The patient's ability to hear the examiner's voice in ordinary conversation is noted. The ability to hear the sound produced by rubbing the thumb and forefinger together is then tested for each ear at distances up to a few centimeters. The farthest distance from either ear at which the ticking of a loud watch or the spoken voice is heard can be measured.

Use a tuning fork vibrating at 256 Hz to test air and bone conduction for each ear (see Table 15–1): In Rinne's test, the vibrating tuning fork is placed on the mastoid process and then in front of the ear. Normally, the fork is heard for several seconds longer when it is placed in front of the ear than

when it is placed on the mastoid. In injury to the cochlear nerve, there may be complete or partial inability to hear the vibrating tuning fork (nerve deafness). When partial hearing remains, air conduction exceeds bone conduction. In disease of the middle ear with impaired hearing, bone conduction of the sound of the tuning fork is better than air conduction (conduction deafness).

In Weber's test, a vibrating tuning fork (256 Hz) is placed on the bridge of the nose or over the vertex of the scalp. Normally, the sound is heard equally well in both ears. In patients with unilateral deafness due to middle ear disease, the sound is heard best in the affected ear.

2. Vestibular nerve—The caloric test is frequently used to evaluate vestibular function. The eardrum is first examined to make certain no perforations exist. The patient is asked to sit with the head tilted slightly forward to test the vertical canals or to lie supine with the head tilted back at an angle of 60 degrees to test the horizontal canals. The examiner slowly and steadily irrigates one external auditory canal with cool (30°C) or warm (40°C) water. Normally, cool water in one ear produces nystagmus on the opposite side; warm water produces it on the same side. (A mnemonic for this is COWS: *c*ool, *o*pposite; *w*arm, *s*ame.) Irrigation is continued until the patient complains of nausea or dizziness or until nystagmus is detected. This normally takes 20–30 seconds. If no reaction occurs after 3 minutes, the test is discontinued.

G. Glossopharyngeal Nerve (IX): Taste over the posterior third of the tongue is tested in a manner similar to that described above for the anterior two-thirds of the tongue. Sensation (usually touch) is tested on the soft palate and pharynx. The pharyngeal response (gag reflex) is tested bilaterally.

H. Vagus Nerve (X): Test the swallowing function by noting the patient's ability to drink water and eat solid food. The pharyngeal wall contraction is observed as part of the gag reflex. Movement of the median raphe of the palate and uvula when the patient says "ah" is recorded. In unilateral paralysis of the vagus nerve, the raphe and uvula move toward the intact side, and the posterior pharyngeal wall of the paralyzed side moves like a curtain toward the intact side. The character, volume, and sound of the patient's voice are recorded. Using a dental mirror, the position of the vocal cords can be observed by indirect laryngoscopy. The resting heart rate and the bradycardia produced by pressure on the eyeball (oculocardiac reflex) or pressure on the carotid sinus may be influenced by lesions involving the vagus nerve.

I. Accessory Nerve (XI): Instruct the patient to rotate his or her head against resistance applied to the side of the chin. This tests the function of the opposite sternocleidomastoid muscle. To test both sternocleidomastoid muscles together, the patient flexes the head forward against resistance placed under the chin. Shrugging a shoulder against resistance is a way of testing trapezius muscle function.

J. Hypoglossal Nerve (XII): Examine the tongue for atrophy and for fasciculations or tremors when it is protruded and when it is lying at rest in the mouth. Note any deviation of the tongue on protrusion; a lesion of the hypoglossal nerve or nucleus causes deviation to the same side.

Motor System

The power of muscle groups of the extremities, neck, and trunk is tested. Where there is an indication of diminished strength, test smaller muscle groups and individual muscles (see Appendix B). Atrophy or hypertrophy of muscles is judged by inspection and palpation and, in the case of the musculature of the extremities, by measuring the circumferences of the limbs. The differences between the circumferences on the 2 sides may be related to the handedness or occupation of the patient. Note abnormal movements, and record the influence upon them of postural and emotional change, intention, and voluntary movements.

Muscle tone (tonus) is judged by palpation of the muscles of the extremities and by passive movements of the joints by the examiner. Carefully describe increased or decreased resistance to passive movement. Note tone alterations, including clasp-knife spasticity, plastic or cogwheel rigidity, spasms, contractures, and hypotonia.

Pendulousness is the motion of a passively displaced extremity when it is permitted to swing freely. It is increased in hypotonia, markedly reduced in rigidity of extrapyramidal origin, and irregular in pattern (though normal or slightly diminished in duration) in spasticity. Note and describe involuntary movements, including tremors, athetosis, chorea, tics, and myoclonus.

Coordination, Gait, & Equilibrium

A. Simple Walking Test: Observe posture, gait, coordinated automatic movements (swinging arms), and ability to walk a straight line and to make rapid turning movements as the patient walks. Record a detailed and full description of the gait.

B. Romberg Test: Have the patient stand with heels and toes together and eyes closed. Increased swaying commonly occurs in patients with dysfunction of cerebellar or vestibular mechanisms. Patients with disease of the posterior columns of the spinal cord may fall when their eyes are closed, although they are able to maintain their position well with the eyes open.

C. Finger-to-Nose and Finger-to-Finger Tests: In the finger-to-nose test, the patient places the tip of a finger on his or her nose. In the finger-to-finger test, the patient attempts to approximate the tips of the index fingers after the arms have been extended forward. Dysmetria, with overshooting of the mark, is often observed in cerebellar disorders.

D. Heel-to-Shin Test: The patient places one heel on the opposite knee and then moves the heel along the shin. Dysmetria, with overshooting the mark, is often observed in cerebellar disorders.

E. Rapidly Alternating Movements: In this test, the patient rapidly flexes and extends the fingers or taps the table rapidly with extended fingers. Test supination and pronation of the forearm in continuous rapid alternation. The inability to perform these movements quickly and smoothly is a feature of dysdiadochokinesia, an indication of cerebellar disease.

Reflexes

The following reflexes are routinely tested, and the response elicited is graded from 0 to 4+ (2+ is normal).

A. Deep Reflexes:

1. Biceps reflex–When the patient's elbow is flexed at a right angle, the examiner places a thumb on the patient's biceps tendon and then strikes the thumb. Normally, a slight contraction of the biceps muscle occurs.

2. Triceps reflex–With the patient's elbow supported in the examiner's hand, the triceps tendon is sharply percussed just above the olecranon. Contraction of the triceps muscle, with extension of the forearm, usually results.

3. Knee reflex–The patellar tendon is located by palpation and tapped lightly with a percussion hammer or fingers. Increase the force of the tapping until contraction of the quadriceps muscle can be elicited. The patient is usually seated on the edge of a table or bed, with the legs hanging loosely. For patients who are bedridden, the knees can be flexed over the supporting arm of the examiner, with the heels resting lightly on the bed.

4. Ankle reflex–This is best elicited by having the patient kneel on a chair, with ankles and feet projecting over the edge of the chair. The Achilles tendon is then struck with a percussion hammer.

B. Superficial Reflexes:

1. Abdominal reflex–With the patient lying supine with relaxed abdominal muscles, stroke the skin of each quadrant of the abdomen briskly with a pin from the periphery toward the umbilicus. Normally, the local abdominal muscles contract, causing the umbilicus to move toward the quadrant stimulated.

2. Cremasteric reflex–In men, stroking the skin of the inner side of the proximal third of the thigh causes retraction of the ipsilateral testicle.

3. Plantar response–With the thigh in slight external rotation, stroke the outer surface of the sole of the foot lightly with a large pin or wooden applicator from the heel toward the base of the little toe and then inward across the ball of the foot. The normal plantar response consists of plantar flexion of all toes, with slight inversion and flexion of the distal portion of the foot. In abnormal responses, there may be extension of the great toe, with fanning and flexion of the other toes (Babinski's reflex).

C. Clonus: Clonus (repeated reflex muscular movements) may be elicited in patients with exaggerated reflexes. Wrist clonus is sometimes elicited by forcible flexion of the wrist. Patellar clonus can be elicited by sudden downward movement of the patella, with consequent clonic contraction of the quadriceps muscle. Ankle clonus is tested by quickly flexing the foot dorsally, producing clonic contractions of the calf muscles.

Sensory System

Sensory examination is a difficult and tiring procedure for both the patient and the examiner. The patient should be well rested and must be reassured and in a cooperative frame of mind before a sensory examination is attempted. Abnormalities, especially of minor degree, should be checked by frequent reexamination. The following modalities are tested and charted.

A. Pain: Test the patient's ability to perceive pinprick or deep pressure.

B. Temperature: To check for the ability to detect and distinguish between warm and cold, use a test tube of warm water and one of cold water.

C. Touch: Test the ability to perceive light stroking of the skin with cotton.

D. Vibration: The patient should be able to feel the buzz of a tuning fork (at a frequency of 128 Hz) applied to the bony prominences. After the tuning fork has been set into maximum vibration, the duration of the patient's perception of the vibration is timed with the base of the fork applied to the malleoli, patellas, iliac crests, vertebral spinous processes, and ulnar prominences.

E. Sense of Position: This is tested by having the patient determine the position of toes and fingers when these are grasped by the examiner. A digit is grasped on the sides, and the patient, with eyes closed, attempts to determine whether it is moved upward or downward. Test the larger parts of the extremities if impairment is demonstrated in the digits.

F. Perception of Passive Motion: Check the patient's ability to perceive passive movements of the extremities, especially the distal portions.

G. Stereognosis: To test the patient's capacity to recognize the forms, sizes, and weights of objects, place a familiar object (eg, a coin, key, or knife) in the patient's hand and ask him or her to identify the object without looking at it.

H. Two-Point Discrimination: The shortest distance between 2 separate points of a compass or calipers at which the patient perceives 2 stimuli is compared for homologous areas of the body. (Normal: finger tips, 0.3–0.6 cm; palms of hands and soles of feet, 1.5–2 cm; dorsum of hands, 3 cm; and shin, 4 cm.)

I. Topognosis: After making sure that the patient's eyes are closed, the examiner touches the patient's body. The patient then points to the spot touched, thereby enabling the examiner to assess the patient's ability to localize tactile sensation. Similar areas of both sides of the body are compared.

EXAMINING NEONATES

The neonatal neurologic examination is usually performed 36–60 hours after birth. Repeat examinations at weekly intervals may be desirable. The examination should be planned so that little stimulation of the infant occurs initially.

GENERAL STATUS

Observe the motor pattern and supine and prone body posture and evaluate the reflexes throughout the examination.

In normal infants, the limbs are flexed, the head may be turned to the side, and there may be kicking movements of the lower limbs. Extension of the limbs can occur with intracranial hemorrhage, opisthotonos with kernicterus, and asymmetry of the upper limbs with brachial plexus palsy. Paucity of movements may occur with brachial plexus palsy and meningomyelocele.

Infants normally become more active and cry during the examination. In cases of anoxia or intracerebral hemorrhage, the infant reacts very little.

THE NEUROLOGIC EXAMINATION

Cranial Nerves

A. Optic Nerve (II): Test the infant's blink response to light. Ophthalmoscopic examination should be made at the end of the examination.

B. Oculomotor (III), Trochlear (IV), and Abducens (VI) Nerves: Check the size, shape, and equality of the pupils and pupillary responses to light. Lateral rotation of the head causes rotation of the eyes in the opposite direction (doll's eye reflex).

C. Trigeminal (V) and Facial (VII) Nerves: The sucking reflex is elicited by placing a finger or nipple between the infant's lips. In the rooting reflex, the infant's mouth will open and turn toward the stimulus if a fingertip touches the infant's cheek.

D. Vestibulocochlear Nerve (VIII): The blink response occurs in reaction to loud noise. To test the labyrinthine reflex, the infant is carried and held up by the examiner, who makes several turns to the right and then to the left. A normal infant will look ahead in the direction of rotation; when rotation stops, the infant will look back in the opposite direction.

E. Glossopharyngeal (IX) and Vagus (X) Nerves: Note the infant's ability to swallow.

Motor System & Reflexes

Spontaneous and induced motor activity are noted. If the infant is inactive and quiet, the Moro reflex (see below) may be used or the infant may be placed in the prone position to induce movement.

A. Incurvation Reflex (Galant's Reflex): With the infant prone, tactile stimulation of the normal thoracolumbar paravertebral zone with a finger produces contraction of the ipsilateral long muscles of the back, so that the head and legs curve towards the stimulated area and the trunk moves away from the stimulus.

B. Muscle Tone: Assess muscle tone by palpating muscles during activity and relaxation. Resistance to passive extension of the elbows and knees is noted.

C. Limb Motion: Determine the infant's ability to move a limb from a given position.

D. Joint Motion: Flex the infant's hip and knee joints to check the pull of gravity when the infant is held head down in vertical suspension.

E. Grasp Reflex: Stimulation of the ulnar palmar surfaces causes the infant to grasp the examiner's hands forcefully.

F. Traction Response: Contraction of shoulder and neck muscles occurs when a normal infant is pulled from the supine to a sitting position.

G. Stepping Response: The normal infant makes stepping movements when held upright with the feet just touching the table.

H. Placing and Supporting Reactions: Drawing the dorsum of the infant's foot across the lower edge of a moderately sharp surface (eg, the edge of the examining table) normally produces flexion at the knee and hip, followed by extension at the hip (placing reaction). If the plantar surface comes in contact with a flat surface, extension of the knee and hip may occur (positive supporting reaction).

I. Moro Reflex (Startle Response): The Moro reflex is present in normal infants. A sudden stimulus (eg, a loud noise) causes abduction and extension of all extremities, with extension and fanning of digits except for flexion of the index finger and thumb. This is followed by flexion and adduction of the extremities.

J. Other Reflexes and Responses: Knee jerk, plantar response (normal response is extensor), abdominal reflex, and ankle clonus are tested with the infant quiet and relaxed.

Sensory System

Withdrawal of the stimulated limb and sometimes also the unstimulated limb may be caused by pinprick of the sole of the foot.

Appendix B: Testing Muscle Function

Muscle testing depends upon a thorough understanding of which muscles are used in performing certain movements. Testing is best performed when the patient is warm, rested, comfortable, attentive, and alone with the examiner. Since several muscles may function similarly, it is not always easy for the patient to contract a single muscle upon request. Positioning or fixation of parts can emphasize the contraction of a particular muscle while other muscles of similar function are inhibited. The effect of gravity must be considered, since it can enhance or reduce certain movements. Testing of individual muscles is useful for evaluating peripheral nerve and muscle function and dysfunction.

Two techniques of testing can be used: active motion against the examiner's resistance and resistance against a movement performed by the examiner. The degree of impairment of muscle function may be difficult to estimate by inspection. It is helpful to palpate the body or tendon of a muscle for evidence of contraction or movement. The normal or least affected muscles should be tested first to gain the cooperation and confidence of the patient. The strength of the muscle tested should always be compared with that of its contralateral muscle.

The strength of various muscles should also be graded and charted. Grading scales of various types are used, eg, minus to $4+$, 0 to 100%, or letter codes such as N for normal, G for good, F for fair, P for poor, T for trace, and O for zero.

See Tables B–1 and B–2 and Figs B–1 to B–54.

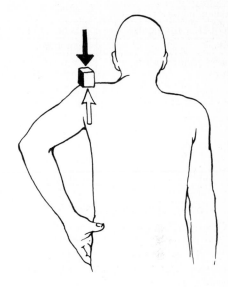

Figure B-1. Trapezius, upper portion (C3, 4; spinal accessory nerve). The shoulder is elevated against resistance.

Table B-1. Grading muscle strength.

Normal	N	5	Complete range of motion against gravity with full resistance
Good	G	4	Complete range of motion against gravity with some resistance
Fair	F	3	Complete range of motion against gravity
Poor	P	2	Complete range of motion with gravity eliminated
Trace	T	1	Evidence of slight contractility. No joint motion
Zero	O	0	No evidence of contractility

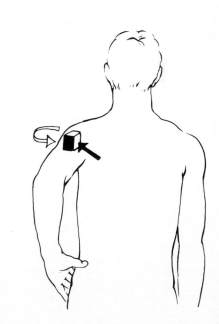

Figure B-2. Trapezius, lower portion (C3, 4; spinal accessory nerve). The shoulder is thrust backward against resistance.

Table B-2. Motor function.*

Action to Be Tested	Muscle	Cord Segment	Nerves	Plexus
Shoulder Girdle and Upper Extremity				
Flexion of neck	Deep neck muscles (stem- ocleidomastoid and trape- zius also participate)	C1–4	Cervical	Cervical
Extension of neck				
Rotation of neck				
Lateral bending of neck				
Elevation of upper thorax	Scaleni	C3–5	Phrenic	
Inspiration	Diaphragm			
Adduction of arm from behind to front	Pectoralis major and minor	C5–8, T1	Pectroal (thoracic; from medial and lat- eral cords of plexus)	Brachial
Forward thrust of shoulder	Serratus anterior	C5–7	Long thoracic	
Elevation of scapula	Levator scapulae	C3–5	Dorsal scapular	
Medial adduction and eleva- tion of scapula	Rhomboids	C4, 5		
Abduction of arm	Supraspinatus	C4–6	Suprascapular	
Lateral rotation of arm	Infraspinatus	C4–6		
Medial rotation of arm	Latissimus dorsi, teres major, and subscapularis	C5–8	Subscapular (from posterior cord of plexus)	
Adduction of arm from front to back				
Abduction of arm	Deltoid	C5, 6	Axillary (from poste- rior cord of plexus)	
Lateral rotation of arm	Teres minor	C4,5		
Flexion of forearm	Biceps brachii	C5,6	Musculocutaneous (from lateral cord of plexus)	
Supination of forearm				
Adduction of arm	Coracobrachialis	C5–7		
Flexion of forearm				
Flexion of forearm	Brachialis	C5,6		
Ulnar flexion of hand	Flexor carpi ulnaris	C7, 8; T1	Ulnar (from medial cord of plexus)	
Flexion of all fingers but thumb	Flexor digitorum profun- dus (ulnar portion)	C7, 8; T1		
Adduction of metacarpal of thumb	Adductor pollicis	C8, T1		
Abduction of little finger	Abductor digiti quinti	C8, T1		
Opposition of little finger	Opponens digiti quinti	C7, 8; T1		
Flexion of little finger	Flexor digiti quinti	C7, 8; T1		
Flexion of proximal phalanx, extension of 2 distal pha- langes, adduction and ab- duction of fingers	Interossei	C8, T1		
Pronation of forearm	Pronator teres	C6, 7	Median (C6, 7 from lat- eral cord of plexus; C8, T1 from medial cord of plexus)	
Radial flexion of hand	Flexor carpi radialis	C6, 7		
Flexion of hand	Palmaris longus	C7, 8; T1		
Flexion of middle phalanx of index, middle, ring, or little finger	Flexor digitorum superfi- cialis	C7, 8; T1		
Flexion of hand				
Flexion of terminal phalanx of thumb	Flexor pollicis longus	C7, 8; T1		
Flexion of terminal phalanx of index or middle finger	Flexor digitorum profun- dus (radial portion)	C7, 8; T1		
Flexion of hand				

(continued)

Table B-2 (cont'd). Motor function.*

Action to Be Tested	Muscle	Cord Segment	Nerves	Plexus
Shoulder Girdle and Upper Extremity (cont.)				
Abduction of metacarpal of thumb	Abductor pollicis brevis	C7, 8; T1	Median (C7, 8 from lateral cord of plexus; C8, T1 from medial cord of plexus)	Brachial
Flexion of proximal phalanx of thumb	Flexor pollicis brevis	C7, 8; T1		
Opposition of matacarpal of thumb	Opponens pollicis	C8, T1		
Flexion of proximal phalanx and extension of the 2 distal phalanges of index, middle, ring, or little finger	Lumbricales (the 2 lateral)	C8, T1		
	Lumbricales (the 2 medial)	C8, T1	Ulnar	
Extension of forearm	Triceps brachii and anconeus	C6–8	Radial (from posterior cord of plexus)	
Flexion of forearm	Brachioradialis	C5, 6		
Radial extension of hand	Extensor carpi radialis	C6–8		
Extension of phalanges of index, middle, ring, or little finger	Extensor digitorum	C7–8		
Extension of hand				
Extension of phalanges of little finger	Extensor digiti quinti proprius	C6–8		
Extension of hand				
Ulnar extension of hand	Extensor carpi ulnaris	C6–8		
Supination of forearm	Supinator	C5–7	Radial (from posterior cord of plexus)	
Abduction of metacarpal of thumb	Abductor pollicis longus	C7, 8; T1		
Radial extension of hand				
Extension of thumb	Extensor pollicis brevis	C7, 8		
Radial extension of hand	Extensor pollicis longus	C6–8		
Extension of index finger	Extensor indicis proprius	C6–8		
Extension of hand				
Trunk and Thorax				
Elevation of ribs	Thoracic, abdominal, and back	T1–L3	Thoracic and posterior lumbosacral branches	Brachial
Depression of ribs				
Contraction of abdomen				
Anteroflexion of trunk				
Lateral flexion of trunk				
Hip Girdle and Lower Extremity				
Flexion of hip	Iliopsoas	L1–3	Femoral	Lumbar
Flexion of hip (and eversion of thigh)	Sartorius	L2, 3		
Extension of leg	Quadriceps femoris	L2–4		
Adduction of thigh	Pectineus	L2, 3	Obturator	
	Adductor longus	L2, 3		
	Adductor brevis	L2–4		
	Adductor magnus	L3, 4		
	Gracilis	L2–4		
Adduction of thigh	Obturator externus	L3, 4		
Lateral rotation of thigh				

(continued)

Table B-2 (cont'd). Motor function.*

Action to Be Tested	Muscle	Cord Segment	Nerves	Plexus
Abduction of thigh	Gluteus medius and minimus	L4, 5; S1	Superior gluteal	Sacral
Medial rotation of thigh				
Flexion of thigh	Tensor fasciae latae	L4, 5		
Lateral rotation of thigh	Piriformis	S1, 2	. . .	
Abduction of thigh	Gluteus maximus	L4, 5; S1, 2	Inferior gluteal	
Lateral rotation of thigh	Obturator internus	L5, S1,	Muscular branches from sacral plexus	
	Gemelli	L4, 5; S1		
	Quadratus femoris	L4, 5; S1		
Flexion of leg (assist in extension of thigh)	Biceps femoris	L4, 5; S1, 2	Sciatic (trunk)	Sacral
	Semitendinosus	L4, 5; S1		
	Semimembranosus	L4, 5; S1		
Dorsal flexion of foot	Tibialis anterior	L4, 5	Deep peroneal	
Supination of foot				
Extension of toes 2–5	Extensor digitorum longus	L4, 5; S1		
Dorsal flexion of foot				
Extension of great toe	Extensor hallucis longus	L4, 5; S1		
Dorsal flexion of foot				
Extension of great toe and the 3 medial toes	Extensor digitorum brevis	L4, 5; S1		
Plantar flexion of foot in pronation	Peroneus longus and brevis	L5, S1	Superficial peroneal	
	Gastrocnemius	L5, S1, 2	Tibial	
Plantar flexion of foot in supination	Tibialis posterior and triceps surae	L5, S1		
Plantar flexion of foot in supination	Flexor digitorum longus	S1, 2		
Flexion of terminal phalanx of toes II–V				
Plantar flexion of foot in supination	Flexor hallucis longus	L5, S1, 2		
Flexion of terminal phalanx of great toe				
Flexion of middle phalanx of toes II–V	Flexor digitorum brevis	L5, S1		
Flexion of proximal phalanx of great toe	Flexor hallucis brevis	L5, S1, 2		
Spreading and closing of toes	Small muscles of foot	S1, 2		
Flexion of proximal phalanx of toes				
Voluntary control of pelvic floor	Perineal and sphincters	S2–4	Pudendal	

*Modified and reproduced, with permission, from JC McKinley.

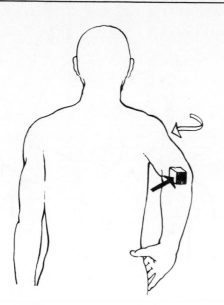

Figure B-3. Rhomboids (C4, 5; dorsal scapular nerve). The shoulder is thrust backward against resistance.

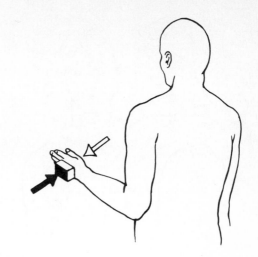

Figure B-5. Infraspinatus (C4–6; suprascapular nerve). With the elbow flexed at the side, the arm is externally rotated against resistance on the forearm.

Note that in all the figures, white arrows indicate the direction of movement in testing the given muscle. Black arrows indicate the direction of resistance, and the blocks show the site of application of resistance.

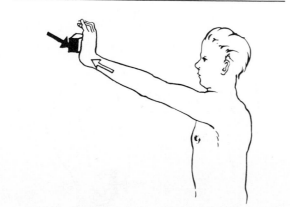

Figure B-4. Serratus anterior (C5–7; long thoracic nerve). The patient pushes hard with outstretched arms; the inner edge of the scapula remains against the thoracic wall. (If the trapezius is weak, the inner edge may move from the chest wall.)

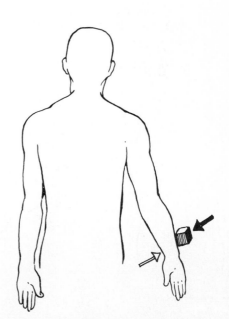

Figure B-6. Supraspinatus (C4–6; suprascapular nerve). The arm is abducted from the side of the body against resistance.

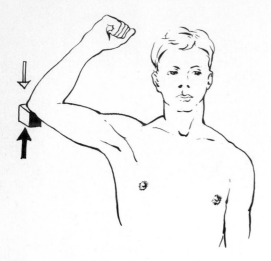

Figure B-7. Latissimus dorsi (C5–8; subscapular nerve). The arm is adducted from a horizontal and lateral position against resistance.

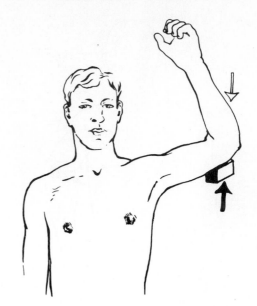

Figure B-9. Pectoralis major, upper portion (C5–8; T1; lateral and medial pectoral nerves). The arm is adducted from an elevated or horizontal and forward position against resistance.

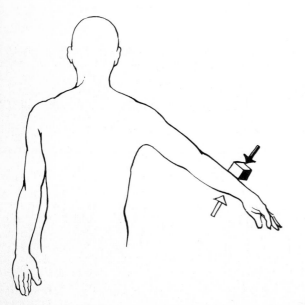

Figure B-8. Deltoid (C5, 6; axillary nerve). Abduction of laterally raised arm (30–75 degrees from body) against resistance.

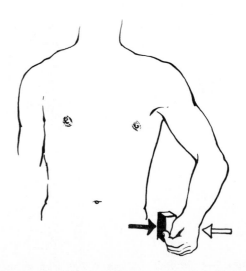

Figure B-10. Pectoralis major, lower portion (C5–8, T1; lateral and medial pectoral nerves). The arm is adducted from a forward position below the horizontal level against resistance.

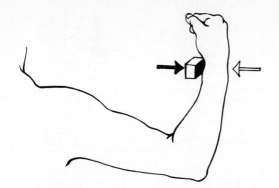

Figure B-11. Biceps (C5, 6; musculocutaneous nerve). The supinated forearm is flexed against resistance.

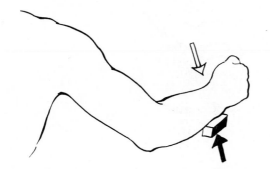

Figure B-12. Triceps (C6-8; radial nerve). The forearm, flexed at the elbow, is extended against resistance.

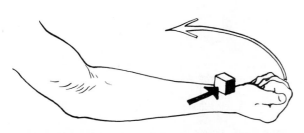

Figure B-13. Brachioradialis (C5, 6; radial nerve). The forearm is flexed against resistance while it is in neutral position (neither pronated nor supinated).

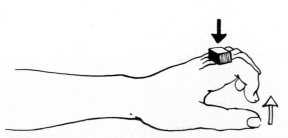

Figure B-14. Extensor digitorum (C7, 8; radial nerve). The fingers are extended at the metacarpophalangeal joints against resistance.

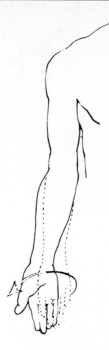

Figure B-15. Supinator (C5-7; radial nerve). The hand is supinated against resistance, with arms extended at the side. Resistance is applied by the grip of the examiner's hand on the patient's forearm near the wrist.

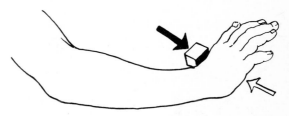

Figure B-16. Extensor carpi radialis (C6-8; radial nerve). The wrist is extended to the radial side against resistance; fingers remain extended.

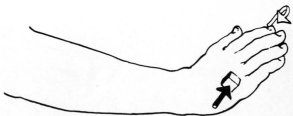

Figure B-17. Extensor carpi ulnaris (C6-8; radial nerve). The wrist joint is extended to the ulnar side against resistance.

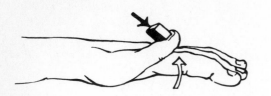

Figure B-18. Extensor pollicis longus (C7, 8; radial nerve). The thumb is extended against resistance.

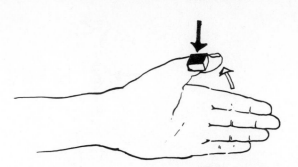

Figure B-21. Abductor pollicis longus (C7, 8; T1; radial nerve). The thumb is abducted against resistance in a plane at a right angle to the palmar surface.

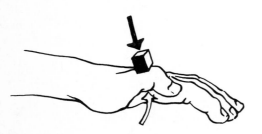

Figure B-19. Extensor pollicis brevis (C7, 8; radial nerve). The thumb is extended at the metacarpophalangeal joint against resistance.

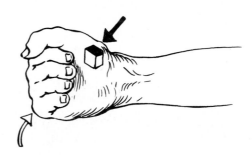

Figure B-22. Flexor carpi radialis (C6, 7; median nerve). The wrist is flexed to the radial side against resistance.

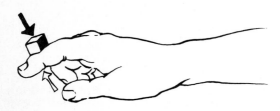

Figure B-20. Extensor indicis proprius (C6–8; radial nerve). The index finger is extended against resistance placed on the dorsal aspect of the finger.

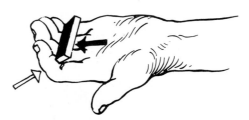

Figure B-23. Flexor digitorum superficialis (C7, 8, T1; median nerve). The fingers are flexed at the first interphalangeal joint against resistance; proximal phalanges remain fixed.

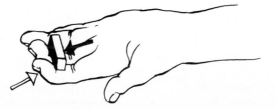

Figure B-24. Flexor digitorum profundus (C7, 8; T1; median nerve). The terminal phalanges of the index and middle fingers are flexed against resistance while the second phalanges are held in extension.

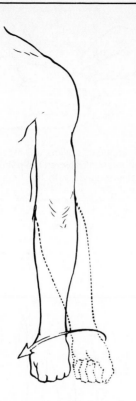

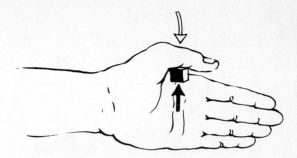

Figure B-28. Flexor pollicis brevis (C7, 8; T1; median nerve). The proximal phalanx of the thumb is flexed against resistance placed on its palmar surface.

Figure B-25. Pronator teres (C6, 7; median nerve). The extended arm is pronated against resistance. Resistance is applied by the grip of the examiner's hand on the patient's forearm near the wrist.

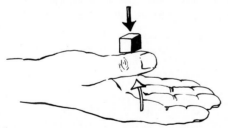

Figure B-26. Abductor pollicis brevis (C7, 8; T1; median nerve). The thumb is abducted against resistance in a plane at a right angle to the palmar surface.

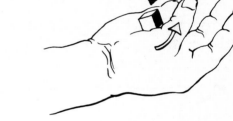

Figure B-29. Opponens pollicis (C8, T1; median nerve). The thumb is crossed over the palm against resistance to touch the top of the little finger, with the thumbnail held parallel to the palm.

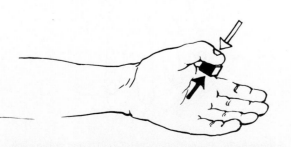

Figure B-27. Flexor pollicis longus (C7, 8; T1; median nerve). The terminal phalanx of the thumb is flexed against resistance as the proximal phalanx is held in extension.

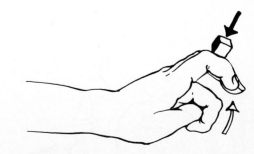

Figure B-30. Lumbricales-interossei, radial half (C8, T1; median and ulnar nerves). The second and third phalanges are extended against resistance; the first phalanx is in full extension. The ulnar has the same innervation and can be tested in the same manner.

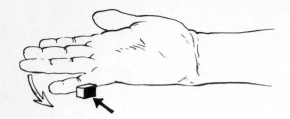

Figure B-31. Flexor carpi ulnaris (C7, 8; T1; ulnar nerve). The little finger is abducted *strongly* against resistance as the supinated hand lies with fingers extended on the table.

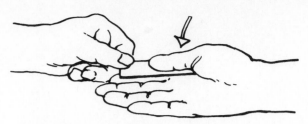

Figure B-34. Adductor pollicis (C8, T1; ulnar nerve). A piece of paper grasped between the palm and the thumb is held against resistance with the thumbnail kept at a right angle to the palm.

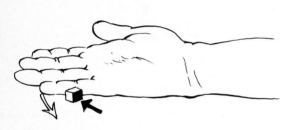

Figure B-32. Abductor digiti quinti (C8, T1; ulnar nerve). The little finger is abducted against resistance as the supinated hand with fingers extended lies on the table.

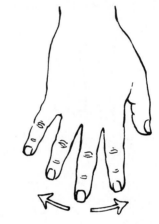

Figure B-35. Dorsal interossei (C8, T1; ulnar nerve). The index and ring fingers are abducted from the midline against resistance as the palm of the hand lies flat on the table.

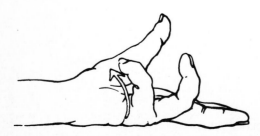

Figure B-33. Opponens digiti quinti (C7, 8; T1; ulnar nerve). With fingers extended, the little finger is moved across the palm to the base of the thumb.

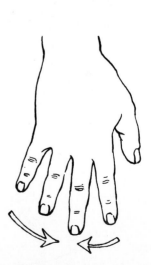

Figure B-36. Palmar interossei (C8, T1; ulnar nerve). The abducted index, ring, and little fingers are adducted to the midline against resistance as the palm of the hand lies flat on the table.

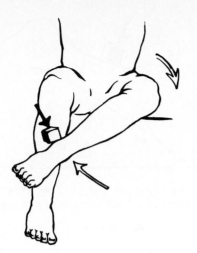

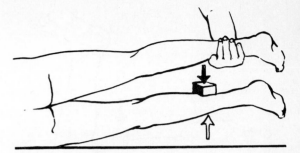

Figure B-40. Adductors (L2–4; obturator nerve). With the patient on one side with knees extended, the lower extremity is adducted against resistance; the upper leg is supported by the examiner.

Figure B-37. Sartorius (L2, 3; femoral nerve). With the patient sitting and the knee flexed, the thigh is rotated outward against resistance on the leg.

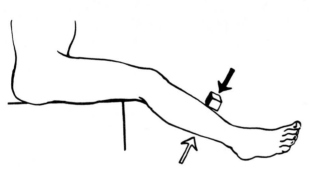

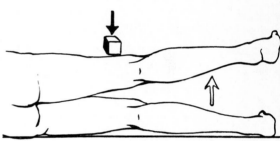

Figure B-41. Gluteus medius and minimus; tensor fasciae latae (L4, 5; S1; superior gluteal nerve). Testing abduction: With the patient lying on one side and the thigh and leg extended, the uppermost lower extremity is abducted against resistance.

Figure B-38. Quadriceps femoris (L2–4; femoral nerve). The knee is extended against resistance on the leg.

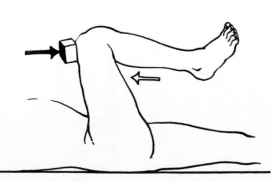

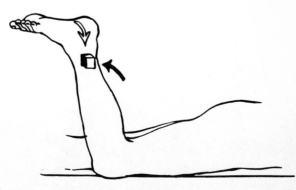

Figure B-39. Iliopsoas (L1–3; femoral nerve). The patient lies supine with the knee flexed. The flexed thigh (at about 90 degrees) is further flexed against resistance.

Figure B-42. Gluteus medius and minimus; tensor fasciae latae (L4, 5; S1; superior gluteal nerve). Testing rotation: With the patient prone and the knee flexed, the foot is moved laterally against resistance.

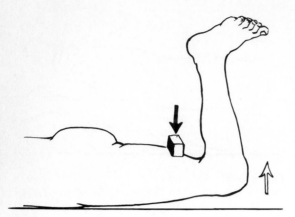

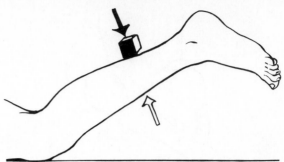

Figure B-43. Gluteus maximus (L4, 5; S1, 2; inferior gluteal nerve). With the patient prone, the knee is lifted off the table against resistance.

Figure B-44. Hamstring group (L4, 5; S1, 2; sciatic nerve). With the patient prone, the knee is flexed against resistance.

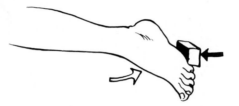

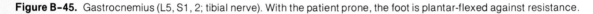

Figure B-45. Gastrocnemius (L5, S1, 2; tibial nerve). With the patient prone, the foot is plantar-flexed against resistance.

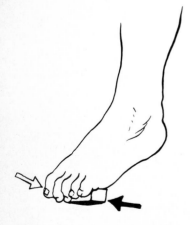

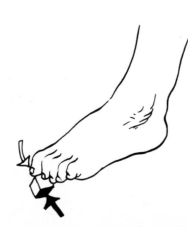

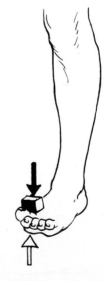

Figure B-46. Flexor digitorum longus (S1, 2; tibial nerve). The toe joints are plantar-flexed against resistance.

Figure B-47. Flexor hallucis longus (L5, S1, 2; tibial nerve). The great toe is plantar-flexed against resistance. The second and third toes are also flexed.

Figure B-48. Extensor hallucis longus (L4, 5; S1; deep peroneal nerve). The large toe is dorsiflexed against resistance.

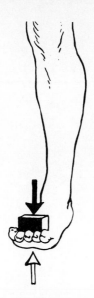

Figure B-49. Extensor digitorum longus (L4, 5; S1; deep peroneal nerve). The toes are dorsiflexed against resistance.

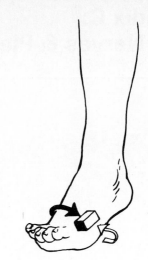

Figure B-51. Peroneus longus and brevis (L5, S1; superficial peroneal nerve). The foot is everted against resistance applied by gripping the foot with the examiner's hand.

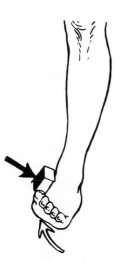

Figure B-50. Tibialis anterior (L4, 5; deep peroneal nerve). The foot is dorsiflexed and inverted against resistance applied by gripping the foot with the examiner's hand.

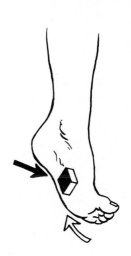

Figure B-52. Tibialis posterior (L5, S1; tibial nerve). The plantar-flexed foot is inverted against resistance applied by gripping the foot with the examiner's hand.

Appendix C:
Spinal Nerves & Plexuses

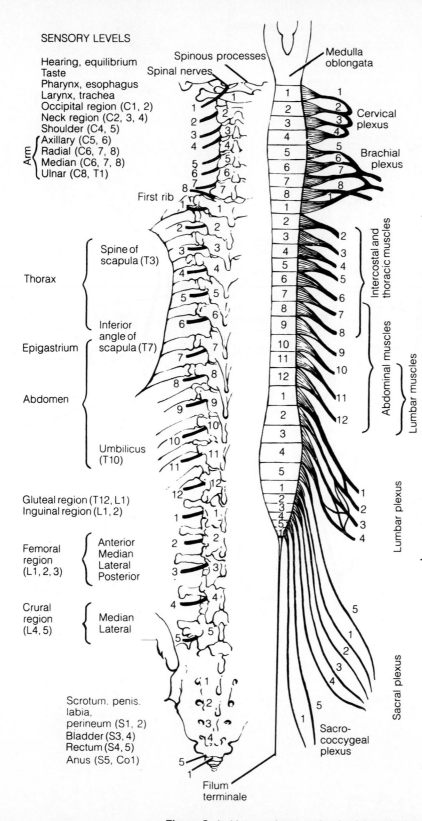

SENSORY LEVELS

Hearing, equilibrium
Taste
Pharynx, esophagus
Larynx, trachea
Occipital region (C1, 2)
Neck region (C2, 3, 4)
Shoulder (C4, 5)

Arm
{
Axillary (C5, 6)
Radial (C6, 7, 8)
Median (C6, 7, 8)
Ulnar (C8, T1)
}

Thorax { Spine of scapula (T3)

Epigastrium { Inferior angle of scapula (T7)

Abdomen {

Umbilicus (T10)

Gluteal region (T12, L1)
Inguinal region (L1, 2)

Femoral region (L1, 2, 3)
{
Anterior
Median
Lateral
Posterior
}

Crural region (L4, 5)
{
Median
Lateral
}

Scrotum. penis.
labia,
perineum (S1, 2)
Bladder (S3, 4)
Rectum (S4, 5)
Anus (S5, Co1)

Spinous processes
Spinal nerves
First rib
Filum terminale

Medulla oblongata
Cervical plexus
Brachial plexus
Intercostal and thoracic muscles
Abdominal muscles
Lumbar muscles
Lumbar plexus
Sacral plexus
Sacro-coccygeal plexus

MOTOR LEVELS

Facial muscles VII
Pharyngeal, palatine muscles X
Laryngeal muscles XI
Tongue muscles XII
Esophagus X
Sternocleidomastoid XI (C1, 2, 3)
Neck muscles (C1, 2, 3)
Trapezius (C3, 4)
Rhomboids (C4, 5)
Diaphragm (C3, 4, 5)
Supra-, infraspinatus (C4, 5, 6)

Deltoid, brachioradialis,
  and biceps (C5, 6)
Serratus anterior (C5, 6, 7)
Pectoralis major (C5, 6, 7, 8)   Arm
Teres minor (C4, 5)
Pronators (C6, 7, 8, T1)
Triceps (C6, 7, 8)

Long extensors of carpi
  and digits (C6, 7, 8)
Latissimus dorsi, teres   Forearm
  major (C5, 6, 7, 8)
Long flexors (C7, 8, T1)

Thumb extensors (C7, 8)
Interossei, lumbricales,   Hand
  thenar, hypothenar (C8, T1)

Iliopsoas (L1, 2, 3)
Sartorius (L2, 3)
Quadriceps femoris (L2, 3, 4)
Gluteal muscles (L4, 5, S1)
Tensor fasciae latae (L4, 5)
Adductors of femur (L2, 3, 4)
Abductors of femur (L4, 5, S1)
Tibialis anterior (L5)
Gastrocnemius, soleus (L5, S1, 2)
Biceps, semitendinosus,
  semimembranosus (L4, 5, S1)
Obturator, piriformis,
  quadratus femoris (L4, 5, S1)
Flexors of the foot,
  extensors of toes (L5, S1)
Peronei (L5, S1)
Flexors of toes (L5, S1, 2)
Interossei (S1, 2)
Perineal muscles (S3, 4)
Vesicular muscles (S4, 5)
Rectal muscles (S4, 5, Co1)

Figure C-1. Motor and sensory levels of the spinal cord.

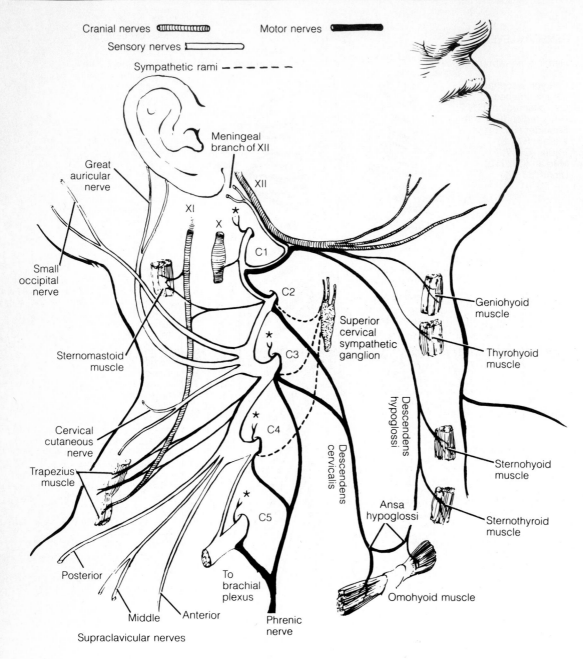

Figure C-2. The cervical plexus.

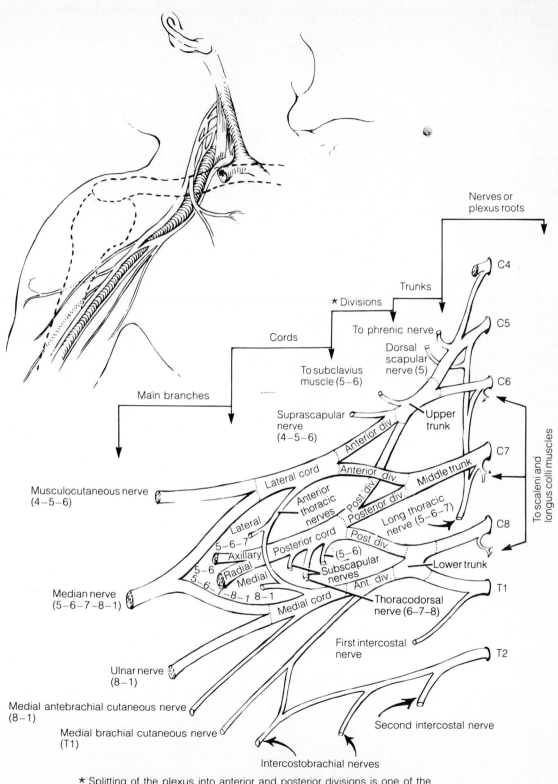

Nerves or
plexus roots

Trunks

★ Divisions

To phrenic nerve

Dorsal
scapular
nerve (5)

Cords

To subclavius
muscle (5–6)

Main branches

Suprascapular
nerve
(4–5–6)

Anterior div.

Upper
trunk

C4

C5

C6

C7

C8

To scaleni and
longus colli muscles

Musculocutaneous nerve
(4–5–6)

Lateral cord

Anterior div.

Anterior
thoracic
nerves

Post. div.

Posterior div.

Middle trunk

Long thoracic
nerve (5–6–7)

Lateral
5–6–7
Axillary

Radial

Posterior cord

Post div.

(5–6)
Subscapular
nerves

Lower trunk

T1

Median nerve
(5–6–7–8–1)

5–6

5–6
5–6
–8–1

Medial

8–1

Medial cord

Ant. div.

Thoracodorsal
nerve (6–7–8)

First intercostal
nerve

T2

Ulnar nerve
(8–1)

Medial antebrachial cutaneous nerve
(8–1)

Medial brachial cutaneous nerve
(T1)

Second intercostal nerve

Intercostobrachial nerves

★ Splitting of the plexus into anterior and posterior divisions is one of the
most significant features in the redistribution of nerve fibers, since it is
here that fibers supplying the flexor and extensor groups of muscles of
the upper extremity are separated. Similar splitting is noted in the lumbar
and sacral plexuses for the supply of muscles of the lower extremity.

Figure C–3. The brachial plexus.

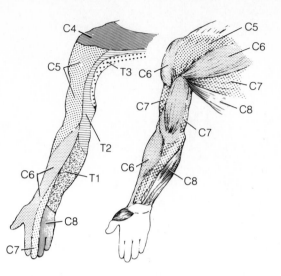

Figure C–4. Segmental innervation of the right upper extremity, anterior view. (Reproduced, with permission, from Inman VT, Saunders JBdeCM: Referred pain from skeletal structures. *J Nerv Ment Dis* 1944;**99:**660.)

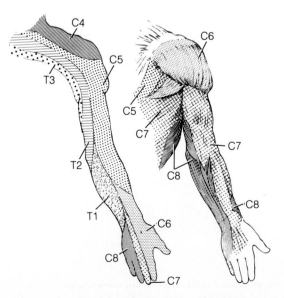

Figure C–5. Segmental innervation of the right upper extremity, posterior view. (Reproduced, with permission, from Inman VT, Saunders JBdeCM: Referred pain from skeletal structures. *J Nerv Ment Dis* 1944;**99:**660.)

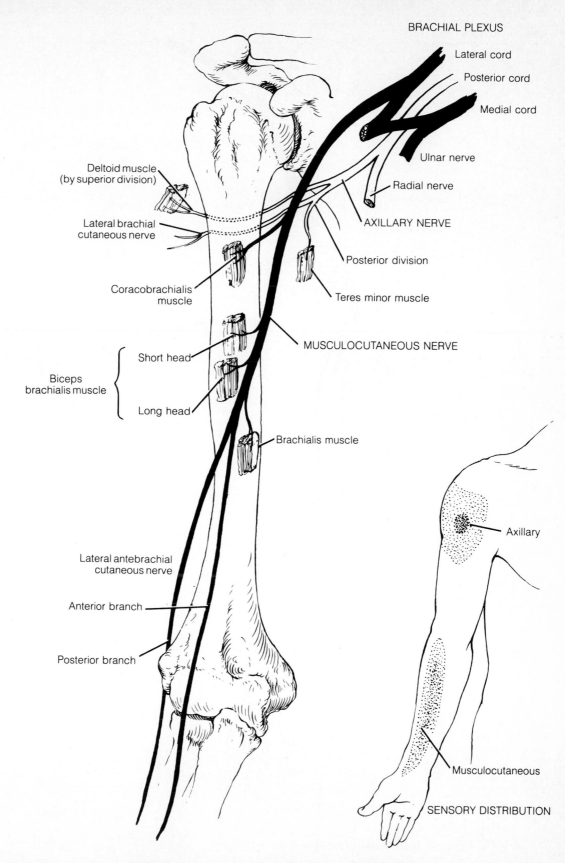

Figure C-6. Musculocutaneous (C5, 6) and axillary (C5, 6) nerves.

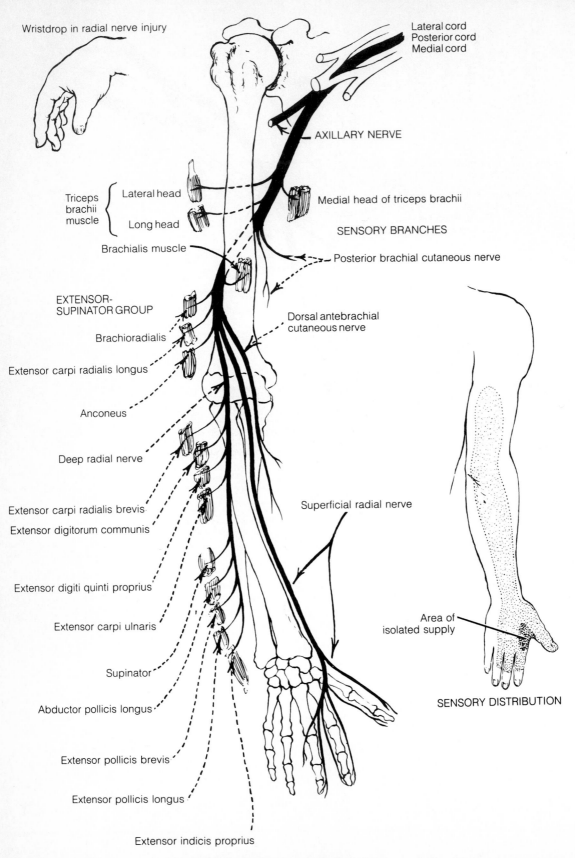

Wristdrop in radial nerve injury

Lateral cord
Posterior cord
Medial cord

AXILLARY NERVE

Triceps brachii muscle { Lateral head / Long head

Medial head of triceps brachii

SENSORY BRANCHES

Brachialis muscle

Posterior brachial cutaneous nerve

EXTENSOR-SUPINATOR GROUP

Dorsal antebrachial cutaneous nerve

Brachioradialis

Extensor carpi radialis longus

Anconeus

Deep radial nerve

Extensor carpi radialis brevis

Extensor digitorum communis

Superficial radial nerve

Extensor digiti quinti proprius

Extensor carpi ulnaris

Supinator

Area of isolated supply

Abductor pollicis longus

SENSORY DISTRIBUTION

Extensor pollicis brevis

Extensor pollicis longus

Extensor indicis proprius

Figure C-7. The radial nerve (C6–8, T1).

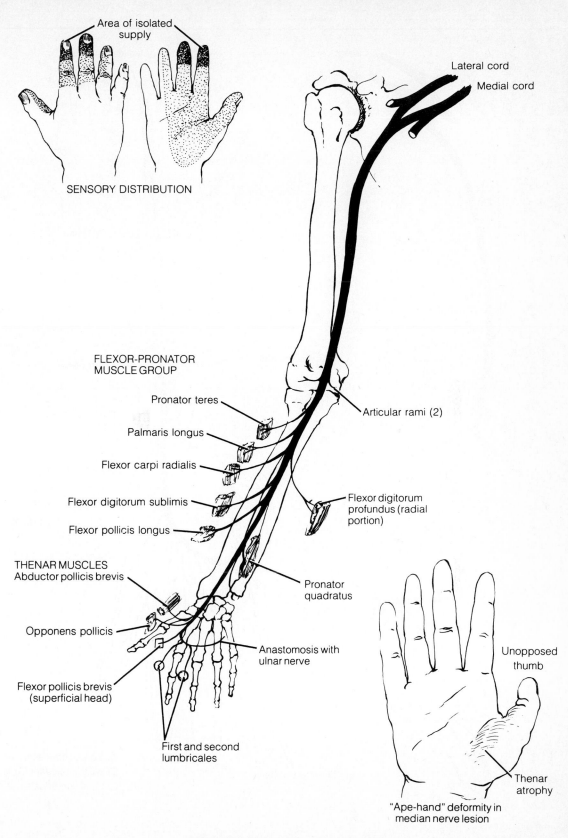

Area of isolated supply

SENSORY DISTRIBUTION

Lateral cord

Medial cord

FLEXOR-PRONATOR
MUSCLE GROUP

Pronator teres

Palmaris longus

Flexor carpi radialis

Flexor digitorum sublimis

Flexor pollicis longus

THENAR MUSCLES
Abductor pollicis brevis

Opponens pollicis

Flexor pollicis brevis
(superficial head)

First and second
lumbricales

Articular rami (2)

Flexor digitorum
profundus (radial
portion)

Pronator
quadratus

Anastomosis with
ulnar nerve

Unopposed
thumb

Thenar
atrophy

"Ape-hand" deformity in
median nerve lesion

Figure C-8. The median nerve (C6–8, T1).

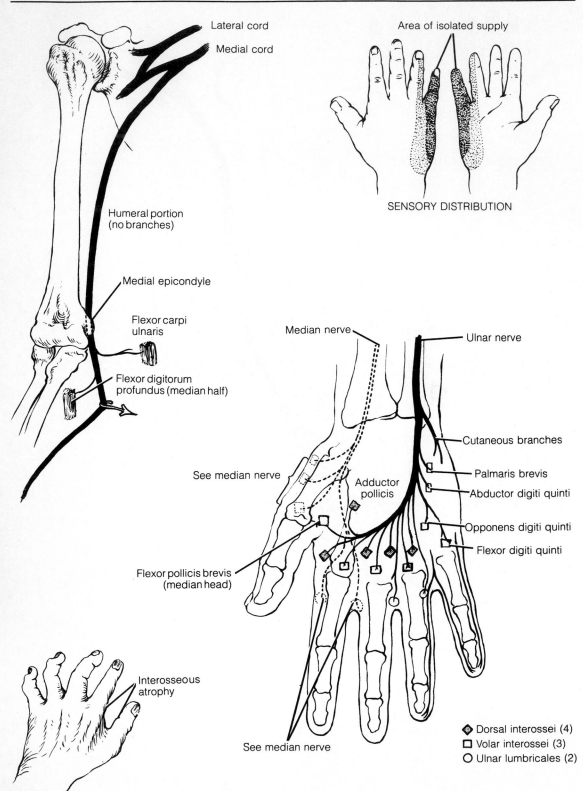

Lateral cord

Medial cord

Area of isolated supply

SENSORY DISTRIBUTION

Humeral portion
(no branches)

Medial epicondyle

Flexor carpi
ulnaris

Flexor digitorum
profundus (median half)

Median nerve

Ulnar nerve

See median nerve

Adductor
pollicis

Cutaneous branches

Palmaris brevis

Abductor digiti quinti

Opponens digiti quinti

Flexor digiti quinti

Flexor pollicis brevis
(median head)

Interosseous
atrophy

See median nerve

◈ Dorsal interossei (4)
☐ Volar interossei (3)
○ Ulnar lumbricales (2)

Clawhand deformity
in ulnar lesions

Figure C–9. The ulnar nerve (C8, T1).

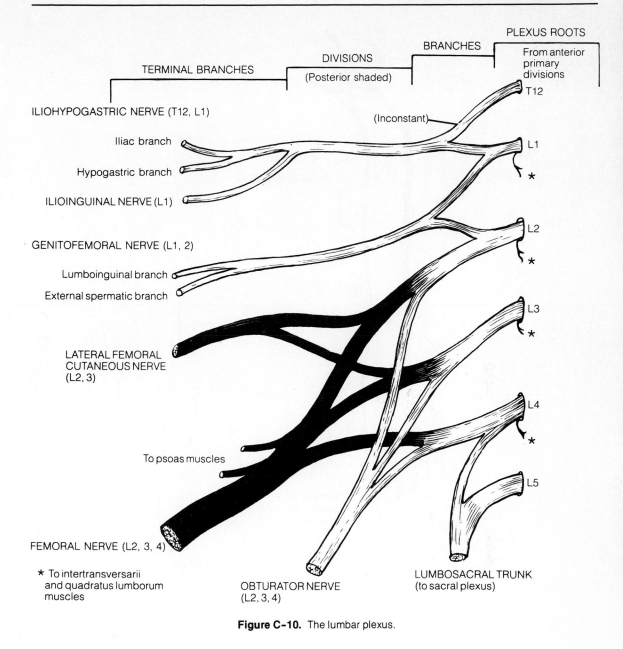

TERMINAL BRANCHES

DIVISIONS
(Posterior shaded)

BRANCHES

PLEXUS ROOTS
From anterior primary divisions

T12

ILIOHYPOGASTRIC NERVE (T12, L1)

(Inconstant)

Iliac branch

L1

Hypogastric branch

*

ILIOINGUINAL NERVE (L1)

GENITOFEMORAL NERVE (L1, 2)

L2

*

Lumboinguinal branch

External spermatic branch

L3

*

LATERAL FEMORAL CUTANEOUS NERVE (L2, 3)

L4

*

To psoas muscles

L5

FEMORAL NERVE (L2, 3, 4)

* To intertransversarii and quadratus lumborum muscles

OBTURATOR NERVE (L2, 3, 4)

LUMBOSACRAL TRUNK (to sacral plexus)

Figure C-10. The lumbar plexus.

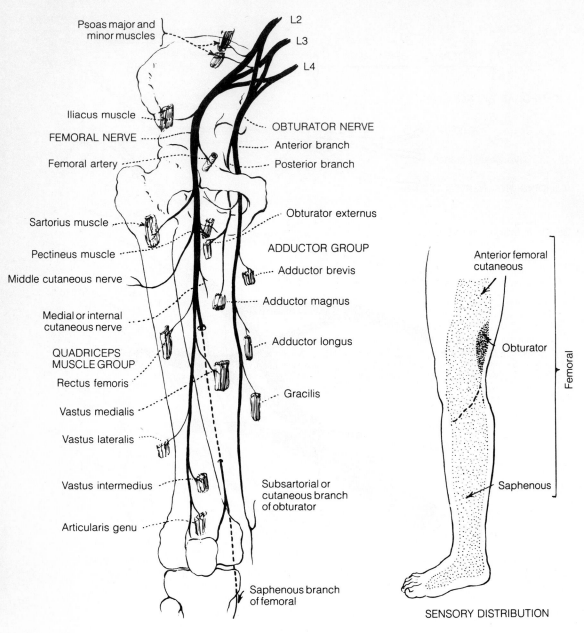

Psoas major and
minor muscles

L2
L3
L4

Iliacus muscle

FEMORAL NERVE

Femoral artery

OBTURATOR NERVE

Anterior branch

Posterior branch

Sartorius muscle

Pectineus muscle

Middle cutaneous nerve

Medial or internal
cutaneous nerve

QUADRICEPS
MUSCLE GROUP

Rectus femoris

Vastus medialis

Vastus lateralis

Vastus intermedius

Articularis genu

Obturator externus

ADDUCTOR GROUP

Adductor brevis

Adductor magnus

Adductor longus

Gracilis

Subsartorial or
cutaneous branch
of obturator

Saphenous branch
of femoral

Anterior femoral
cutaneous

Obturator

Femoral

Saphenous

SENSORY DISTRIBUTION

Figure C–11. The femoral (L2–4) and obturator (L2–4) nerves.

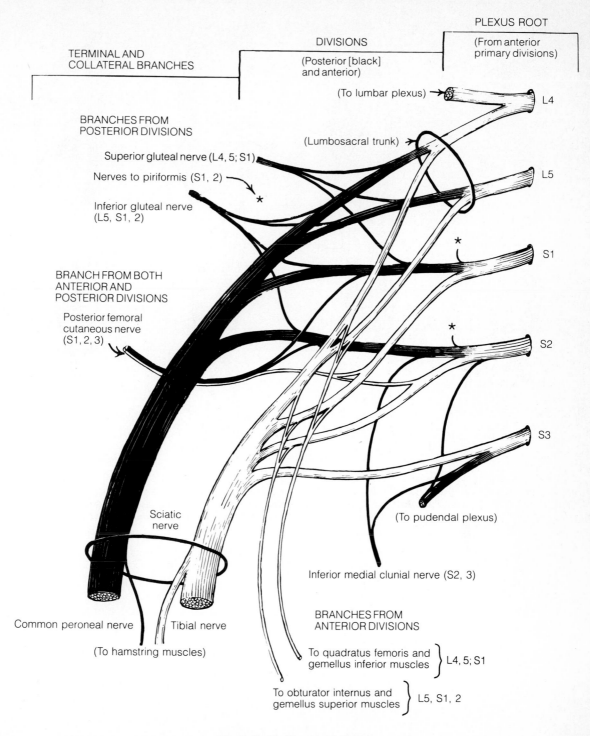

PLEXUS ROOT

(From anterior primary divisions)

DIVISIONS

(Posterior [black] and anterior)

TERMINAL AND COLLATERAL BRANCHES

(To lumbar plexus)

L4

BRANCHES FROM POSTERIOR DIVISIONS

(Lumbosacral trunk)

Superior gluteal nerve (L4, 5; S1)

L5

Nerves to piriformis (S1, 2)

*

Inferior gluteal nerve (L5, S1, 2)

*

S1

BRANCH FROM BOTH ANTERIOR AND POSTERIOR DIVISIONS

Posterior femoral cutaneous nerve (S1, 2, 3)

*

S2

S3

Sciatic nerve

(To pudendal plexus)

Inferior medial clunial nerve (S2, 3)

Common peroneal nerve

Tibial nerve

(To hamstring muscles)

BRANCHES FROM ANTERIOR DIVISIONS

To quadratus femoris and gemellus inferior muscles } L4, 5; S1

To obturator internus and gemellus superior muscles } L5, S1, 2

Figure C–12. The sacral plexus.

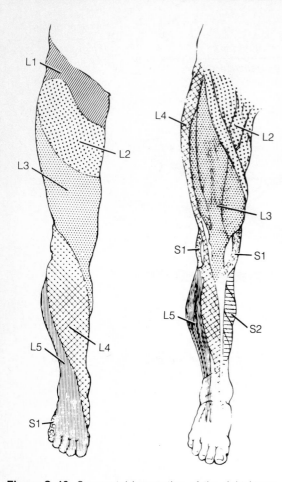

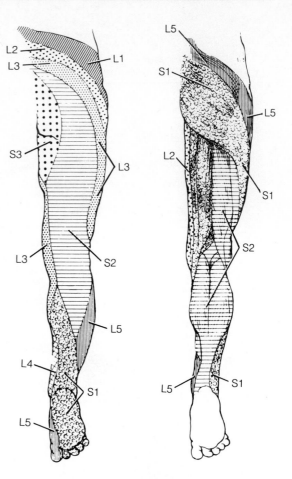

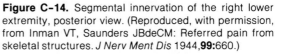

Figure C-13. Segmental innervation of the right lower extremity, anterior view. (Reproduced, with permission, from Inman VT, Saunders JBdeCM: Referred pain from skeletal structures. *J Nerv Ment Dis* 1944;**99:**660.)

Figure C-14. Segmental innervation of the right lower extremity, posterior view. (Reproduced, with permission, from Inman VT, Saunders JBdeCM: Referred pain from skeletal structures. *J Nerv Ment Dis* 1944,**99:**660.)

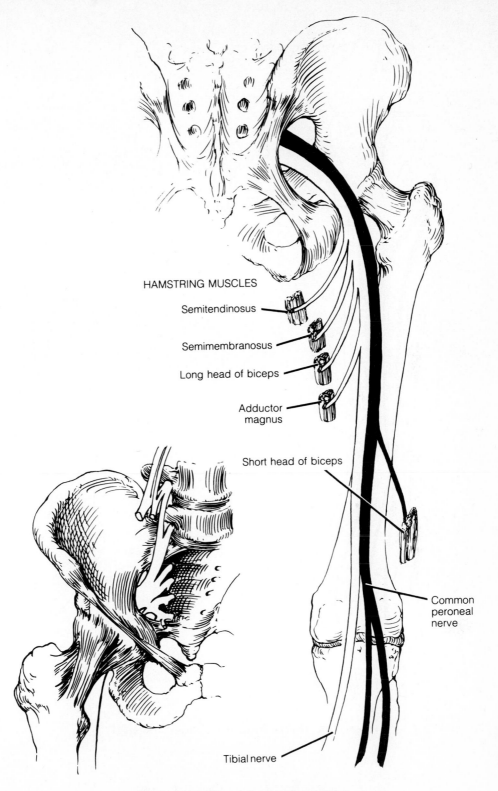

HAMSTRING MUSCLES

Semitendinosus

Semimembranosus

Long head of biceps

Adductor
magnus

Short head of biceps

Common
peroneal
nerve

Tibial nerve

Figure C–15. The sciatic nerve (L4, 5; S1–3).

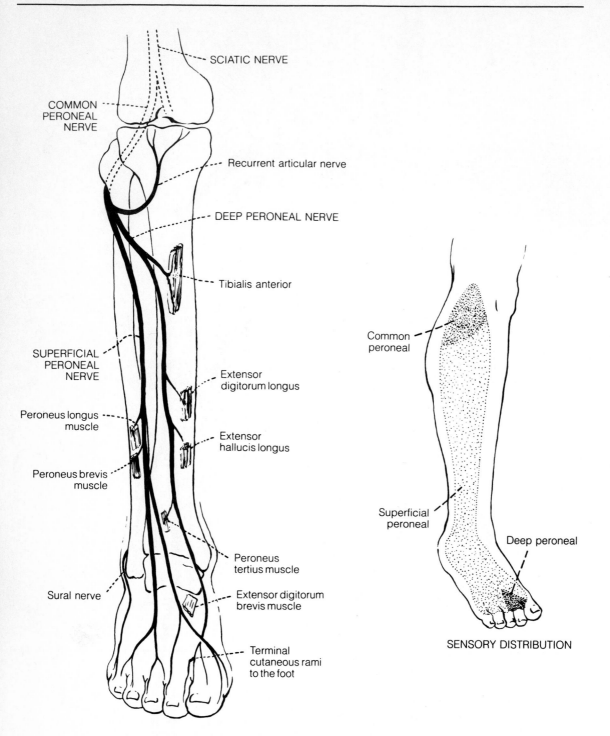

SCIATIC NERVE

COMMON
PERONEAL
NERVE

Recurrent articular nerve

DEEP PERONEAL NERVE

Tibialis anterior

SUPERFICIAL
PERONEAL
NERVE

Extensor
digitorum longus

Peroneus longus
muscle

Extensor
hallucis longus

Peroneus brevis
muscle

Peroneus
tertius muscle

Sural nerve

Extensor digitorum
brevis muscle

Terminal
cutaneous rami
to the foot

Common
peroneal

Superficial
peroneal

Deep peroneal

SENSORY DISTRIBUTION

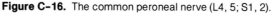

Figure C–16. The common peroneal nerve (L4, 5; S1, 2).

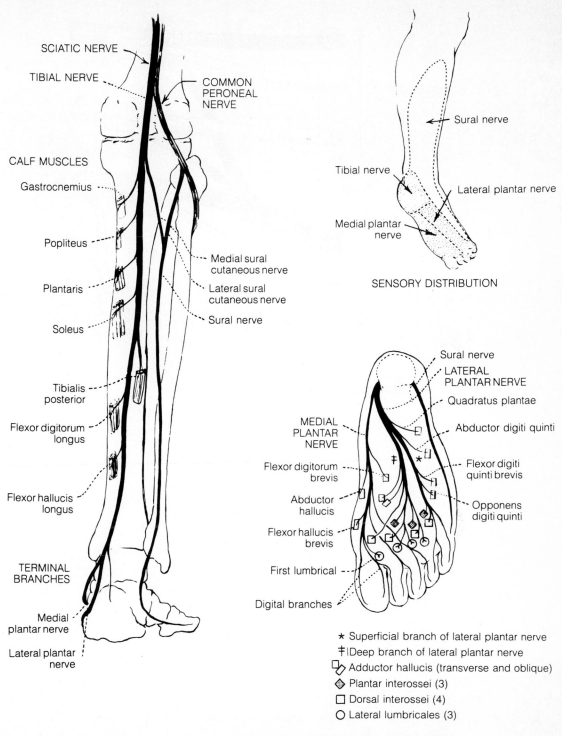

SCIATIC NERVE

TIBIAL NERVE

COMMON PERONEAL NERVE

CALF MUSCLES

Gastrocnemius

Popliteus

Plantaris

Soleus

Tibialis posterior

Flexor digitorum longus

Flexor hallucis longus

TERMINAL BRANCHES

Medial plantar nerve

Lateral plantar nerve

Medial sural cutaneous nerve

Lateral sural cutaneous nerve

Sural nerve

Sural nerve

Tibial nerve

Lateral plantar nerve

Medial plantar nerve

SENSORY DISTRIBUTION

Sural nerve

LATERAL PLANTAR NERVE

Quadratus plantae

Abductor digiti quinti

Flexor digiti quinti brevis

Opponens digiti quinti

MEDIAL PLANTAR NERVE

Flexor digitorum brevis

Abductor hallucis

Flexor hallucis brevis

First lumbrical

Digital branches

★ Superficial branch of lateral plantar nerve

‡ Deep branch of lateral plantar nerve

⬗ Adductor hallucis (transverse and oblique)

◈ Plantar interossei (3)

☐ Dorsal interossei (4)

○ Lateral lumbricales (3)

PLANTAR VIEW OF THE FOOT

Figure C–17. The tibial nerve (L4, 5; S1–3).

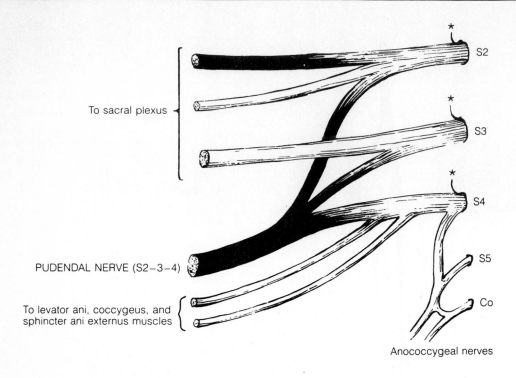

To sacral plexus

PUDENDAL NERVE (S2–3–4)

To levator ani, coccygeus, and
sphincter ani externus muscles

S2

S3

S4

S5

Co

Anococcygeal nerves

* Visceral branches

Figure C–18. The pudendal and coccygeal plexuses.

Appendix D:
Questions & Answers

QUESTIONS

Section I: Chapters 1, 2, and 3
In the following questions, select the single best answer.

1. A spike initiated in the initial segment of a motor neuron propagates in both directions (ie, both out along the axon and back into the soma)—
   A. always.
   B. sometimes.
   C. never.
2. In a motor neuron at rest, an excitatory synapse produces an EPSP of 15 mV, and an inhibitory synapse produces an IPSP of 5 mV. If both the EPSP and IPSP occur simultaneously, then the motor neuron would—
   A. depolarize by about 10 mV.
   B. depolarize by about 15 mV.
   C. change the potential by less than 10 mV.
3. The equilibrium potential for chloride in motor neurons is ordinarily nearest the—
   A. equilibrium potential for sodium.
   B. resting potential.
   C. reversal potential for the EPSP.
4. An axon in an absolute refractory period is unable to conduct another action potential for about one millisecond after an action potential passes because—
   A. it takes that long for ion pumps to restore K^+ to the cell's interior.
   B. the spike takes that long to reach the end of the axon.
   C. sodium channels take that long to recover from inactivation.
5. The cerebrum consists of the—
   A. thalamus and basal ganglia.
   B. telencephalon and midbrain.
   C. telencephalon and diencephalon.
   D. brain stem and prosencephalon.
   E. cerebellum and prosencephalon.
6. The somatic nervous system innervates the—
   A. blood vessels of the skin.
   B. blood vessels of the brain.
   C. muscles of the heart.
   D. muscles of the body wall.
   E. muscles of the viscera.

7. Microglial cells are also called—
   A. astrocytes.
   B. collateral cells.
   C. oligodendrocytes.
   D. lymphocytes.
   E. rod cells.
8. Synaptic vessels with a dense core contain—
   A. catecholamine.
   B. GABA.
   C. substance P.
   D. endorphin.
   E. glutamic acid.
9. The peripheral nervous system—
   A. includes the spinal cord.
   B. is sheathed in fluid-filled spaces enclosed by membranes.
   C. includes cranial nerves.
   D. does not include spinal nerves.
   E. is surrounded by bone.
10. The only one of the following substances normally not found in nervous tissue of a newborn is—
    A. water.
    B. inorganic salts.
    C. iron.
    D. lipids.
    E. calcium.

In the following questions, one or more answers may be correct. Select—
   A if 1, 2, and 3 are correct;
   B if 1 and 3 are correct;
   C if 2 and 4 are correct;
   D if only 4 is correct;
   E if all are correct.
11. A spinal motor neuron in an adult—
    1. maintains its membrane potential via the active transport of sodium ions.
    2. synthesizes protein only in the cell body but transmits newly formed protein.
    3. does not synthesize DNA for mitosis.
    4. does not regenerate its axon following section of its peripheral portion.
12. The myelin sheath is—
    1. produced within the central nervous system by oligodendrites.
    2. produced within the peripheral nervous system by Schwann (neurilemma) cells.

3. interrupted periodically by the nodes of Ranvier.
4. composed of spirally wrapped plasma membrane.

13. Most materials synthesized in the cell body move along the axon to synaptic terminals by a process involving—
1. extracellular fluid movement.
2. action potentials.
3. hydrostatic pressure gradients.
4. axoplasmic transport.

14. Astrocytes—
1. may function as a sink for extracellular K^+.
2. are interconnected by gap junctions.
3. can proliferate to form a scar following an injury.
4. migrate to the central nervous system from bone marrow.

15. The cell body of most neurons—
1. cannot divide in the adult.
2. is the main site of protein synthesis in the neuron.
3. is the site of the cell nucleus.
4. invariably has a volume greater than that of the axon.

16. Most synaptic terminals of axons that form chemical synapses in the central nervous system contain—
1. synaptic vesicles.
2. presynaptic densities.
3. neurotransmitter(s).
4. rough endoplasmic reticulum.

17. Cells that form myelin include—
1. Schwann cells.
2. astrocytes.
3. oligodendrocytes.
4. some neurons in the central nervous system.

18. In axoplasmic transport—
1. some macromolecules move away from the cell body at rates of several centimeters per day.
2. mitochondria move along the axon.
3. microtubules seem to be involved.
4. some types of molecules move toward the cell body at rates of 80–150 mm per day.

19. The subdivision of the brain stem includes the—
1. metencephalon.
2. diencephalon.
3. midbrain.
4. medulla spinalis.

20. A ganglion is defined as a—
1. part of the basal ganglia.
2. group of nerve cell bodies within the hypothalamus.
3. layer of similar cells in the cerebral cortex.

4. group of nerve cell bodies outside the neuraxis.

21. The nerve conduction velocity is higher in—
1. myelinated fibers than in unmyelinated fibers.
2. pain and temperature fibers than in proprioceptive fibers.
3. somatic motor fibers than in efferents to muscle spindles.
4. preganglionic fibers than in pain and temperature fibers.

22. Neurotransmitters found in the brain stem include—
1. acetylcholine.
2. norepinephrine.
3. dopamine.
4. serotonin.

23. The cell layer around the central canal of the spinal cord—
1. is called the ventricular zone.
2. is the same as the pia.
3. encloses cerebrospinal fluid.
4. is called the marginal zone.

24. Norepinephrine is found in the—
1. sympathetic nervous system.
2. locus ceruleus.
3. lateral tegmentum of the midbrain.
4. neuromuscular junction.

25. Decussations are—
1. aggregates of tracts.
2. fiber bundles in a spinal nerve.
3. horizontal connections crossing within the central nervous system from left to right.
4. vertical connections crossing within the central nervous system from left to right or vice versa.

Section II: Chapters 4 and 5

In the following questions, select the single best answer.

1. The spinothalamic tract—
   A. contains axons that respond to noxious stimulation.
   B. contains axons that respond to innocuous stimulation.
   C. terminates in part in the ventroposterolateral nucleus of the thalamus.
   D. contains only axons originating in laminas I and V of the dorsal horn.

2. A patient complains of unsteadiness. Examination shows a marked diminution of position sense, vibration sense, and stereognosis in all extremities. He is unable to stand without wavering for more than a few seconds when his eyes are closed. There are no other findings. The lesion most likely involves the—

A. lateral columns of the spinal cord, bilaterally.
B. inferior cerebellar peduncles, bilaterally.
C. dorsal columns of the cord, bilaterally.
D. spinothalamic tracts, bilaterally.

3. The lateral column of the spinal cord contains the—
A. lateral corticospinal tract.
B. direct corticospinal tract.
C. cuneate tract.
D. Lissauer's tract.
E. Gracile tract.

4. The alar plate is separated from the basal plate by the—
A. central canal.
B. mantle layer.
C. lamina terminalis.
D. dorsal root ganglion.
E. ependyma.

5. The following fiber systems in the spinal cord are descending tracts except for the—
A. rubrospinal tract.
B. ventrolateral tract.
C. corticospinal tract.
D. tectospinal tract.
E. medial longitudinal lemniscus.

6. A sign of an upper motor lesion in the spinal cord is—
A. severe muscle atrophy.
B. hyperactive deep tendon reflexes.
C. flaccid paralysis.
D. absence of pathologic reflexes.
E. absence of withdrawal responses.

7. The following fiber systems in the spinal cord are ascending tracts except for the—
A. cuneate tract.
B. ventral spinocerebellar tract.
C. spinothalamic tract.
D. spinoreticular tract.
E. reticulospinal tract.

8. The spinal subarachnoid space normally—
A. lies between the pachymeninx and the arachnoid.
B. lies between the pia and the arachnoid.
C. ends at the cauda equina.
D. communicates with the peritoneal space.
E. is adjacent to the vertebrae.

9. The subclavian artery gives rise directly to the—
A. lumbar radicular artery.
B. great ventral radicular artery.
C. anterior spinal artery.
D. vertebral artery.

10. The nucleus dorsalis (of Clarke) in the spinal cord—
A. receives contralateral input from dorsal ganglia.
B. terminates at the L2 segment.
C. terminates in the midbrain.
D. terminates in the ipsilateral cerebellum.

E. receives fibers from the external cuneate nucleus.

In the following questions, one or more answers may be correct. Select—
A if **1, 2,** and **3** are correct;
B if **1** and **3** are correct;
C if **2** and **4** are correct;
D if only **4** is correct;
E if all are correct.

11. Fine diameter dorsal root axons of L5 on one side terminate in the—
1. marginal layer of the ipsilateral dorsal horn.
2. ipsilateral substantia gelatinosa.
3. ipsilateral lamina V of the dorsal horn.
4. ipsilateral nucleus dorsalis (of Clarke).

12. Cells in lamina V of the dorsal horn respond to—
1. visceral afferent inputs.
2. noxious tactile stimulation.
3. nonnoxious tactile stimulation.
4. auditory stimulation.

13. A-delta and C peripheral afferent fibers—
1. terminate in laminas I and II of the dorsal horn.
2. excite lamina IV neurons in the dorsal horn.
3. terminate in lamina V of the dorsal horn.
4. convey the sensation of light touch.

14. Axons of dorsal root ganglion cells of L5 on the right side synapse with cells in the right—
1. gracile nucleus.
2. cuneate nucleus.
3. nucleus dorsalis.
4. external cuneate nucleus.

15. The long-term consequences of a left hemisection of the spinal cord at midthoracic level would include—
1. loss of voluntary movement of the left leg.
2. loss of pain and temperature sensation in the right leg.
3. diminished position and vibration sense in the left leg.
4. diminished deep tendon reflexes in the left leg.

16. In humans, the spinothalamic tract—
1. carries information from the ipsilateral side of the body.
2. exhibits topographic organization.
3. arises principally from neurons of the same side of the cord.
4. mediates information about pain and temperature.

17. The spinothalamic tract of the left side of the spinal cord—
1. arises primarily from neurons of the left spinal gray matter.
2. arises primarily from neurons of the right spinal gray matter.

3. terminates principally in nuclei of the right thalamus.
4. terminates principally in nuclei of the left thalamus.

18. Large-diameter dorsal root axons of one side of L5 terminate in the—
    1. marginal layer of the ipsilateral dorsal horn.
    2. ipsilateral nucleus gracilis.
    3. ipsilateral nucleus cuneatus.
    4. ipsilateral nucleus dorsalis (of Clarke).

19. The fibers carrying information from the spinal cord to the cerebellum—
    1. can arise from Clarke's column cells (nucleus dorsalis).
    2. represent the contralateral body half in the dorsal spinocerebellar tract.
    3. can arise from cells of the external cuneate nucleus.
    4. are important elements in the conscious sensation of joint position.

20. In patients with spasticity associated with a suprasegmental lesion, the—
    1. stretch reflex threshold is lowered.
    2. blocking of fusimotor innervation to the spastic muscles diminishes the spasticity.
    3. inverse myotatic (clasp-knife) reflex can be more readily evoked than in normal subjects.
    4. firing threshold of motor neurons innervating spastic musculature is lowered.

21. Gamma efferent motor neurons—
    1. are located in the intermediolateral cell column of the spinal cord.
    2. cause contraction of intrafusal muscle fibers.
    3. provide vasomotor control to blood vessels in muscles.
    4. are modulated by axons in the vestibulospinal tract.

22. The dorsal column system of one side of the spinal cord—
    1. is essential for normal 2-point discrimination on that side.
    2. arises from both dorsal root ganglion cells and dorsal horn neurons.
    3. synapses upon neurons of the ipsilateral dorsal column.
    4. consists primarily of large, myelinated, rapidly conducting axons.

23. The dorsal spinocerebellar tract of one side—
    1. carries information arising from the ipsilateral body half.
    2. contains axons of ipsilateral dorsal root ganglion cells.
    3. terminates in the ipsilateral cerebellum.
    4. is a major pathway for the conscious sensation of joint position (proprioception).

24. The left seventh cervical nerve passes through an intervertebral foramen between—
    1. C7 and C8.
    2. T1 and T2.
    3. C7 and T1.
    4. C6 and C7.

25. The intermediolateral horn is found in spinal cord segments—
    1. L1 and L2.
    2. S2 to S4.
    3. T1 and T2.
    4. C1 to C4.

Section III: Chapters 6 through 11

In the following questions, select the single best answer.

1. Examination of a patient revealed a drooping left eyelid, external strabismus of the left eye, loss of the pupillary light reflex in the left eye, and weakness of the limbs and lower facial muscles on the right side. A single lesion most likely to produce all these signs would be located in the—
   A. medial region of the left pontomedullary junction.
   B. basomedial region of the left cerebral peduncle.
   C. superior region of the left mesencephalon.
   D. dorsolateral region of the medulla on the left side.
   E. periaqueductal gray matter on the left side.

2. A neurologic syndrome is characterized by loss of pain and thermal sensibility on the left side of the face and on the right side of the body from the neck down; partial paralysis of the soft palate, larynx, and pharynx on the left side; and ataxia on the left side. This syndrome could be expected from thrombosis of the—
   A. basilar artery.
   B. right posterior inferior cerebellar artery.
   C. left posterior inferior cerebellar artery.
   D. right superior cerebellar artery.
   E. left superior cerebellar artery.

3. Hemiplegia and a somatosensory deficit on the right side of the body may be caused by occlusion of the—
   A. left middle cerebral artery.
   B. right anterior cerebral artery.
   C. left posterior cerebral artery.
   D. left superior cerebellar artery.
   E. anterior communicating artery.

4. If the oculomotor nerve (III) is sectioned, each of the following may result except for—
   A. partial ptosis.
   B. abduction of the eyeball.
   C. dilation of the pupil.

D. impairment of lacrimal secretion.

E. paralysis of the ciliary muscle.

5. Structures in the ventromedial regions of the medulla receive their blood supply from the—

A. posterior spinal and superior cerebellar arteries.

B. vertebral and anterior spinal arteries.

C. posterior spinal and posterior cerebral arteries.

D. posterior spinal and posterior inferior cerebellar arteries.

E. posterior and anterior inferior cerebellar arteries.

6. The efferent axons of the cerebellar cortex arise from—

A. Golgi cells.

B. fastigial nucleus cells.

C. granule cells.

D. Purkinje cells.

E. pyramidal cells.

7. You are recording electrical activity at the cortical surface with a monopolar electrode using a distant electrode as reference. With this arrangement, a positive wave at the cortical surface could represent—

A. pyramidal cell hyperpolarization near the cortical surface.

B. pyramidal cell action potentials near cortical layer IV.

C. pyramidal cell hyperpolarization near cortical layer IV.

D. stellate cell depolarization near cortical layer IV.

E. stellate cell action potentials.

8. The only one of the following structures not involved in the pathways for control of pupil size is the—

A. hypothalamus.

B. spinal cord.

C. optic nerve.

D. ciliary ganglion.

E. oculomotor nerve.

9. A lesion in the nucleus of cranial nerve IV could produce a deficit in the—

A. upward gaze in the ipsilateral eye.

B. upward gaze in the contralateral eye.

C. downward gaze in the contralateral eye.

D. downward gaze in the ipsilateral eye.

10. In a shivering patient who has chills and cutaneous vasoconstriction associated with an infectious disease, body temperature is likely to be—

A. rising.

B. falling.

C. elevated but stable.

D. normal and stable.

In the following questions, one or more answers may be correct. Select—

A if **1, 2,** and **3** are correct;

B if **1** and **3** are correct;

C if **2** and **4** are correct;

D if only **4** is correct;

E if all are correct.

11. The ventrolateral nucleus of the thalamus—

1. receives axons from neurons in the globus pallidus.

2. projects axons to the motor cortex (area 4).

3. receives axons from neurons in the red nucleus.

4. receives axons from cells in the motor cortex (area 4).

12. The ventroposterior medialis nucleus of the thalamus—

1. receives axons from neurons located in the contralateral cuneate nucleus of the medulla.

2. receives axons of neurons located in area 4 on the medial surface of the ipsilateral cerebral hemisphere.

3. contains neurons that respond to olfactory stimuli applied ipsilaterally.

4. contains neurons whose axons project to the somatosensory cortex of the ipsilateral cerebral hemisphere.

13. The vagus nerve contains–

1. visceral afferent fibers.

2. visceral efferent fibers.

3. branchial efferent fibers.

4. somatic efferent fibers.

14. Lesions of the cerebral cortex on one side can result in a deficit in—

1. contralateral (not ipsilateral) nerve III.

2. ipsilateral (not contralateral) ambiguous nucleus.

3. contralateral (not ipsilateral) motor (nerve) V.

4. contralateral (not ipsilateral) nerve XII.

15. The trigeminal nuclear complex—

1. has somatic afferent components.

2. participates in certain reflex responses of cranial muscles.

3. has a branchial efferent component.

4. receives projections of axons coursing with nerve X.

16. The nucleus solitarius—

1. serves visceral functions, none of which are consciously perceived.

2. gives rise to preganglionic parasympathetic axons.

3. mediates pain arising from the heart during myocardial ischemia.

4. receives axons running with nerve VII.

17. The somatosensory cortex projects to the—

1. striatum.

2. ventrolateral nucleus of the thalamus.

3. dorsal column nuclei.

4. vestibular nuclei.

18. A lesion restricted to the left medullary pyramid—
    1. produces contralateral spastic hemiplegia.
    2. results in a disturbance of postural muscles, principally on the right.
    3. results in prominent muscle atrophy of the right limbs.
    4. results in a deficiency of fine movements of the right hand.

19. If cranial nerve nuclei originating from the basal plate failed to develop, absent nuclei would include the—
    1. nucleus ambiguous.
    2. principal nucleus of nerve V.
    3. abducens nucleus (VI).
    4. nucleus solitarius.

20. Principal components of the blood-brain barrier to macromolecules include—
    1. astrocytes.
    2. dural cells.
    3. endothelial cells.
    4. arachnoid cells.

21. The anatomic basis of the consensual light reflex is—
    1. reticulotectal projections to the nuclei of the oculomotor nerve (III).
    2. the projection of each optic nerve (II) to both pretectal nuclei.
    3. corticobulbar connections to the nuclei of the oculomotor (III) and abducens (IV) nerves.
    4. bilateral pretectal projections to the Edinger-Westphal nuclei.

22. A healthy 25-year-old man had an episode of blurred vision and difficulty in walking. Physical examination showed nystagmus, a right temporal visual field defect, impaired balance with loss of vibration sensation on the right, bilateral hyperactive deep tendon reflexes with a Babinski sign on the right, and paresthesias of the right arm. Three years later (at age 28), the man was admitted to the hospital with an influenzalike illness accompanied by dysarthria, weakness in both legs, tremor, and urinary incontinence. The clinical features are consistent with—
    1. subacute combined degeneration.
    2. postinfectious encephalomyelitis.
    3. neurosyphilis.
    4. multiple sclerosis.

23. In the case described in question 22, lumbar puncture and examination of the patient's cerebrospinal fluid are likely to reveal—
    1. normal cerebrospinal fluid pressure.
    2. a mildly increased mononuclear cell count.
    3. an elevated IgG concentration.
    4. a low glucose concentration.

24. Which of the following statements concerning cerebellar Purkinje cells is/are correct?
    1. They provide all known efferent axons from the cerebellar cortex.
    2. Their axons project to the red nucleus via the superior cerebellar peduncle.
    3. They receive excitatory input from mossy fibers.
    4. They receive no vestibular input.

25. Axon pathways that decussate before they terminate include the—
    1. optic nerve (II) fibers from the temporal retina.
    2. fasciculus gracilis.
    3. fasciculus cuneatus.
    4. olivocerebellar fibers

Section IV: Chapters 12 through 21

In the following questions, select the single best answer.

1. Surgical removal of both carotid bodies without disturbing the receptors of the carotid sinus would result in—
    A. hypertension caused by the loss of baroreceptors.
    B. hypotension caused by the loss of baroreceptors.
    C. a loss of hypoxia-induced hyperventilation because of the removal of chemoreceptors.
    D. augmentation of hypoxia-induced hyperventilation because of the removal of chemoreceptors.

2. In a single cortical column of area 17, all orientation-selective cells have a similar—
    A. optimal stimulus orientation.
    B. eye preference.
    C. approximate receptive field location.
    D. A and C.
    E. A, B, and C.

3. A lesion of the right frontal cortex (area 8) produces—
    A. double vision (diplopia).
    B. impaired gaze to the left.
    C. impaired gaze to the right.
    D. dilated pupils.
    E. no disturbances of the oculomotor system.

4. In the autonomic nervous system, acetylcholine (through its action on muscarinic receptors) produces all the following changes except—
    A. depolarization of smooth muscle.
    B. hyperpolarization of smooth muscle.
    C. depolarization of cardiac muscle.
    D. hyperpolarization of cardiac muscle.
    E. increased secretion by the salivary glands.

5. Giving tryptophan orally to a patient may be helpful for intractable pain because—

A. it prevents the depletion of serotonin in the raphe-spinal terminals in the spinal dorsal horn.

B. it increases the effect of periaqueductal gray-matter stimulation upon neurons of the nucleus raphe magnus.

C. it can be used to overcome some of the tolerance that builds up with repeated electrical stimulation in the periaqueductal gray matter.

D. A and C.

E. A, B, and C.

6. Biochemical and physiologic changes associated with normal aging include—

A. a decrease in total DNA because of a decrease in glia.

B. a decrease in cortical choline acetyltransferase levels.

C. an increase in short-term memory capacity.

D. a decrease in the cerebral synthesis of dopamine and norepinephrine.

E. an increase in speed of recovery from brain damage.

7. REM sleep is typically accompanied by—

A. slow eye movements.

B. spindles on the electroencephalogram.

C. decreased cerebral blood flow and body temperature.

D. vivid dream images.

8. Retrograde amnesia can be produced in animals by—

A. stimulation of the ventromedial hypothalamus.

B. stimulation of the caudate putamen.

C. electroconvulsive shock.

D. all of these.

9. Which of the following statements about the auditory system is not true?

A. Fibers of the cochlear nerve are purely afferent.

B. The cochlear nuclei have multiple representations of the cochlea; ie, they exhibit tonotopic organization.

C. The lateral lemniscus carries information from both ears.

D. It has a major synaptic relay in the midbrain.

E. It has a major synaptic relay in the thalamus.

10. A right-handed patient with a complete lesion of the corpus callosum would demonstrate—

A. hemiplegia.

B. aphasia.

C. a failure to correctly name objects placed in the right hand.

D. schizophrenia.

E. none of the above.

In the following questions one or more answers may be correct. Select—

A if **1, 2,** and **3** are correct;

B if **1** and **3** are correct;

C if **2** and **4** are correct;

D if only **4** is correct;

E if all are correct.

11. Which of the following statements concerning aqueous humor is/are correct?

1. It is formed by the ciliary processes.

2. It drains from the posterior chamber through the pupil to the anterior chamber.

3. Its production determines intraocular pressure and thus maintains the shape and relationships of the cornea and retina for proper vision.

4. It nourishes the lens and part of the cornea.

12. Auditory stimuli normally cause impulses to pass through the—

1. trapezoid body.

2. inferior olivary nucleus

3. medial geniculate nucleus

4. medial lemniscus.

13. Hair cells of the macula of the utricle are stimulated by—

1. slight rotatory movements (angular accelerations) of the body.

2. movements of the otoliths.

3. displacement of the cupula.

4. changes in head position (eg, tilting).

14. The principal neurotransmitter(s) released by synaptic terminals of sympathetic axons is/are—

1. epinephrine.

2. norepinephrine.

3. acetylcholine.

4. gamma-aminobutyric acid.

15. A hypothalamic center that inhibits feeding behavior is located in the—

1. ventromedial nucleus.

2. dorsomedial nucleus.

3. lateral nucleus.

4. anterior nucleus.

16. An increase in heart rate can result from—

1. increased parasympathetic nerve activity.

2. decreased parasympathetic nerve activity.

3. increased sympathetic nerve activity.

4. decreased sympathetic nerve activity.

17. Assuming there is no edema or distortion of the brain, coma can be caused by—

1. liver disease.

2. a bilateral pontine infarction.

3. a bilateral midbrain tegmentum lesion.

4. a unilateral hypothalamic lesion.

18. Deep levels (stages III and IV) of slow-wave sleep are associated with—

1. a slow-frequency, high-amplitude electroencephalogram.

2. vivid visual imagery.

3. increased brain oxygen consumption.
4. a loss of postural muscle tone.

19. A normal person who is isolated and deprived of all cues about what time it is will—
    1. sleep the usual number of hours, but fall asleep several times during a 24-hour period.
    2. sleep for 8 hours at his usual bedtime but go directly to REM sleep.
    3. have relatively less REM and relatively more slow-wave sleep.
    4. have an almost normal sleep-wakefulness pattern, but become progressively out of phase with people who know what time it is.

20. Neurofibrillary tangles and senile plaques are found in—
    1. the substantia nigra of patients with Parkinson's disease.
    2. the hippocampus of normal 80-year-old people.
    3. young adults with multiple sclerosis.
    4. patients with senile dementia, Alzheimer type.

21. A bilateral lesion of the amygdala—
    1. increases the incidence of aggressive behavior.
    2. produces Wallerian degeneration in sympathetic neurons.
    3. produces Klüver-Bucy syndrome.
    4. produces anterograde amnesia.

22. The opiate antagonist naloxone reportedly reverses such pain control procedures as—
    1. hypnosis.
    2. acupuncture.
    3. spinal tractotomy.
    4. placebo administration.

23. Stimulation of the left vestibular nucleus produces—
    1. smooth eye movements to the left, followed by rapid jumps in the eye position back to the right.
    2. smooth eye movements to the right, followed by rapid jumps in the eye back to the left.
    3. movements of the right eye only.
    4. conjugate movements of both eyes.

24. Destruction of the lower cervical and upper thoracic ventral roots on the left side leads to a—
    1. constricted right pupil.
    2. dilated right pupil.
    3. constricted left pupil.
    4. dilated left pupil.

25. Following transection of a peripheral nerve, the—
    1. axons and Schwann cells distal to the cut undergo degeneration and disappear.
    2. sensory axons distal to the cut survive, but motor axons degenerate.
    3. motor neurons whose axons were cut degenerate and disappear.
    4. surviving axons of the proximal stump will send out new growth cones to attempt regeneration.

ANSWERS

Section I

1. B	6. D	11. A	16. A	21. B
2. C	7. E	12. E	17. B	22. E
3. B	8. A	13. D	18. B	23. B
4. A	9. C	14. A	19. A	24. A
5. C	10. E	15. E	20. D	25. D

Section II

1. A	6. B	11. A	16. C	21. C
2. C	7. E	12. B	17. C	22. E
3. A	8. B	13. A	18. C	23. B
4. C	9. D	14. B	19. B	24. D
5. B	10. D	15. E	20. E	25. A

Section III

1. B	6. D	11. E	16. D	21. C
2. C	7. D	12. D	17. B	22. D
3. A	8. C	13. E	18. D	23. B
4. D	9. D	14. D	19. B	24. B
5. B	10. A	15. D	20. B	25. D

Section IV

1. C	6. D	11. E	16. D	21. C
2. E	7. D	12. B	17. B	22. C
3. B	8. A	13. C	18. D	23. C
4. C	9. B	14. A	19. D	24. D
5. A	10. C	15. C	20. C	25. D

Index

Page numbers in **bold** indicate a major discussion.

examination of, 266
extension, 37, **145**
extensor, 38
extensor plantar, **37**
  testing for, **39**
flexion, 37, **145**
flexor, 37–38
Galant's, 268
grasp, 268
incurvation, 268
jaw, **37**, **145**
knee, examination of, 266
light, 37, **145**
Moro, 268
nasal, **37**, **145**
oculocardiac, **37**, **145**
Oppenheim, **37**
patellar, 37, **145**
periosteoradial, 37, **145**
pharyngeal, **37**, 82, **145**
plantar, **37**, **145**
  examination of, 266–267
postsynaptic, 38
pupillary light, 77
  path of, **78**
rectal, **37**, **145**
spinal, 37–38
superficial, **37**, **145**
  examination of, 266–267
triceps, 37, **145**
  examination of, 266
types of, 36–37
uvular, **37**, **145**
vestibulo-ocular, 76, 176
visceral, **37**, **145**
wrist, **37**, **145**
Refraction, 161
  errors of, 161–163
Refractory period, 19
REM sleep, 180
Repolarization, 19
Resting membrane potential,
  18–19
Reticular formation, 57, 179–183
Reticular nucleus, 89
Reticular system, ascending, **179**
Reticulospinal system, 34
  function and location in cord,
  34
Reticulospinal tract, 147
Retina, **159**
Retrobulbar neuritis, 163
Retrograde amnesia, 211
Retrograde transport, 8
Rhinencephalon, 184
Rhombencephalon, 55, **56**
Rhomboid fossa, 115
Rigidity, gamma, 38
Rods, 158, **159**
  phototransduction in, se-
  quence of events in, **160**
Roentgenography, 50, 223

Romberg test, 266
Rubrospinal tract, 34, 147
  function and location in cord,
  34

Saccades, 76
Saccule, 176
Sacral plexus, **293**
Sagittal sinuses, 134
Salts, in nervous tissue, 14
Schwannoma, 40
Sciatica, 247
Scleroderma, 198
Sclerosis
  amyotrophic, 22, 247
  multiple, 249
    cerebrospinal fluid findings
    in, **245**
    demyelinization in, **250**
    lesions of, **249**
    posterolateral, 41
Scotomas, 162–163
  hearing, 173
Seasickness, 177
Seizures
  absence (petit mal), 211–212
  myoclonic, 212
  psychomotor, 191
  tonic-clonic (grand mal), 212
Sella turcica, 125–126
Semicircular canals, 176
Semicoma, 179
Senile dementia, 217–218, 262
  plaques in, **218**
Senile plaques, 216, **216**
Sensation, 152–154
Sensorimotor area, 109, **109**
Sensorimotor cortex, 143, **144**
Sensory ataxia, 177
Sensory deficits, 154
Sensory ganglia, 199
Sensory homunculus, **109**
Sensory neurons, numerical clas-
  sifications for, **20**
Sensory nuclei, 90
Sensory pathways, 154
Sensory system, examination of,
  267
Septal area, 184, 188
  function of, 189–190
Septum lucidum, 188
Serotonin, 24, 156
  areas of concentration of, **23**
Serotoninergic pathways, 57
Shock, spinal, 41, 198
Short-term memory, 190, 211
Sigmoid sinuses, 134
Single photon emission com-
  puted tomography, 233–
  234, **233**
Sinuses
  carotid, 81

cavernous, 131, 134
occipital, 127
petrosal, 134
  inferior, 127
sagittal, 134
sigmoid, 134
sphenoparietal, 134
straight, 131, 134
transverse, 127, 134
venous, 130, 133–134
Skull, 123–127
  basal view of, **124, 125, 126**
  lateral view of, **123**
Sleep, 180–181
  rapid eye movement, 180
  slow-wave, 180
  stages of, **182**
Snellen card test, **162**
Solids, in neural tissue, 11–14
Solitary nucleus, 62
Solitary tract, 62
Soluble fraction, structure and
  function of, **8**
Soma, 6
Somatesthetic area, **109**
Somatosensory cortex, primary,
  154
Somatosensory systems, 152–157
Somatostatin, 202
Somatotopic distribution, 154
Somatotopic organization, 34, **35**
Somnambulism, 181
Special senses, 152
Speech, 208–211
Sphenoparietal sinuses, 134
Spina bifida, 27, 47
Spina bifida occulta, 47, **48**
Spinal cord, 1, **2, 3**, 27–42
  ascending fiber systems in, **35**
  cervical, cross section of, **45**
  circulation in, 44–46
  descending fiber systems in, **34**
  development of, 27–28, **27**
  disorders of, 40–42
  dorsal segments of, cordotomy
    of, **155**
  external anatomy of, 28–29, **28**
  function in autonomic nervous
    system, 200
  imaging of, 50–52
  inhibition in, **22**
  internal divisions of, 31–33
  investing membranes of, 43
  lesions of
    localization of, 39–40
    types of, 40
  motor and sensory levels of,
    283
  relationships of, **29, 44**
  segment of, **31**
  stimulation of, pain relief and,
    155–156